Behavioral Principles in Communicative Disorders

Applications to Assessment and Treatment

Christine A. Maul, PhD, CCC-SLP
Brooke R. Findley, MA, CCC-SLP, BCBA
Amanda Nicolson Adams, PhD, BCBA

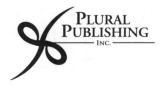
PLURAL
PUBLISHING
INC.

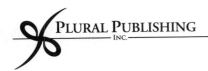

5521 Ruffin Road
San Diego, CA 92123

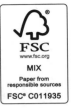

e-mail: info@pluralpublishing.com
Website: http://www.pluralpublishing.com

Library of Congress Cataloging-in-Publication Data

Maul, Christine A., author.
  Behavioral principles in communicative disorders : applications to assessment and treatment / Christine A. Maul, Brooke R. Findley, Amanda Nicolson Adams.
       p. ; cm.
  Includes bibliographical references and index.
  ISBN 978-1-59756-788-6 (alk. paper)—ISBN 1-59756-788-4 (alk. paper)
  I. Findley, Brooke R., author. II. Adams, Amanda Nicolson, author. III. Title.
  [DNLM: 1. Communication Disorders—diagnosis. 2. Communication Disorders—therapy. 3. Behavior Control—methods. 4. Behavioral Symptoms. 5. Behaviorism. WM 475]
  RC423
  616.85'5—dc23
                                                                    2015029454

Contents

Preface

Welcome to *Behavioral Principles in Communicative Disorders: Applications to Assessment and Treatment*. This book is an uncommon text in that it bridges two disciplines in one practical, application-focused volume. This interdisciplinary feature has shaped a valuable and unique contribution to the current available selection of textbooks for training in communicative disorders and in the field of applied behavior analysis (ABA). The authors of this book have presented information that is comprehensive while remaining focused on the goal of being truly applied. The book is geared toward speech-language pathologists (SLPs) but should also be useful to professionals in other disciplines, such as ABA and special education.

Therefore, this textbook can be considered an interdisciplinary introduction to behavior analysis and contains more than enough technical information to challenge even the most serious ABA student, including those pursuing the credential of board certified behavior analyst (BCBA). However, it is written primarily to speak to those who are in training for a career in communicative disorders by including examples relevant and pertinent to this discipline. In an ever-changing and increasingly interdisciplinary atmosphere, a textbook of this kind is appropriate and timely.

The authors of this book represent this professional diversity both in training and in specialized experience. The authors include two doctoral-level SLPs, a doctoral-level BCBA, and a combination SLP/BCBA. All authors have experience as university faculty (three in communicative disorders, one in psychology),

and all authors have practical experience working in clinical settings in a variety of capacities. Prior to entering the university setting, Christine A. Maul served as an SLP in the public schools, with a specialty in serving children and young adults with severe developmental and intellectual disabilities. She has been a faculty member in the Department of Communicative Disorders and Deaf Studies at California State University, Fresno (CSUF) for 17 years, as a lecturer and currently as an assistant professor. As part of her duties, she supervises students performing clinical practicum at the CSUF Speech, Language, and Hearing Clinic, where individuals across the life span with a wide range of communicative disorders are served. Brooke R. Findley serves as an SLP in a rural school district and part-time lecturer at CSUF. After becoming an SLP, she recognized the value in pursuing further education in the field of ABA and is currently also certified as a behavior analyst. Her areas of professional interest include verbal behavior, cultural and linguistic diversity, and educational leadership. She is currently pursuing a doctoral degree in Educational Leadership at CSUF. Amanda Adams started as a director for agencies providing autism services and then served as the lead behavior analyst for a large school district before accepting a faculty position in the psychology department at CSUF. In her 8 years at CSUF, she was the coordinator for the ABA master's program and the founder of the Fresno State autism center. She is now the CEO and executive director of the California Autism Center. In addition, another doctoral-level SLP, Frances Pomaville, also an assistant professor at CSUF, stepped forward to write the chapter on verbal behavior to help us meet our deadline. She did a thorough job with a difficult topic, and we are grateful for her contribution. We would also like to thank graduate student assistant Victoria Riley who gave us much help in putting together the glossary.

The focus of this textbook is on behavioral principles derived from learning theory, as discovered by the work of behavioral scientists, chief among them B. F. Skinner. The authors admittedly share a significant bias toward the behavioral viewpoint presented in this text. Although we acknowledge the contributions of other approaches, it was our intent in writing this text to present basic behavioral principles and propose ways in which those principles can effectuate positive change in communicative behaviors. It is not within the scope of the text to thoroughly examine the great theoretically oriented debates that have spun around behaviorism, particularly the cognitive-linguistic versus the behavioral viewpoints. Such theoretical discussion regarding other approaches is largely omitted from this text due to our desire to maintain a clinically oriented focus on behavioral principles.

We also acknowledge that bias against behaviorism still exists in many modern-day circles, although we find this to be unfortunate. Criticisms regarding behaviorism were easier to understand before the 1980s, before we had a body of research supporting the applied extensions of the basic and theoretical work resulting from Skinner's research. In the 1960s, the use of behavioral techniques in applied settings increased, improving outcomes in people with mental and developmental disabilities. Then, in the 1970s and 1980s, the methodology to empirically validate

behavioral techniques progressed, and the number of scientific publications demonstrating the value of those techniques consequently increased. Currently, the evidence supporting the application of behavioral principles to effectuate change in human behavior is vast, and people seeking to improve their communicative behaviors should have access to treatment that incorporates those principles. In writing this textbook, it was our intent to present material specifically focused on empirically validated behavioral techniques that have shown efficacy in enhancing clinicians' skills and clients' outcomes.

In addition to our advocacy for the science of behaviorism, we also share a dedication to putting professional territorialism behind us and embracing interdisciplinary collaboration to provide the best evidence-based services possible to the people we serve. This is a highly personal devotion among the authors of this book, one of whom is the parent of a young man with autism and mental illness. Participating in clinical intervention techniques not only as a professional but also as a parent may be one of the most profound ways of experiencing the importance of scientific collaboration in maximizing outcomes for a loved one. This is a measure of success that can be achieved only if theoretical turf battles are abandoned in favor of interdisciplinary collaboration among professionals dedicated to pursuing common goals within an evidence-based framework. Our clinical fields are experiencing a shift, and professionals from complimentary disciplines (SLP, school psychology, BCBA, special education teachers, etc.) are working together more than ever before. This is happening not only in public schools but also, to an increasing degree, within the private sector. Being knowledgeable about the valuable methods and techniques used by our colleagues in neighboring fields of practice is extremely helpful in strengthening our own practice as clinicians and, more important, will be of benefit to the clients we serve. We hope that you find this book to be challenging, informative, and useful in your professional growth and clinical work.

—Amanda Nicolson Adams,
PhD, BCBA
California Autism Center,
Fresno, California

Contributors

Amanda Nicolson Adams, PhD, BCBA
CEO, Executive Director
California Autism Center and Learning Group
Fresno, California

Brooke R. Findley, MA, CCC-SLP, BCBA
Lecturer
Department of Communicative Disorders and Deaf Studies
California State University, Fresno
Fresno, California

Christine A. Maul, PhD, CCC-SLP
Assistant Professor
Department of Communicative Disorders and Deaf Studies
California State University, Fresno
Fresno, California

Frances Pomaville, PhD, CCC-SLP
Assistant Professor and Speech-Language Pathologist
Department of Communicative Disorders and Deaf Studies
California State University, Fresno
Fresno, California
Chapter 2

To M. N. Hegde

CHAPTER 1

Introduction to Behaviorism

Chapter Outline

- Why Should SLPs Learn the Principles of Behaviorism and How to Apply Them?
- Definition and History of Behaviorism
    - Early Behavioral Scientists
        - Pavlov (1849–1936)
        - Watson (1878–1958)
        - B. F. Skinner (1904–1990)
- Principles of Behaviorism
    - Operant Conditioning and Respondent Conditioning
    - Positive and Negative Reinforcement
    - Differential Reinforcement
    - Positive and Negative Punishment
    - Stimulus Discrimination and Generalization
- Behavior Modification: The Early Days
- Philosophical Underpinnings
- Early Experimentation in Behavior Modification
- Applied Behavior Analysis
    - Definition of ABA
    - Who Are Board Certified Behavior Analysts (BCBAs)?
    - How Can SLPs and BCBAs Collaborate?

Why Should SLPs Learn the Principles of Behaviorism and How to Apply Them?

Speech-language pathologists (SLPs) are in the business of changing communicative behaviors in the clients that they serve. SLPs seek to establish new communicative behaviors in their clients, rehabilitate communicative behaviors that may have been lost, strengthen and maintain existing communicative behaviors, and, often simultaneously, decrease communicative behaviors that are undesirable. SLPs are ethically charged to engage in evidence-based practice to achieve these goals, taking into consideration scientific evidence reported in peer-reviewed journals, the preferences of their clients, and their own clinical expertise (American Speech-Language-Hearing Association, 2005). The well-researched principles of behaviorism, therefore, are highly relevant to the field of speech-language pathology because it is a science that has resulted in an evidence-based, systematic set of methods applied to modify the behaviors of others. On that basis alone, it is beneficial for SLPs to have knowledge of those methods and understand how they can be applied in the assessment and treatment of their clients. However, there are other good reasons why SLPs should know and apply principles of behaviorism.

> SLPs are ethically charged to engage in _____-_____ _____.

Clients served by SLPs often present with accompanying behavioral difficulties. In the adult population, behavior problems are a frequently occurring effect of stroke and traumatic brain injury (TBI). Also, the comorbidity of speech-language difficulties and social emotional behavior disorders (SEBDs) in children has been well documented. It has been reported that 21.6% of the child and adolescent populations in the United States exhibit behaviors that warrant the diagnosis of some type of psychiatric disorder (Carter et al., 2010). Among children who are diagnosed with language disorders, there is a much higher prevalence of SEBD; estimates by various researchers range between 50% and 70% (Redmond & Rice, 1998). Therefore, SLPs working in all settings are likely to encounter behavioral difficulties in a significant percentage of the clients they attempt to help. Often behavior problems must be addressed before clients can fully benefit from treatment.

It is also becoming increasingly likely for SLPs to be asked to take part in collaborative, multidisciplinary efforts to help children overcome behavioral difficulties that may impede their access to educational curriculum (Bopp, Brown, & Mirenda, 2004). In particular, SLPs may be called upon to work closely with board certified behavior analysts (BCBAs) who are experts in discovering and describing problem behaviors in children and adults and then writing behavior plans to address those problems. BCBAs have special expertise in **applied behavior analysis** (ABA), a systematic set of methods designed to discover aspects of a person's environment that contribute to problem behavior through **functional behavior assessment** (FBA). In addition, BCBAs are experts in applying ABA principles to build and shape new behaviors that may be nonexistent or deficient in clients who do not necessarily exhibit problem behaviors. SLPs can therefore collaborate with BCBAs in assisting clients with a wide range of communicative difficulties, with or without accompanying behavior disorders. This chapter ends with a further discussion of the origin of applied behavior analysis and professional collaboration between SLPs and BCBAs.

> Clients with behavioral difficulties will benefit from collaboration between SLPs and _____-_____ _____-_____.

Finally, although principles of ABA are more closely associated with assessment and intervention for children with autism and other severe disabilities, those principles have much broader application to the entire gamut of types of communicative disorders, levels of severity, and behaviors that simply interfere with the delivery of therapy. SLPs who understand the principles of ABA can address problems as critical as helping a nonverbal individual obtain a system of communication to as mild as helping a child stay in seat during therapy.

In summary, SLPs should learn and apply principles of behaviorism because (a) there is a well-established evidence base for the efficacy of methods based on behaviorism, (b) many clients on SLPs' caseloads are likely to exhibit challenging behaviors, (c) there is an increasing need for SLPs to collaborate with BCBAs in providing assessment and intervention for children with behavior disorders, and (d) the principles of behaviorism are broadly applicable across types and levels of severity of communicative disorders.

Definition and History of Behaviorism

Behaviorism as a philosophy is grounded in the principles of **empiricism** and **determinism**. These principles are not compat-

ible with **mentalism**, another widely held philosophy that emphasizes assumed internal processes such as thought and perception as the key to understanding why human beings behave the way they do.

Empiricism is the belief that knowledge can be derived only from sensory experiences—from that which can be seen, heard, touched, tasted, or smelled. Therefore, direct observation is inextricably necessary in establishing a knowledge base. It is a well-founded principle of behaviorism that human behavior must be defined in terms of that which can be observed and measured. For example, it is not acceptable to a behaviorist to describe a behavior as an internal emotional event, such as joy. A behaviorist would instead describe and quantify behaviors that might indicate the person is joyful, such as smiling, laughing, jumping up and down, or making cheering noises.

Empiricists also do not accept an idea simply because it appears to be logical, well argued, or coherent. They insist on putting ideas to the empirical test, a scientific experiment arranged to directly experience the truth or untruth of a statement or hypothesis. Principles of behaviorism have been thoroughly examined through empirical research, most often utilizing single-case research design methodology, which is described in more depth in Chapter 9.

> The belief that knowledge can be derived only from sensory experiences is called _____.

Determinism is the belief that nothing that happens in the world is haphazard. Determinists believe that there is a systematic order in which phenomena relate to each other. Every effect has a cause, and it is possible through scientific experimentation to discover, understand, and exert control over a cause-effect relationship.

> The belief that every effect has a cause is called _____.

The philosophical concepts of empiricism and determinism demand explanations of human behavior that cannot be derived from a mentalistic viewpoint. Mentalism is the belief that humans act the way they do because of internal, unobservable phenomena, such as mind, thought, and free will. There are a myriad of other hypothetical constructs that mentalistic authors have set forth. Freud (1949), for example, described id, ego, and super ego as the prime determinants of human behavior. Chomsky (1965) proposed an internal language acquisition device (LAD) as the mechanism by which children acquire language. Modern-day authors have proposed many models showing how the brain processes information in much the same way as a computer does without the neurological data to prove such processes (e.g., Schyns, Gosslin, & Smith, 2009). All of these are examples of hypothetical constructs that do not lend themselves to observation and measurement and therefore cannot be subjected to empirical testing. Behavioral scientists therefore argue that, although such constructs may be a part of the human experience, they do not contribute much to a functional understanding of why human beings behave the way they do.

> The belief that humans act the way they do because of internal, unobservable phenomena is called _____.

Early Behavioral Scientists

Behavioral principles have been in operation since the beginning of the history of humankind. In response to the conditions of their environments, humans learn to seek shelter when it is cold, to hunt and to farm in order to obtain food, to run in times of danger, to swim instead of drown, and so forth. Parents teach their children by praising them when they are behaving in a desirable way and by punishing them when they are not. People repeat behaviors that result in rewards such as a paycheck from a boss, a kiss from a spouse, a hug from a child, or a smile from a friend.

Although these are everyday occurrences that are taken for granted by the general public, the way in which behavioral principles shape our lives was not fully described or understood until scientists began to systematically study how living organisms respond to environmental stimuli. Three scientists who contributed to the founding of behavioral science were Ivan Pavlov (1849–1936), John B. Watson (1878–1958), and B. F. Skinner (1904–1990).

Pavlov (1849–1936)

To understand Pavlov's pioneering work, it is necessary to distinguish between an **unconditioned stimulus**, which elicits an unconditioned response, and a **conditioned stimulus**, which elicits a conditioned response. Unconditioned stimuli automatically elicit an unconditioned response; living organisms, including human beings, react to certain stimuli in certain ways from birth, and those reactions persist throughout the life span. For example, the presentation of good food elicits salivation, touching a hot plate elicits a rapid removal of the hand, experiencing pain elicits moaning, pollen in the air elicits sneezing, and so forth. In each of these examples, there is an unconditioned stimulus (such as pollen) and an unconditioned response (such as sneezing).

Pavlov established that it is possible to elicit an unconditioned response to neutral stimuli that do not ordinarily elicit such a response. In his classic experiments, he presented a variety of neutral stimuli, most famously the sound of a bell, prior to the presentation of food to a dog. The food, the unconditioned stimulus, elicited the dog's salivation. However, after repeated pairings of the bell tone with presentation of the food, the dog salivated upon hearing the bell. At that point, the tone became a **conditioned stimulus** and the dog's salivation became a **conditioned response** (Figure 1–1).

Pairing a neutral stimulus to an unconditioned stimulus to eventually elicit an unconditioned response by presentation of the neutral stimulus alone is currently referred to as **respondent conditioning**. "Pavlov's dog" became an icon for the

establishment of a set of behavioral techniques based on respondent conditioning, which, when applied ethically, can help people overcome irrational fears, such as fear of flying, or cease undesirable habits, such as smoking or excessive alcohol consumption. This type of respondent conditioning, also called Pavlovian or **classical conditioning**, has limited application to the treatment of communicative disorders. However, Display Box 1–1 shows an example of the importance of understanding the concept of respondent conditioning.

Watson (1878–1958)

Watson was the mentalist's biggest foe. He soundly denounced the idea that scientific inquiry in the field of psychology should be concerned with unobservable mental states (e.g., thought, mood, dreams, theoretical constructs of consciousness, etc.). He proposed instead that studies be conducted solely to discover the causes of observable behavior, with the ultimate

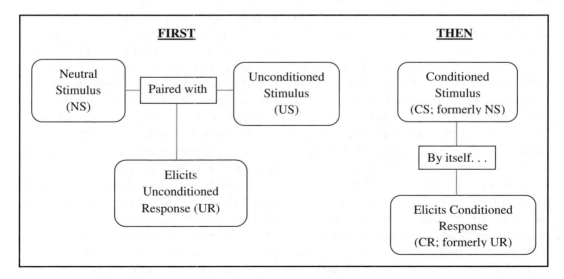

Figure 1–1. The process of respondent conditioning.

Display Box 1–1. Keep Those White Coats in the Closet!

Although respondent conditioning has little application to the treatment of communicative disorders, it is beneficial for clinicians to understand how people can have reflexive, conditioned reactions to stimuli that would not ordinarily elicit such reactions. For example, fear responses from a child may be elicited by a clinician wearing a white lab coat. Previous trips to the doctor's office, in which people often wearing white coats administer vaccinations, may have conditioned the children to react in such a manner. Similarly, the mere sight of a tongue depressor may elicit a backward jerk of the head or even a gag reflex in clients who have previously experienced oral facial examinations.

Based on the schematic given in Figure 1–1, identify the unconditioned stimuli and the unconditioned responses, leading to the conditioned stimuli and conditioned responses described here.

goal of devising methods by which human behavior can be predicted and controlled. His ideas formed the foundation for behaviorism as a purely objective natural science leading to understanding the relationships between environmental stimuli and responses of living organisms to those stimuli.

Watson was a colorful character with strong opinions that led him in various directions, most notably into animal behavior, childrearing, and marketing. In his most controversial experiment, he applied the Pavlovian principle of respondent conditioning to an 11-month-old child, dubbed "Little Albert," presenting a furry little white rat to the child simultaneously with the disturbingly loud noise of an iron rod clanging (Watson & Rayner, 1920). Albert had exhibited no previous fear of the rat, but he understandably reacted with fear to the clang of the iron rod. After several simultaneous presentations of the two stimuli, the child began to exhibit fearful reactions to the presentation of the rat alone and also to other animals and objects that had any kind of resemblance to the rat. Thus, Watson proved that fear could be a conditioned response that could generalize to related objects. Watson did not attempt to de-condition Little Albert, and because the little boy died at the age of 6 from hydrocephalus, it was not possible to determine what effect this experiment might have had on his life. This type of experimentation, coupled with Watson's penchant for strongly worded hyperbolic statements, discredited him and the newly proposed science of behaviorism in the eyes of many. Display Box 1–2 presents one of Watson's most controversial statements.

Display Box 1–2. Watson's "Dozen Infants" Quote

Watson wrote in the area of childrearing, advocating for a type of emotionally detached style of parenting in which children would be regarded and treated as young adults. He was so convinced of the possibilities of molding children through control of environmental stimuli that he went so far as to propose a 20-year moratorium on pregnancies to give behavioral scientists time to gather data to propose the most efficient way to raise children. One of his most widely quoted statements (Watson, 1928) indicated his fervent belief in the power of behavioral parenting:

> Give me a dozen healthy infants, well-formed, and my own specified world to bring them up in, and I'll guarantee to take any one at random and train him to become any type of specialist I might select—doctor, lawyer, artist, merchant-chief and, yes, even beggar-man and thief. (p. 104)

For more information on Watson's writings on childrearing, refer to Houk (2000).

In the Little Albert experiment, what were the unconditioned stimulus, the neutral stimulus, and the unconditioned response? What eventually became the conditioned stimulus and the conditioned response?

B. F. Skinner (1904–1990)

Behaviorism as a science did not exist until B. F. Skinner addressed human behavior as observable, measurable events that could be explained through discovery of the causes of those behaviors. Through his experiments with laboratory animals, mostly rats and pigeons, Skinner discovered patterns of behavior caused by responses to environmental stimuli. He devised the Skinner box, although Skinner did not like the term *Skinner box* to describe the device he invented. He preferred terms such as *lever box* or *operant conditioning chamber*. Figure 1–2 provides a schematic of a Skinner box.

The Skinner box was a cage containing a lever that, when pressed, would dispense a morsel of food. A rat running around the cage would eventually accidentally depress the lever—a behavior that was rewarded, or reinforced, by the presentation of food. Skinner observed that the rat's lever-pressing behavior would then increase, as a result of having received the food. This learning process, in which a behavior is increased through a reinforcing event, is one component of

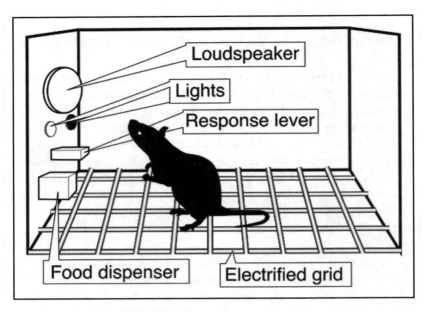

Figure 1–2. The Skinner box.

what Skinner called **operant conditioning**. This was but one of many principles of behaviorism established through this type of experimental manipulation of antecedent and consequence events causing a change in animal behavior.

> The learning process in which a behavior is increased through a reinforcing event is one component of what Skinner called _____.

Principles of Behaviorism

Through many and repeated experiments, Skinner demonstrated patterns of animal behavior that are considered foundational principles of behaviorism. These broad principles are briefly described here. In later chapters, these principles

are discussed in more detail and applications to clinical practice, with examples, are given.

Operant Conditioning and Respondent Conditioning

Operant conditioning is the primary process through which Skinner believed people learn to behave the way that they do. Through operant conditioning, behavior is shaped and maintained by the consequences that immediately follow the behavior. Consequences alter the frequency of the occurrence of behavior either by increasing the behavior through **reinforcement** or decreasing, or often entirely eliminating, a behavior through **punishment**. From birth, human beings encounter a myriad of consequences on the way to becoming persons who behave the way they do. A small infant may curl his lips in a reflexive response to passing

Introduction to Behaviorism

gas, but the attention adults in the environment shower upon him quickly results in the infant learning the social smile—an example of reinforcement. A toddler may reach up to touch a hot stove burner and may either experience the pain that comes from touching it or be saved by a sharp "No!" and redirection from his parent, resulting in decreased or eliminated stove-top touching—an example of punishment.

Operant conditioning is distinguished from respondent conditioning, because the behaviors that are learned through operant conditioning are a result of an individual's previous interactions and exposure to consequences, while behaviors elicited through respondent conditioning are reflexive (recall Pavlov's experiment with the salivating dog). Respondent behaviors occur because of past associations that people have made with antecedent events. A particular song that was sung at a loved one's funeral may elicit crying behavior whenever a person hears it in the future. The sight of a particular breed of dog may cause a person's heart to race if he or she has been bitten by that breed in the past. Operant behaviors, on the other hand, are nonreflexive behaviors learned through past encounters with consequences. Reflexive behaviors elicited through respondent conditioning are few and finite, while responsive behaviors evoked through operant conditioning are many and infinitely varied.

> The process by which behavior is shaped and maintained through consequences that immediately follow the behavior and alter the frequency of the occurrence of the behavior is called _____ _____.

Positive and Negative Reinforcement

The observation that specific animal behaviors could be increased through presentation of food immediately after the performance of the behavior established the principle of **reinforcement**, the process of strengthening and increasing the frequency of a behavior. A **reinforcer** is an event that follows a behavior and results in increasing that behavior. There are many different types of reinforcers, and an event that may be reinforcing to one person may not be reinforcing to another. A young child who loves art might work hard to gain access to the opportunity to paint, while a child who loves sports might not find that activity to be desirable and will not work to gain access to it.

> The process of strengthening and increasing a behavior is called _____.

> An event that follows a behavior and results in increasing that behavior is called a _____.

Behaviors increase through **positive reinforcement** or **negative reinforcement**. The concept of positive reinforcement is straightforward and easy to understand. Positive reinforcement occurs when a reinforcer is presented right after a behavior has occurred, resulting in the increase of that behavior. For example, if an adolescent mows the lawn at home and his parent presents him with a plate of warm, fresh-baked cookies as a reward right after he's finished, his lawn-mowing behavior is likely to increase because that behavior has been positively reinforced. Positive reinforcement, then, has to do with the *presentation* of a stimulus.

> Positive reinforcement has to do with stimulus _____.

Negative reinforcement is harder to understand and is often confused with punishment, which, as will soon be explained, is not at all the same as negative reinforcement. Remember that the process of reinforcement serves to *increase* a behavior. Negative reinforcement increases a behavior by removing or postponing an event that a person finds to be aversive. People seek to escape from situations they find to be unpleasant or avoid them altogether. Behaviors that allow them to escape or avoid an unpleasant situation are likely to be repeated, as a result of negative reinforcement. For example, if cold air is blowing into a house, a person is likely to shut the window. The cold air is blocked, or removed, and the window-shutting behavior has been negatively reinforced. Turning down the volume on a radio blasting loud music is a negatively reinforced behavior, as is taking an aspirin to relieve headache pain. Negative reinforcement, then, has to do with the *withdrawal* of a stimulus following a person's behavior that results in escape or avoidance of an aversive, or unpleasant, situation.

> Negative reinforcement has to do with stimulus _____.

The difference between positive and negative reinforcement might be further explained by looking again at the illustration of the Skinner box. When the caged rat depressed the lever and immediately received food, he was *positively* reinforced through the *presentation* of the food stimulus, and his lever-pressing behavior increased. Notice, however, that the floor of the Skinner box consisted of an electric grid. Skinner ran another set of experiments in which he introduced a steady electric current along this grid that could be interrupted by depressing the lever. The rats in these experiments understandably found the induced electric shock to be highly aversive and quickly learned to depress the lever to cause the cessation of the electric current. In this case, the lever-pressing behavior was *negatively* reinforced through the *withdrawal* of a stimulus, the electric shock.

The principle of reinforcement is not dependent upon subjective feelings. For example, a boss may deliver warm verbal praise to a frequently late employee who arrives to work on time one day, and they both may have pleasant feelings about giving and receiving that praise. However, if the employee's behavior of being punctual does not increase, then no matter how well both the boss and the employee might feel about the praise, it is not reinforcing the employee's punctual behavior, and the boss should find some other way to address the problem. Remember that inherent in the description of a reinforcer is that it results in the increase of the behavior; if it does not, then it cannot be considered to be a reinforcer.

Also, the principle of reinforcement applies to all behaviors, both desirable and undesirable. If an adolescent, for example, is given praise and acceptance by his peers for smoking, and as a result his smoking behavior increases, then the smoking behavior has been reinforced. Similarly, if parents cannot help but laugh when a toddler utters a naughty word, then that may serve as a reinforcer for the utterance of the naughty word, and the toddler will gleefully repeat it.

Differential Reinforcement

Differential reinforcement occurs when only a specified response is reinforced and another specified response is given no reinforcement. For example, let us suppose a parent is fed up with a 4-year-old's whiney voice. The wise parent might choose to withhold reinforcement from the child when the child is using the whiney voice, but the moment a child uses a more well-modulated voice, the parent warmly says, "Oh! What a nice big girl voice!" and pays attention to what the child is saying. If this is done consistently, the frequency of the production of the whiny voice will be extinguished, or eliminated, and production of the more well-modulated voice will increase.

The appropriate application of the principle of differential reinforcement would serve to increase a desirable behavior through reinforcement and decrease an undesirable behavior by withholding reinforcement. However, recall that principles of behaviorism apply across all behaviors, desirable or undesirable. So, for example, if a child is being raised in a household in which finishing homework behavior is not reinforced but watching television is, the child will learn to not complete homework assignments and to join the family in front of the television instead. When applied appropriately, however, differential reinforcement is an effective technique and is discussed further in Chapter 8 on decreasing undesirable behaviors.

> Differential reinforcement occurs when a specified response is _____ and another specified response is _____.

Positive and Negative Punishment

The word **punishment** is fraught with unsavory connotations to most people. It may bring up images of spankings, harsh words, restraints, solitary confinement, and so forth. In some areas of the United States, the word no longer is applied to procedures necessary to address behavior problems in school children. Similarly, advocates for the disabled have fought against the use of punishment in the treatment of behavioral disorders in people with developmental disability and/or mental illness.

However, in the clinical sense of the word, punishment simply means that some contingency placed on a behavior has resulted in a *decrease* of a specified behavior. This is the critical difference distinguishing punishment from negative reinforcement—two terms that are often confused. Punishment results in the *decrease* of a behavior; negative reinforcement results in the *increase* of a behavior.

> Negative reinforcement results in a behavior _____.

> Punishment results in a behavior _____.

Just as in the principle of reinforcement, there is **positive punishment** and **negative punishment**. Positive punishment occurs when a stimulus is delivered right after a behavior is exhibited and results in the decreased frequency of that behavior. For example, if a young child starts to run into the street, a parent might speak very sharply, saying, "No! Do not run into the street without looking both ways!" If the child's behavior of impulsively running into the street is decreased, or hopefully ceases altogether, then the parent's sharp words have served as positive punishment. *Presentation* of a stimulus right after a behavior is exhibited that results in a decrease of that behavior is positive punishment.

> Positive punishment involves stimulus _____.

Negative punishment occurs when a stimulus that is present in a person's environment is withdrawn right after a behavior is exhibited, again resulting in a decreased occurrence of that behavior. For example, if two siblings are sitting in front of the television set, watching their favorite show, and start fighting with each other, a parent might go over and turn off the television. If withdrawing the television show results in a decrease in fighting behavior, then that behavior has been negatively punished. *Withdrawing* a stimulus right after a behavior is exhibited, if it results in the decrease of that behavior, is negative punishment.

> Negative punishment involves stimulus _____.

Again, just as in the principle of reinforcement, punishment is not dependent upon subjective feelings. An event might appear to be punishing, but if it does not result in the decrease of a behavior, then it is not. For example, a teacher might feel that making students who misbehave during recess stand against the fence is a punishment (a type of negative punishment called *time-out*, which is discussed further in Chapter 8). However, if the same students end up standing against the fence every recess, then the misbehavior is not decreasing, and isolating them in that way cannot be said to be punishment. Remember that inherent in the definition of a punisher is that it results in the *decrease* of a behavior; if it does not, then it cannot be called a punisher.

Stimulus Discrimination and Generalization

Stimulus discrimination and stimulus generalization are two opposite concepts. Discrimination occurs when a response is given to a specific **discriminative stimulus**, annotated S^D, because the response has been given past reinforcement in the presence of that stimulus. The ringing of a telephone, for example, is an S^D for picking up the phone behavior. A red light is an S^D for stopping the car behavior. An outstretched hand is an S^D for handshaking behavior.

Stimulus generalization, on the other hand, occurs when the same response is given in the presence of stimuli that are similar to the antecedent S^D but are not entirely the same. For example, a toddler may say the word *ball* when presented with a big rubber ball at home but quickly learns that that response is also reinforced when he says the word *ball* in the presence of basketballs, tennis balls, soccer balls, baseballs, and so forth.

For various reasons, sometimes people fail to appropriately discriminate and generalize. The toddler, for example, who learns to call his mother "Mommy" but then applies that word to every woman he meets has not yet learned that only his own mommy is the S^D that should evoke that title. Similarly, a child who learns the word *dog* in reference to the family pet but fails to produce the word in the presence of any other dog has failed to properly generalize. Also, sometimes when children learn a new grammatical structure, they may overgeneralize, producing such charming errors as *foots* or *eated*.

A toddler who calls all women "Mommy" has failed to appropriately _____.

A child who names only the family pet as a dog, but no other dog is so named has failed to appropriately _____.

Behavior Modification: The Early Days

Behavioral principles are embedded in the everyday lives of human beings. Behavioral scientists did not invent behavioral principles; they simply discovered them through repeated, well-constructed experiments. People alter their behavior in response to countless day-to-day encounters with various stimuli that serve to either reinforce or punish. These principles, in other words, are in operation whether or not the environment is deliberately manipulated by a person to cause a change in the behavior of another person.

Having discovered the principles, however, behavioral scientists went quite a bit further in investigating ways in which human behavior could be modified, not by chance encounter of consequences in the natural environment, but by purposeful manipulation of the environment. Through repeated experimentation, a set of methods emerged that came to be called **behavior modification**; the application of well-researched, empirically based principles of behaviorism by a person or persons to either increase or decrease a specified human behavior in another person. Early behavioral scientists emphasized the importance of defining behaviors in terms that could be observed and measured, subsequently addressing those behaviors through behavior modification procedures, and keeping track of progress through careful collection of data.

It was believed that, if best applied, behavior modification should increase behaviors considered to be desirable and decrease behaviors considered to be undesirable, therefore resulting in an increased quality of life for the person undergoing treatment. The worthiness of such goals would appear to be above reproach; however, behavior modification generated quite a bit of controversy in the early days, the residue of which still exists to some extent in the present day. Controversy regarding the application of behavior modification was centered on at least two factors: (a) the sometimes hyperbolic expression of the philosophical underpinnings of behaviorism, which was often at odds with cherished beliefs held by many, and (b) the nature of early experimentation to establish behavior modification procedures.

Philosophical Underpinnings

"Behaviorism is not the science of human behavior; it is the philosophy of that science" (Skinner, 1974, p. 3). What follows is a necessarily brief and simplified explanation of some of the philosophical underpinnings that came to be associated with behaviorism, often creating much controversy. For a deeper understanding, readers are encouraged to read the original sources, because Skinner was not just a scientist—he was a prolific and eloquent writer.

Skinner's explanations of the philosophy of behaviorism directly challenged beliefs embedded in American tradition—belief in concepts such as freedom, free will, human dignity, and religious belief. He denied the cherished notion that humankind is capable of exercising free will to change the world, stating, "A person does not act upon the world, the world acts upon him" (Skinner, 1971, p. 202). The quest for freedom was explained by the concept of negative reinforcement; revolutions occurred because human beings sought to escape from aversive conditions, not because they were motivated by "a will to be free" (Skinner, 1971, p. 39). Human dignity was described as dependent upon giving credit to a person for something he or she has done. More credit is given when human accomplishments are believed to have no definite cause—when a person's behavior is attributed only to that person and not to some identifiable cause. Therefore, Skinner argued against the concept of human dignity as discouraging to developing an understanding of the causes of human behavior. Finally, Skinner was an atheist, and, for many, behaviorism was linked to arguments against the existence of God. Display Box 1–3 presents a quote from Skinner on the origins of his atheism. For a more thorough understanding of Skinner's controversial, but well-considered, viewpoints, refer to his book, *Beyond Freedom and Dignity* (1971).

Skinner believed that the implementation of his ideas would result in a much improved world. He lived during a time when grave concerns were just emerging regarding overpopulation, the threat of nuclear war, and the pollution of our environment. He pointed out that the ills of our society could not be addressed through technological advancements—humankind was the source of the world's problems, and until the behavior of humans changed, little could be accomplished in moving human society forward. He therefore called for a "behavioral technology"—the application of behavioral principles to create a society in which humankind could live in harmony with their environment and with each other (Skinner, 1971, p. 3). He called for a better way to change humankind other than through the usual punishments society metes out—corporal punishment, imprisonment, and so forth. If it is accepted that human behavior is controlled by the environment, then it should be possible to create an environment that would not evoke punishable behavior—this is actually the principle behind the modern-day concept of **positive behavior support**, a technique that is discussed in Chapter 8. Skinner (1948) described an experimental society incorporating behavioral principles in his utopian novel, *Walden 2*, so entitled as homage to the idyllic life depicted in Thoreau's much earlier work. Aspects of Skinner's vision of a utopian society, such as the extinguishment of competitiveness, and the abolition of the nuclear family in favor of communal childrearing, again provoked much debate.

Display Box 1–3. Skinner and Atheism

Skinner was a self-avowed atheist, which added to the controversy that often surrounded his ideas. He believed that no explanation for a phenomenon was better than a poor explanation for a phenomenon, such as the belief that a deity was the cause. He described the emergence of his atheism in a brief autobiography, in which he described how his grandmother told him of hell "by showing me the glowing bed of coals in the parlor stove" (Boring & Linzey, 1967, p. 391). Later, a teacher, Miss Graves, who Skinner described as a liberal but staunch Christian, suggested to him that some people interpreted the Bible's accounting of miracles as figurative rather than literal. Skinner related the following: "Within a year I had gone to Miss Graves to tell her that I no longer believed in God. 'I know,' she said, 'I have been through that myself.' But her strategy misfired: I never went *through* it" (Boring & Linzey, 1967, p. 391).

Early Experimentation in Behavior Modification

The nature of early experimentation in establishing the principles upon which behavior modification is based also contributed to the public's distrust of behavioral methods. Perhaps the description of Watson's "Little Albert" experiment foreshadowed the sometimes extreme lengths to which early behavioral scientists went to demonstrate the effectiveness of behavior modification techniques (Watson & Rayner, 1920). Experimentation was conducted on a wide range of human behaviors, among them communicative difficulties, which later became known as speech and language disorders. Behavioral techniques were also developed to assist in the remediation of problem behaviors in children and adults with intellectual disability and mental illness, populations with

which the SLP often comes into contact. A brief description of some of the experiments in these areas is mentioned here; this type of experimentation and relevant ethical issues are discussed in more depth in Chapter 10.

Stuttering, which later came to be known as a fluency disorder, was an observable, measurable behavior that lent itself nicely to early experiments in behavioral modification. Flanagan, Goldiamond, and Azrin (1958, 1959) conducted a series of two experiments to demonstrate that stuttering was an act that could be manipulated by bringing it under stimulus control. Participants in the first experiment were three males, ages 15, 22, and 37, who stuttered. The stimulus consisted of a high-pitched, loud tone (e.g., 6000 Hz, 105 dB). The participants wore headphones, and the experimenter had access to a switch that, when depressed, activated the noise stimulus. There were two conditions in which the stimulus was presented: (a) the *aversive* condition and (b) the *escape* condition. For the aversive condition, the experimenter administered a 1-second blast of the noise stimulus to the participant whenever the participant began to stutter. Data collected indicated that under this condition, the frequency of stuttering decreased. For the escape condition, the noise was presented constantly through the participants' headphones when the participants spoke fluently and ceased only when participants began stuttering. Data collected indicated that under the escape condition, stuttering increased.

In the aversive condition (Flanagan et al., 1958), the frequency of stuttering decreased due to _____ punishment.

In the escape condition (Flanagan et al., 1958), the frequency of stuttering increased due to _____ reinforcement.

The second experiment (Flanagan et al., 1959) was conducted in much the same way, but participants were typically fluent speakers, and the aversive stimulus used was electric shock. The participants were given printed passages to read, while they were subjected to a persistent, ongoing electric shock. Because no one is perfectly fluent, every now and then a participant would stutter, and the shock would cease. The participants then began to stutter frequently to escape the electric shock. The researchers then reversed the experiment, ceasing the electric shock when participants spoke fluently and turning the shock back on when participants stuttered. The participants then

began to speak fluently, which was, of course, no problem for them as they were normally fluent speakers. Results of these two experiments demonstrated that frequency of stuttering could be manipulated through application of the behavioral principles of negative reinforcement and positive punishment.

Lovaas, Schaeffer, and Simmons (1965) also investigated the use of electric shock as a negative reinforcer to increase social interaction in children diagnosed with autism. Display Box 1–4 provides a description of behaviors commonly exhibited by people with autism. Participants were 5-year-old identical twins with a diagnosis of *childhood schizophrenia*, a past term applied to children with autism, which is no longer used. Results indicated that it was possible to compel the children to approach previously ignored adults and to reduce their self-stimulatory behaviors to avoid the painful, incessant shock the researchers administered. The researchers also stated that, because the adults were associated with cessation of the shock stimulus, the children also learned to display affection toward them.

Lovaas went on to become the principal investigator of the effectiveness of behavioral treatment for children with autism. His most famous and influential work was a longitudinal study of the application of an intense (e.g., 40 hours a week) behavior modification program with an experimental group of 19 young children with autism with a mean chronological age (CA) of 35 months at the beginning of the experiment (Lovaas, 1987). A control group of 40 children, with a mean CA of 41 months at the beginning of the experiment, was given a less intensive program of under 10 hours of behavior modification a week. The treatment administered was centered on dis-

---

Display Box 1–4. Behaviors Characteristic of Autism Spectrum Disorder (ASD)

Children with ASD were participants in much of the early research conducted to establish behavioral modification techniques. Behaviors associated with autism range from mild to severe and include the following:

- Lack of eye contact
- Stereotypical behaviors (e.g., hand flapping, spinning, rocking, posturing, etc.)
- Rigid adherence to routines
- Hypo- or hyper-reaction to sensory stimuli
- Ritualistic behaviors (e.g., lining up objects, picking leaves off of bushes or lint off of rugs, etc.)
- Severe impairments in social interaction and communication
- Intense preoccupations with specific objects or activities
- Echolalic speech

This list is not at all inclusive of every characteristic that might be seen in people with ASD. Every person with autism presents with a unique combination of symptoms; it is a very heterogenous disorder.

For a full explanation of diagnostic criteria for ASD, see the *Diagnostic and Statistical Manual of Mental Disorders, Fifth Edition* (DSM-5; American Psychiatric Association, 2013).

---

crete trial therapy (see Chapter 5). The entire program was described in detail in a teaching manual (Lovaas et al., 1980) and included use of aversive procedures "as a last resort," including "the delivery of a loud 'no' or a slap on the thigh contingent upon the presence of an undesirable behavior" (Lovaas, 1987, p. 5). Results were that, of the children in the experimental group, nine children (47% of the total in the experimental group) were enrolled in general education classrooms, and had successfully completed first grade by the end of the experiment. All these children also scored in the average or above-average range in intelligence quotient (IQ) testing. These children were described as having "recovered" from autism (p. 7). Eight children in the experimental group were placed in special education classrooms, with a mean IQ score of 70, indicating a mild degree of intellectual disability. Only two of the children in the experimental group were classified as "profoundly mentally retarded," to use the terminology of the day, and were placed in classrooms for severely disabled children with autism, intellectual disability, or both (p. 6).

The success of the children in Lovaas's experimental group, who received 40 hours of behavior modification treatment a week over 2 years, contrasted sharply with the progress made by the 40 children in the control group, who received less than 10 hours of such treatment over the same period of time. At the end of the experiment, only 2% of those children had achieved "normal educational and intellectual functioning"; 45% were classified as "mildly retarded," served in classrooms for children with language delays; and 53% were "severely retarded," served in classrooms for children with profound intellectual disabilities (p. 3). Lovaas extrapolated the results of his study to claim that, if parents got their children to him as early as possible, preferably before 3½ years of age, they had a 50% chance of seeing their child recover from autism.

Lovaas's study was groundbreaking and the first to suggest something other than a totally bleak prognostic outlook for children with autism. However, the study was not without its critics. Schopler, Short, and Mesibov (1989) pointed out flaws in the methodology of the study in the following areas: (a) lack of data documenting specific outcomes, (b) biased participant selection, (c) the intellectual level of the participants, and (d) the manner in which participants were assigned to either the experimental or control groups. Outcome measures consisted only of the subjective judgment of school personnel that the recovered children were indistinguishable from other children; the usual baseline and probe data regarding specific social and communicative behaviors were not reported. Participant selection was biased in favor of high-functioning children with autism, as evidenced by Lovaas's own measurements of intellectual level and by the fact that children

from 40 to 46 months were excluded from the study unless they exhibited echolalic speech, a characteristic of children with autism that often indicates a better prognostic profile. Finally, Schopler et al. (1989) questioned the equivalency of the control group and experimental group, pointing out that families of participant children who had specific challenges such as divorce, personal problems, or the level of severity of the child were offered the less intensive treatment; thus, the children in the control groups came from families that were highly dissimilar to the families of children in the experimental group. Due to these methodological flaws, it was concluded that it was "not possible to determine the effects of this intervention" (p. 164).

Lovaas, Smith, and McEachin (1989, p. 167) delivered a rebuttal to these criticisms, stating that the use of control groups and pretreatment and follow-up measures "safeguarded" their study from the methodological flaws described by Schopler et al. (1989). Furthermore, results of a 4-year follow-up study indicated that the gains the children in the experimental high-intensity intervention group made had been maintained over time (McEachin, Smith, & Lovaas, 1993). In contrast, the children in the control low-intensity intervention program continued to function at a much lower level than children in the experimental group. These results sparked a resurging interest in intensive behavioral treatment to address the social and communicative deficits in children with autism. Regardless of previous controversy over philosophical underpinnings of behaviorism, it was recognized that techniques generated from the science of behavior work. As one commentator stated, "To be opposed to behavior modification is to be opposed to the law of gravity" (Stolz, Wienckowski, & Brown, 1975, p. 1027).

Throughout the 1990s, modifications were made to traditional rigid and sometimes aversive behavioral modification procedures. For example, previous research had indicated that behavioral modification was more effective if children with autism were taught in natural environments with an emphasis on generalization of taught behaviors. Techniques such as incidental teaching (Hart & Risley, 1975), natural language paradigm (Koegel, O'Dell, & Koegel, 1987), and pivotal response training (Koegel & Frea, 1993) were developed to embed behavioral principles in the child's natural environment. It was during this time that applied behavior analysis, firmly rooted in the principles of behaviorism, also developed and is presently considered to be an effective, evidence-based approach in treating children with autism.

Applied Behavior Analysis

The science of applied behavior analysis (ABA) has received much current recognition, particularly because it has generated a set of methods that have been shown to be an efficacious way to improve the behavior and communication skills of children with autism spectrum disorder (ASD; Beavers, Iwata, & Lerman, 2013; Virues-Ortega, 2010). Although most well-known for the treatment of ASD, the methods have broad applicability to problem behaviors that may be exhibited by any human being, including difficulties with communication skills and undesirable behaviors that may get in the way of getting help with those difficulties. Therefore, it is beneficial for SLPs to

have at least some knowledge of the well-researched science of ABA.

Definition of ABA

ABA is a science resulting in a set of methods in which the principles of behavior are applied in a systematic way to effectuate a change in the behaviors of human beings. The purpose of ABA includes identification of clearly defined problem behaviors, functional assessment to discover environmental variables and contingencies that may be contributing to the establishment and continuation of problem behaviors, and intervention based on ongoing data collection and multidisciplinary consultation.

ABA can be further conceptualized by individually considering its three components. As the name implies, ABA is (a) *applied*, (b) *behavioral*, and (c) *analytic*. Although these components were originally described in the context of conducting scientific research (Baer, Wolf, & Risley, 1968), they may also be applied to conducting assessment and treatment of communicative disorders.

ABA is an applied science because it goes far beyond the mere discovery of behavioral principles; instead, ABA results in a set of methods that are then applied to effectuate behavior change in individuals. ABA scientists are not concerned with changing just any behavior. They seek to change specific behaviors that, when created or improved, will affect an individual's life in a socially significant, positive way. They are also concerned with behaviors that, when modified in a large number of individuals, will result in a better, more peaceful, humane society. Furthermore, the behaviors ABA scientists study are given **operational**

definitions that make it possible to directly observe and measure behaviors, preferably in natural settings.

> Giving an operational definition for a behavior makes it possible for the behavior to be _____ and _____.

Similarly, SLPs seek to apply treatment to effectuate improvement in communicative behaviors that will result in the most benefit to clients in their day-to-day environments. They begin with a target behavior that has been given an operational definition, so that they may observe and measure the behavior to determine baseline, or starting, levels and to keep track of how the client is progressing. For example, an SLP might begin treatment by teaching requesting behaviors to a nonverbal 3-year-old boy, thereby empowering the child to have his basic needs met. A patient who has had a stroke may need to relearn the names of common objects, and the SLP might start with those objects that the patient needs to perform basic daily hygiene, such as a toothbrush, comb, and shaver.

The analytic component of research in ABA refers to the success an experimenter experiences when control over a behavior is achieved. Control occurs when researchers gain the ability to increase, decrease, stop, or start a behavior through the application of the experimental variable. Certain research designs, which are described in Chapter 9, have been employed to demonstrate control of behavior change during carefully conducted scientific experiments testing ABA principles and techniques. SLPs performing routine clinical treatment do not typically exert the same caution and care as scientists do to establish control

over a behavior. They do, however, seek to increase, decrease, stop, or start communicative behaviors in their clients through application of various treatment techniques. When SLPs are successful in effectuating such change in their clients, they establish their accountability as clinicians. However, they cannot claim that their treatment methods alone were responsible for their clients' behavior changes, because efficacy of treatment methods can be shown only through carefully constructed scientific experimentation.

> When researchers are able to increase, decrease, stop, or start a behavior through application of the experimental variable, they are said to have established _____.

ABA, then, is a science resulting in a set of methods. Three components—applied, behavioral, and analytic—have been described as delineating characteristics of ABA. Cooper, Heron, and Heward (2007) summarized the definition of ABA by stating,

> **Applied behavior analysis** is the science in which tactics derived from the principles of behavior are applied systematically to improve socially significant behavior, and experimentation is used to identify the variables responsible for behavior change. (p. 20)

Who Are Board Certified Behavior Analysts (BCBAs)?

Board certified behavior analysts (BCBAs) are experts in the application of applied behavior analysis. To become a BCBA, a person must fulfill requirements as set forth by the Behavior Analyst Certification Board (BACB). Requirements include:

- Completion of a master's degree in behavior analysis, education, or psychology **or** completion of a degree program including a BACB-approved course sequence
- Completion of 270 classroom hours of graduate-level coursework in specific areas related to behaviorism, before being allowed to sit for the BACB Certification Examination
- Passage of the BACB Certification Examination
- Completion of supervised experience
- Approval of application to the BACB

Previously, a degree in speech-language pathology qualified a person to take the additional coursework necessary to become a BCBA, and consequently there are some SLP-BCBA working professionals, such as the second author of this textbook. As of January 2016, degrees in speech-language pathology will no longer be accepted by the BACB (Behavior Analyst Certification Board, 2014). Students wishing to become combination SLP-BCBAs will need to complete two master's degree programs: one in speech-language pathology and one in special education, applied behavior analysis, or psychology. There is also a possibility that university faculty will develop curriculum for a degree in speech-language pathology that will include a BACB-approved course sequence.

BCBAs are qualified professionals who conduct functional behavior assessments (FBAs) to discover the antecedent stimuli that may trigger undesirable behavior and the manner in which those behaviors are reinforced and maintained. After conducting the FBA, BCBAs analyze the data collected and use that analysis as the basis for behavior intervention plans (BIPs). BCBAs may supervise and monitor implementation of the BIP, periodically holding meetings with significant others in the person's natural environment to discuss the effectiveness of the BIP and to brainstorm adjustments, if necessary. Although conducting an FBA is outside of an SLP's Scope of Practice, it is still valuable for SLPs to have some knowledge of the principles of FBA; therefore, FBA is discussed in more detail in Chapter 4.

BCBAs are perhaps known best for their work with children with ASD, but BCBAs work in many settings, performing a variety of services. They might train service animals, consult with big corporations regarding employee productivity or consumer preferences, or work with nonprofit agencies seeking ways to end violence (Reinforcement Unlimited, 2014). However, SLPs are most likely to encounter BCBAs in public school settings where children with autism and other diagnoses, including severe behavioral challenges, may end up on both of their caseloads. Also, often children with autism receive home-based ABA therapy, supervised by a BCBA, and services between professionals working with the child at school and at home should be coordinated.

How Can SLPs and BCBAs Collaborate?

There are many ways in which the expertise and scope of practice of an SLP and a BCBA overlap. SLPs and BCBAs work with people who have the same diagnoses, such as ASD, intellectual disability, and SEBD. In the schools, SLPs and BCBAs can collaborate with each other by being aware of the goals they may have for the children on their caseloads. The SLP can work with the BCBA by suggesting ways in which speech and language development can be addressed during ABA therapy. The BCBA can work with the SLP by suggesting ways to reduce undesirable behaviors that may prevent a child from benefiting from speech and language therapy. And, as previously mentioned, SLPs and BCBAs can collaborate to shape new communicative behaviors in a wide range of clients, including those who do not have a behavior disorder.

Finally, analysis of FBA data may reveal that an undesirable behavior is occurring because a person has no other means to effectively communicate with others. Working hand in hand, SLPs and BCBAs can intervene to teach people more socially acceptable means to communicate the same functions and purposes as an undesirable behavior. This can be accomplished far more easily if professionals have at least some knowledge of the principles and methods employed both in the field of speech-language pathology and in the field of applied behavior analysis. If we speak each other's language and understand the value of each other's approaches, the children and adults we serve will be more likely to receive the maximum benefit of our combined efforts.

Chapter Summary

1. Speech-language pathologists (SLPs) should learn and apply principles of behaviorism because:
   a. There is a well-established evidence base for the efficacy of methods based on behaviorism.
   b. Many clients on SLPs' caseloads are likely to exhibit challenging behaviors.
   c. There is an increasing need for SLPs to collaborate with BCBAs in providing assessment and intervention in the public schools for children with behavior disorders.
   d. The principles of behaviorism are broadly applicable across types and levels of severity of communicative disorders.
   e. BCBAs and SLPs can also collaborate to shape new behaviors in a wide range of clients, including those who do not exhibit behavior disorders.
2. Behaviorism is grounded in the concepts of *determinism* and *empiricism*.
3. Notable behaviorists include Pavlov (1849–1936), Watson (1878–1958), and Skinner (1904–1990).
4. Principles of behaviorism were established through repeated experimentation and include:
   a. Respondent and operant conditioning
   b. Positive and negative reinforcement
   c. Differential reinforcement
   d. Positive and negative punishment
   e. Stimulus generalization and discrimination
5. *Behavior modification* is the application of well-researched, empirically based principles of behaviorism by a person or persons to either increase or decrease a specified human behavior in another person.
6. Controversy has surrounded behavior modification due to the philosophical underpinnings of behaviorism and the nature of early experimentation to establish behavioral principles.
7. Applied behavior analysis is a science resulting in a set of methods in which

the principles of behavior are applied in a systematic way to effectuate a change in the behaviors of human beings.

8. Board certified behavior analysts (BCBAs) are professionals who are qualified to conduct functional behavior assessments (FBAs) and design and implement behavior intervention plans (BIPs).

9. SLPs and BCBAs can collaborate by:
   a. Informing each other of the goals they have for clients they have in common
   b. The SLP suggesting ways in which speech and language development can be supported during ABA therapy
   c. The BCBA suggesting ways in which undesirable behaviors might be reduced so that a person can benefit from speech and language therapy
   d. Working together to teach an alternative communicative behavior that serves the same functions and purposes of an undesirable behavior

   c. Positive punishment and negative punishment
   d. Discrimination and generalization

4. Describe the early controversy over behavioral modification techniques. Identify arguments for and against the statement, "To be opposed to behavior modification is to be opposed to the law of gravity" (Stolz et al., 1975, p. 1027).

5. Discuss the relevance of the three components of ABA to the field of speech-language pathology.

6. A speech-language pathologist (SLP) in the public schools has on her caseload a 5-year-old child with autism with minimal oral language. She has put together a comprehensive treatment plan but finds that the child exhibits several behaviors, such as incessant hand flapping and frequent out-of-seat behavior, that interfere with delivery of therapeutic services. The child also receives at-home ABA therapy after school. How can the SLP collaborate with the ABA therapist to maximize the child's potential to achieve oral language goals?

Application Exercises

1. Explain the rationale for the statement, "Speech-language pathologists are in the business of changing behavior."
2. Write one of many possible examples of respondent conditioning that may inadvertently occur in the context of speech and language therapy.
3. Distinguish between:
   a. Respondent and operant conditioning
   b. Positive reinforcement and negative reinforcement

References

American Psychiatric Association. (2013). *Diagnostic and statistical manual of mental disorders* (5th ed.). Arlington, VA: Author.

American Speech-Language-Hearing Association. (2005). *Evidence-based practices in communicative disorders* [Position statement]. Retrieved from http://www.asha.org/policy

Baer, D. M., Wolf, M. M., & Risley, T. R. (1968). Some current dimensions of applied behavior analysis. *Journal of Applied Behavior Analysis, 1*, 91–97.

Beavers, G. A., Iwata, B. A., & Lerman, D. C. (2013). Thirty years of research on the functional analysis of problem behavior. *Journal of Applied Behavior Analysis, 46*, 1–21.

Behavior Analyst Certification Board. (2014). *Standards for board certified behavior analysts (BCBAs).* Retrieved October 20, 2014, from http://bacb.com/index.php?page=158

Bopp, K. D., Brown, K. E., & Mirenda, P. (2004). Speech-language pathologists' roles in the delivery of positive behavior support for individuals with developmental disabilities. *American Journal of Speech-Language Pathology, 13,* 5–19.

Boring, E. G., & Linzey G. (1967). *A history of psychology in autobiography* (Vol. 5). New York, NY: Appleton-Century-Crofts.

Carter, A. S., Wagmiller, R. J., Gray, S. A. O., McCarthy, K. J., Horwitz, S. M., & Briggs-Gowan, M. J. (2010). Prevalence of DSM-IV disorder in a representative, healthy birth cohort at school entry: Sociodemographic risks and social adaptation. *Journal of the American Academy of Child and Adolescent Psychiatry, 49*(7), 686–698.

Chomsky, N. (1965). *Aspects of the theory of syntax.* Cambridge, MA: MIT Press.

Cooper, J. O., Heron, T. E., & Heward, W. L. (2007). *Applied behavior analysis* (2nd ed.). Upper Saddle River, NJ: Pearson Education.

Flanagan, B., Goldiamond, I., & Azrin, N. (1958). Operant stuttering: The control of stuttering behavior through response-contingent consequences. *Journal of the Experimental Analysis of Behavior, 1,* 173–177.

Flanagan, B., Goldiamond, I., & Azrin, N. (1959). Instatement of stuttering in normally fluent individuals through operant procedures. *Science, 130,* 979–981.

Freud, S. (1949). *The ego and the id.* London, UK: Hogarth Press.

Hart, B., & Risley, T. R. (1975). Incidental teaching of language in the preschool. *Journal of Applied Behavior Analysis, 8,* 411–420.

Houk, S. (2000). *"Psychological care of infant and child": A reflection of its author and his times.* Retrieved August 29, 2013, from http://www.mathcs.duq.edu/~packer/DevPsych/Houk2000.html

Koegel, R. L., & Frea, W. D. (1993). Treatment of social behavior in autism through the modification of pivotal social skills. *Journal of Applied Behavior Analysis, 26,* 369–377.

Koegel, R. L., O'Dell, M. C., & Koegel, L. K. (1987). A natural language paradigm for non-verbal autistic children. *Journal of Autism and Developmental Disabilities, 18,* 525–538.

Lovaas, O. I. (1987). Behavioral treatment and normal educational and intellectual functioning in young autistic children. *Journal of Consulting and Clinical Psychology, 55,* 3–9.

Lovaas, O. I., Ackerman, A. B., Alexander, D., Firestone, P., Perkins, J., & Young, D. (1980). *Teaching developmentally disabled children: The me book.* Austin, TX: Pro-Ed.

Lovaas, O. I., Schaeffer, B., & Simmons, J. Q. (1965). Building social behavior in autistic children by use of electric shock. *Journal of Experimental Research in Personality, 1,* 99–109.

Lovaas, O. I., Smith, T., & McEachin, J. J. (1989). Clarifying comments on the young autism study: Reply to Schopler, Short, and Mesibov. *Journal of Consulting and Clinical Psychology, 57,* 165–167.

McEachin, J. J., Smith, T., & Lovaas, O. I. (1993). Long-term outcome for children with autism who received early intensive behavioral treatment. *American Journal on Mental Retardation, 97,* 359–372.

Redmond, S. M., & Rice, M. L. (1998). The socioemotional behaviors of children with SLI: Social adaptation or social deviance? *Journal of Speech, Language, and Hearing Research, 41,* 688–700.

Reinforcement Unlimited. (2014). *What is BCBA anyway?* Retrieved October 20, 2014, from http://www.behavior-consultant.com/whatisbcba.htm

Schopler, E., Short, A., & Mesibov, G. (1989). Relation of behavioral treatment to "normal functioning": Comment on Lovaas. *Journal of Consulting and Clinical Psychology, 57,* 162–164.

Schyns, P. B., Gosselin, F., & Smith, M. L. (2009). Information processing algorithms in the brain. *Trends in Cognitive Science, 13,* 20–26.

Skinner, B. F. (1948). *Walden Two* (Rev. 1976 ed.). Indianapolis, IN: Hackett.

Skinner, B. F. (1971). *Beyond freedom and dignity.* New York, NY: Alfred A. Knopf.

Skinner, B. F. (1974). *About behaviorism.* New York, NY: Vintage Books.

Stolz, S. B., Wienckowski, L. A., & Brown, B. S. (1975). Behavior modification: A perspective on critical issues. *American Psychologist, 30,* 1027–1048.

Virues-Ortega, J. (2010). Applied behavior analytic intervention for autism in early childhood: Meta-analysis, meta-regression, and dose-response meta-analysis of multiple outcomes. *Clinical Psychology Review, 30*, 387–399.

Watson, J. B. (1928). *Psychological care of infant and child*. New York, NY: W. W. Norton.

Watson, J. B., & Rayner, R. (1920). Conditioned emotional reactions. *Journal of Experimental Psychology, 3*, 1–14.

CHAPTER 2

Verbal Behavior

Frances Pomaville

Chapter Outline

- Definition of Verbal Behavior
- Acquisition of Verbal Behavior
- Functional Units of Verbal Behavior
    - Mand
    - Tact
    - Echoic Behavior
    - Intraverbal Behavior
    - Textual Behavior
    - Transcription
- Autoclitics: The Behavioral Explanation of Rules of Grammar
    - Descriptive Autoclitics
    - Quantifying Autoclitics
    - Qualifying Autoclitics
    - Autoclitic Mands
    - Grammatic Tags and Verbal Ordering
- Multiple Causation: Complex Verbal Operants
- Implications for Assessment and Treatment of Communicative Disorders

---

In Chapter 1, the concept of behaviorism, its underlying principles, and its influence on the field of speech-language pathology were discussed. Operant conditioning, the process by which behavior is shaped and maintained through the manipulation of antecedent or consequence events, was also described. Skinner (1957) believed that operant conditioning shapes the way people behave and that language is just another learned behavior; he therefore coined the term **verbal behavior** to replace the cognitive-linguistic term **language**.

Definition of Verbal Behavior

Many behaviors alter or change the environment through physical actions intended to achieve a desired result. For example, a hungry child might walk toward the refrigerator and open it to obtain an apple. The child's behavior directly changes the environment in order to achieve the ultimate consequence (obtaining an apple). If he gets the desired snack, his actions are reinforced. What if, instead of walking over and opening the refrigerator, the child simply says, "I want an apple," and his mother hands him an apple? In this case, the first effect made is on the behavior of another person. The child has acted indirectly upon the environment, from which the ultimate consequence of his behavior (the apple) emerges. This child engaged in a behavior of producing a certain pattern of sounds that resulted in his mother bringing him an apple. The apple reached the child as a result of a complex series of events that included the behavior of both the speaker and the listener.

Skinner (1957) proposed that this type of behavior, which is effective only through the mediation of other people, was unique, and he called it **verbal behavior**, defined as "behavior reinforced through the mediation of other persons" (p. 2). In other words, verbal behavior involves interactions between the speaker and listener, whereby the speaker gains access to reinforcement and controls the environment through the behavior of the listener (Cooper, Heron, & Heward, 2007). Skinner (1957) further described the combined behaviors of the speaker and listener, such as those of the child and mother in the example above, as a **verbal episode**.

> Behavior reinforced through the mediation of other persons is
> _____ _____ .

> The combined behaviors of the speaker and listener is a
> _____ _____ .

Vocal behavior is the most common form of verbal behavior. However, by defining verbal behavior as behavior reinforced through the mediation of other persons, no one form, mode, or medium can be specified. Based on this definition, any movement capable of affecting another organism may be verbal. This includes vocal behavior (i.e., speech), audible behavior other than speech (e.g., clapping your hands to summons someone), written languages, gestural languages (e.g., sign language or pointing), or tactile languages in which the speaker stimulates the skin of the listener, such as fingerspelling into the palm of a person who is deaf and blind.

The concept of verbal behavior therefore redefines units of language and how those units should be documented. In traditional linguistic analysis, vocal behavior is often described and analyzed in terms of structured units of various sizes. Standard units include morphemes, words, phrases, clauses, and sentences. Traditional linguistic analysis typically involves documenting vocal behavior by creating an acoustic recording or by transcribing a language sample. Such procedures allow the listener or reader to construct a facsimile of the original behavior, but they do not result in analysis of the actual response, because the actual response was made by a different person, at a different time, under different conditions.

The true conditions responsible for a specific response may not be captured by traditional units of verbal behavior or by a traditional linguistic transcription. For example, a transcription may show that a child says "milk," but it will not indicate if this utterance occurred because the child is naming a picture of milk, because the child wants some milk, or because the child is imitating the speech of another person. This is problematic in behavioral analysis because the conditions responsible for a specific response, and the ability to predict or control that response, require knowledge of these details.

In order to more accurately describe verbal behavior, Skinner (1957) coined the term **operant** to describe a unit of verbal behavior that is functionally related to one or more independent variables. The term *operant* is similar to the term *response*, and these terms are sometimes used interchangeably. Responses are instances of behavior that can be observed, but operants go beyond that by specifying the effect that a behavior characteristically (although not always) has upon the environment, as well as the variables that control that behavior.

A unit of behavior functionally related to one or more independent variables is an _____.

As noted earlier, traditional linguistic analysis involves describing and analyzing vocal behavior in terms of structured units such as morphemes, words, phrases, or sentences. A verbal operant, however, is based on its functional unity and the effect that it has; it can be as small as a single sound or intonation or as large as a sentence or more. The identification of verbal operants requires the study of a speaker's behavior. Skinner (1957) defined the term **verbal repertoire** as a collection of verbal operants that can be assigned to an individual. In other words, individuals have responses of various forms that typically appear in their behavior given a specific set of conditions. These responses describe potential behaviors of the speaker.

A collection of operants (behaviors) observed under specific circumstances and assigned to an individual is called a _____
_____.

Once an operant is observed and identified, clinicians will attempt to predict the likelihood that it will occur again given the same or similar circumstances. Skinner (1957) referred to this as the **probability of response**. Given a specific set of circumstances, some parts of an individual's verbal repertoire are more likely to occur than others. The relative probability of a behavior being emitted given a specific set of circumstances is called its **strength**. The following features contribute to determining the strength of a response:

- If a response is emitted at all, the operant is considered strong.
- If the response is emitted in a new, unusual, or ambiguous circumstance, the operant is

considered even stronger (i.e., generalization is occurring).

■ The relative speed of a response is considered an indicator of strength. Strong verbal behavior will result in a rapid response.

■ The energy level of a response (its relative pitch, loudness, or intonation) contributes to the operant's strength and meaning. Display Box 2–1 provides examples of effects of energy level on strength and meaning.

■ The immediate repetition of a response can increase its strength. For example, "No, no, no!" may be stronger than a single "No!" In addition, energy and repetition can be combined to increase the response strength even more.

■ The overall frequency with which a response appears relative to a large sample of verbal behavior may be another indicator of strength; however, it should be evaluated in terms of the individual speaker and the communication contexts in which the responses occurred (Display Box 2–2).

All of these features can influence the strength of a response. However, these features are all affected by the circumstances in which they occur and by conditions of reinforcement; therefore, they need to be evaluated in context. For example, an individual may speak with more energy and repetition when in a noisy environment or when speaking to a person with hearing loss. Therefore, the operant strength cannot be inferred on the bases of the loudness of the voice or the number of repetitions alone. The strength of the operant would be determined by whether the speaker, using the same energy level and repetition pattern,

---

Display Box 2–1. Effects of Energy Level on Response Strength and Meaning

■ An energetic "No!" is more likely to evoke a response (e.g., stopping the child from touching a hot stove) than a timid "no," which might easily be ignored or overcome by competing environmental stimuli.

■ In written verbal behavior, the energy of the response may be indicated by the size of the letters, underlining, pressure of the pen, or even the use of emojies.

■ Variations in energy level can change the meaning of a response. For example, the question, "Who is jumping?" evokes the response, "The BOY is jumping," which infers that the boy is the important element. In contrast, the question, "What is the boy doing?" evokes the response, "The boy is JUMPING," which infers that jumping is the important element.

Display Box 2–2. Response Frequency

A response frequency alone (measurement of the dependent variable, or the effect) does not tell us that all instances of the response are instances of the same operant. A high frequency of response may be a reflection of frequently occurring controlling variables (independent variables, or causes). For example, a little girl sees a ball and says "ball." If she is just labeling or identifying the ball, this response is classified as a tact. If she is requesting the ball because it is out of reach and she wants to play with it, this response is classified as a mand. If the child imitates the clinician's model of the word *ball*, it is an echoic. Although linguistically these responses are represented by the same word (*ball*), the causes of the responses are different. Therefore, each response represents a different cause-effect relationship and different operants. Response frequency is concerned with the number of times a specified operant occurs, not the number of times a *word* occurs. A detailed description of these concepts is presented later in the chapter (see Functional Units of Verbal Behavior).

---

would exhibit the same response given the same set of circumstances.

A functional analysis of verbal behavior involves trying to predict and control the probability that a verbal response of a given form will occur at a given time. This verbal response would be the dependent variable, and the conditions or events that result in predicting or controlling that response are the independent variables. Independent variables that control verbal behavior include (a) motivating variables, (b) discriminative stimuli, and (c) consequences. Motivating variables include a state of deprivation or an aversive stimulus. Discriminative stimuli include objects, persons, or events in the environment that evoke a specific response. Consequences include primary or social reinforcement or punishment.

> A strong operant that is likely to occur given the same or similar circumstances is said to have a high _____ ____ _____.

Acquisition of Verbal Behavior

In the simplest sense, Skinner (1957) viewed verbal behavior acquisition as a process of operant conditioning in which the child is motivated by some factor (e.g., hunger) to produce a response (e.g., pointing or vocalizing) that is subsequently reinforced (e.g., the child is fed). Once the parent or listener reinforces a response, that response is more likely to become part of the child's verbal repertoire. When many instances of a response are reinforced, that operant will increase in strength and is more likely to be repeated and maintained.

Speech-language pathologists are concerned with ways to facilitate the acquisition of verbal behavior. In order to do so, two important considerations must be addressed: (a) how to facilitate the learning of a new verbal behavior that has not yet emerged, and (b) once a desired behavior does occur, what can be done to increase the probability that it will recur with the frequency needed to strengthen it?

Principles of behaviorism do not support the idea that children have an innate knowledge of adult forms of verbal behaviors just waiting to emerge. Therefore, in the initial stages of learning a new verbal behavior, any response that vaguely resembles the desired target behavior is often reinforced. Then, as the behavior begins to appear more frequently, reinforcement may be contingent on a closer approximation to the desired behavior, until the desired end behavior is achieved. This is referred to as reinforcement of **successive approximations**. In this way, complex verbal behaviors, such as vocal communication, can be shaped over time. "A child acquires verbal behavior when relatively unpatterned vocalizations, selectively reinforced, gradually assume forms which produce appropriate consequences in a given verbal community" (Skinner, 1957, p. 31).

Giving reinforcement contingent on increasingly more accurate productions of a target behavior is called

_____ _____ .

After a verbal behavior is acquired, reinforcement becomes important for the maintenance of that behavior. If, for some reason, reinforcement stops, then the operant will weaken, and it is possible that the behavior will be reduced in frequency or even disappear, a process called **extinction**. Therefore, through the application of operant reinforcement, the probability that a certain response will occur can be controlled. An effective reinforcer applied across many instances increases the probability that a desired verbal behavior will occur, thus increasing its frequency of occurrence. Remember, as discussed in Chapter 1, this can occur through application of a reinforcing stimulus (positive reinforcement) or removal of an aversive stimulus (negative reinforcement). Likewise, one way to decrease the probability that an undesired verbal behavior will occur, thus decreasing its frequency of occurrence, is to eliminate whatever is reinforcing that behavior.

In addition to identifying what reinforces a verbal behavior after it occurs, identifying the cause or motivation behind the initial performance of a behavior is also very important. This can help to discover environmental manipulations or motivating factors that can be used to increase the probability that a verbal behavior will occur. After all, the behavior has to occur before it can be reinforced.

Establishing operations (Michael, 1988), a concept that was later redefined as **motivating operations** (MOs) (Laraway, Snycerski, Michael, & Poling, 2003; Display Box 2–3 gives examples of motivating operations), are variables that affect the probability that a specific verbal behavior will occur. They are most often described in the context of teaching mands but can also be used with other verbal behaviors.

Display Box 2–3. Examples of Motivating Operations (MOs)

One way to increase a child's motivation to respond is through **deprivation**.

- If using food as a reinforcer for teaching mands, a hungry child will be more motivated to produce the verbal behavior of saying "hungry" in order to receive food (the reinforcer) than a child who is not hungry; therefore, use meal time or snack time to work on this target behavior.
- Brief deprivation (Williams & Greer, 1993) is when an item is made visible but is only obtainable with an acceptable verbal behavior, after it has not been available for a short time. For example, if the clinician and child are blowing bubbles, the clinician may place the bubbles out of reach and wait for the child to request them.
- Interrupted chain (McGee, Krantz, Mason, & McClannahan, 1983; Michael, 1982) is when items that are needed to complete a sequence or chain of behaviors are removed until the child requests them (e.g., withholding several pieces of a puzzle the child wants to complete).
- Incidental or captured moment (Hart & Risely, 1975) is when desired objects are placed in the natural environment such that the child cannot access them without the mediation of another person. For example, if the desired verbal behavior is for the child to vocalize or gesture "truck" in order to obtain a toy truck, the toy trucks would be placed on a shelf the child cannot reach without assistance.

Another environmental manipulation that can be used to increase motivation to produce a desired verbal behavior is the introduction of an **aversive stimulus**. For example, if a clinician discovers that there is a certain toy that makes a sound that is upsetting to the child, the clinician might use that sound to motivate the child to vocalize or gesture "stop," which would then be reinforced by turning the sound off (i.e., removal of the aversive stimulus).

Motivating operations can increase the probability of a response in two ways. First, MOs can momentarily alter the reinforcing effectiveness of a stimulus, as might occur by creating a state of deprivation or introducing an aversive stimulus. Second, MOs can change the frequency of behaviors that were previously reinforced by a specific activity, object, or event by creating multiple opportunities for that behavior to occur (more than might naturally occur in that environment; Greer & Ross, 2008).

_____ _____ are variables that affect the probability that a specific verbal behavior will occur, such as creating a state of deprivation or introducing an aversive stimulus.

Once a verbal behavior is established, it is important to vary the circumstances in which it occurs, as well as the stimuli used to evoke it. This will further increase the strength of the response. For instance, if a child has learned the verbal behavior *ball*, this behavior will be strengthened by exposing the child to a variety of balls, including different colors, sizes, or even shapes (e.g., a football vs. a tennis ball). In order to strengthen the verbal behavior *stop*, a parent or clinician might vary the aversive circumstances by using tickling (assuming that tickling is aversive to the child) in addition to introducing an aversive sound. Reinforcing the desired verbal behavior, while exposing the child to a variety of stimuli and conditions, increases the probability that the behavior will generalize, thus potentially improving communication even more.

To understand verbal behavior acquisition it is necessary to consider (a) the antecedents that evoke verbal behaviors,

(b) the communication behaviors themselves, and (c) the consequences of those behaviors (i.e., how the listener reacts). Earlier, a verbal episode was defined as the combined behaviors of the speaker and the listener. Therefore, based on Skinner's definition of verbal behavior, it is necessary to consider both the behavior of the speaker and the behavior of the listener to analyze how the behavior of the listener is responsible for reinforcing or punishing the behavior of the speaker. In addition, environmental conditions may be contributing to the probability that a behavior will occur. It is through the analysis and consideration of these factors that the acquisition of verbal behavior is explained.

Functional Units of Verbal Behavior

As described above, Skinner (1957) focused on the cause and effects of human communication. He analyzed and described verbal behaviors in terms of (a) their evoking stimuli, also called **antecedents**; (b) the communication behaviors themselves; and (c) the consequences of those behaviors. This is often described as a three-term contingency:

$(A \rightarrow B \rightarrow C)$, where A = Antecedent, B = Behavior, and C = Consequence

Antecedent conditions might include some state of deprivation or aversive stimulation, referred to earlier as a motivating operation (MO); some aspect of the environment that stimulates a response; or the verbal behavior of others. Consequences are the result following the behavior and may be direct and tangible, such as receiving an item that is requested, or social and educational, such as specific praise or a big smile.

> In the three-term contingency (**A→B→C**), **A** stands for the _____, **B** stands for the _____, and **C** stands for the _____.

Instead of linguistically grouping verbal behaviors into structures such as words and sentences, Skinner (1957) grouped them based on their corresponding antecedent and consequence stimuli and called these cause-effect relationships **functional units**. Skinner described the following functional units of verbal behavior: mands, tacts, echoics, intraverbals, autoclitics, textuals, and transcriptions. Table 2–1 provides a description of these verbal behaviors based on their typical antecedents and consequences.

Mand

Skinner (1957) defined a **mand** as a verbal operant "in which the response is reinforced by a characteristic consequence

Table 2–1. Functional Units of Verbal Behavior

Antecedent	Behavior	Consequence
A state of deprivation or an aversive stimulus	MAND	Primary reinforcement that reduces deprivation or aversive stimuli
An environmental object or event	TACT	Social reinforcement
Verbal behavior of another person	ECHOIC	Social reinforcement
The speaker's or another person's prior speech	INTRAVERBAL	Social reinforcement
Primary verbal behaviors that are enhanced by secondary verbal behaviors (autoclitics), which provide additional information	AUTOCLITIC	Social reinforcement
Printed stimuli or oral speech for dictated writing	TEXTUALS	• Social reinforcement • Conditioned generalized reinforcement • Primary reinforcement such as getting paid for spontaneous writing
An auditory verbal stimulus	TRANSCRIPTIONS	• Social reinforcement

Source: Hegde and Maul (2006); Hegde and Pomaville (2013).

and is therefore under the functional control of relevant conditions of deprivation or aversive stimulation" (pp. 35–36). Mands include verbal behaviors such as commands, demands, requests, and questions (interrogatives). They make up many everyday verbal behaviors and help facilitate early language development. When a child realizes that he or she can obtain a desired item or action (e.g., food or a hug) by acting in a certain way, the foundation for communication is established.

> A _____ is a verbal operant in which the reinforcing consequence is typically specified and the antecedent is a state of deprivation or an aversive stimulus.

The antecedent for a mand is a motivational state caused by conditions of deprivation or exposure to aversive stimuli. Motivational operations that serve as antecedents to mands include hunger, thirst, pain, discomfort, and sex drive. A unique feature about mands is that they typically specify the desired reinforcement (i.e., what they want the listener to provide or do). Because of this, it is often easier for the listener to react in a way that will reinforce the speaker's verbal response. Typical consequences of mands include receiving the requested item (positive reinforcement) or removal of an aversive stimulus (negative reinforcement). In addition, mands are typically reinforced by primary or unconditioned reinforcers, which were defined in Chapter 1 as reinforcers that are biological in nature and don't depend on past experience (e.g., receiving food or drink or getting away from something that is dangerous or uncomfortable). Table 2–2 provides examples of mands along with their antecedents and consequences.

Environmental factors can also influence the production of mands and may contribute to the antecedent events that evoke a specific mand. For example, if an individual is feeling cold (an aversive stimulus), environmental factors may influence whether that individual asks for a sweater or tells someone to turn the heater on. An individual playing outside may request a sweater, whereas a person inside a cold room may ask for the heater to be turned on.

Table 2–2. Mands

Antecedent	Behavior	Consequence
Hunger (deprivation)	Child says, "I want a cookie."	The child receives a cookie (positive reinforcement)
The child wants a toy ball (deprivation)	Child signs "ball."	The child receives the ball (positive reinforcement)
One child is feeling threatened by another child (aversive stimuli)	The first child says, "Go away!"	The *threatening* child goes away (negative reinforcement)

As mentioned earlier, mands generally specify the desired reinforcement. This, combined with knowledge of the environmental factors involved, often makes the motivation behind the mand obvious, and the listener is able to respond readily without questioning the speaker's motivation. There may be times, however, when the motivation behind a mand is not so clear. For example, if a child asks his mother for lunch money even though he was already provided with enough money to cover lunches for the week, the parent might ask, "Why?" Thus, the parent is requesting (manding) additional information to which the child might respond, "I lost it."

There are some mands that become generalized; that is, they may be used across many different states of deprivation in combination with other behaviors that help to clarify their meaning. For example, emphatic expressions such as *Now!* or *Here!* might be used to get the listener's attention even though the reinforcer is not clearly stated in the mand itself. The mand *please* is commonly used to request something without further specification of the desired reinforcer. Environmental circumstances and dynamic properties such as intonation or the energy level of the mand might contribute to the listener's understanding and response to these types of generalized mands.

Skinner (1957) also described several additional classes of mands that are distinguished in terms of the listener's behavior. With these mands, the listener may experience positive consequences that the speaker does not participate in, yet they remain reinforcing to the speaker as well. Examples of this type of mand include giving advice, warning, or permission to others. When the mand results

in positive reinforcement for the listener, it is called *advice* (e.g., "Turn right on Fourth Street"). When the mand results in the listener escaping some aversive stimulus, it is called a *warning* (e.g., "Look out!"). When the mand cancels some restraint that is interfering with a behavior the listener was already inclined to complete, it is called *permission* ("It's OK—go for it").

Over time, individuals may begin to use mands even when characteristic reinforcement of the behavior is unlikely or impossible, called **extended stimulus control**. Examples of extended stimulus control involving mands occur when an individual yells "stop!" as a car is about to crash on the television or when people mand the behavior of untrained animals, dolls, or small babies. The *listeners* in these examples are not capable of reinforcing the mand in the characteristic way. Yet, the listener or situation is similar enough to ones in which the behavior was previously reinforced that it controls the response.

Mands make up some of the earliest developing verbal behaviors and may provide a foundation for learning to communicate. Initially, when a baby cries from hunger, it is a reflexive mand, but if the baby is reinforced by being fed, it may create the foundation for learning more complex patterns of response over time. Later, the child may be taught to say a word such as *milk* when feeling thirsty. As the child gets older, *I want milk please* or a more subtle mand such as *I'm thirsty* might be reinforced and learned. The pattern of response that achieves the desired reinforcement is dependent upon the reinforcing practices of the listener and verbal community. In this way, verbal behaviors develop to match those of others in the child's environment.

Tact

Skinner (1957) defined a **tact** as "a verbal operant in which a response of given form is evoked (or at least strengthened) by a particular object or event or property of an object or event" (pp. 81–82). Tacts often name, comment on, reference, or describe objects or events in the environment. They provide a way for the speaker to share experiences with others.

> A _____ often names, comments on, references, or describes objects or events in the environment.

Tacts differ from mands in several ways. Tacts are not caused by a state of motivation associated with deprivation or the desire to avoid an aversive stimulus. Tacts do not specify their own reinforcers, and the consequences of tacts are not primary reinforcers. It is notable that the controlling stimuli for tacts are nonverbal. The antecedents for tacts are events, people, or objects (discriminative environmental stimuli) that the speaker wants to name or comment on. The consequence of a tact is social (secondary) reinforcement; therefore, a listener or audience is critical. Typical social reinforcers might include a head nod, smile, or expression of agreement from the listener. Increased attention from the listener may also be socially reinforcing. Table 2–3 provides examples of tacts along with their antecedents and consequences.

In Chapter 1, a discriminative stimulus was defined as a stimulus that evokes a specific response because that response has been given past reinforcement in the presence of that stimulus. For example, a mother points to the family dog and says "dog," and the child then repeats "dog" (this is an imitated response or echoic that is discussed later in the chapter). The mother is very excited and declares, "Yes, dog!" thus reinforcing the echoic. However, later that day, the child points to the dog and declares "dog" without a model, which again evokes smiles and praise from his mother. The family dog has become a discriminative stimulus for the verbal behavior *dog* because it was reinforced earlier, and the unprompted declaration of "dog" is a tact that was then reinforced once again with social reinforcement from the mother. Each time this verbal episode is repeated, the response is strengthened, and the probability that seeing the family dog will evoke the tact *dog* increases.

The more a novel stimulus (e.g., another dog in the neighborhood) resem-

Table 2–3. Tacts

Antecedent	Behavior	Consequence
The child sees a ball or a picture of a ball	Child says "ball"	The listener responds, "Yes, that's right!"
The child sees a very large dog	Child signs "big dog"	The listener responds, "Wow, that is a big dog!"
The child hears a dog barking	Child says "doggie barking"	The listener responds, "Yes, I hear it too."

bles the original stimulus, the higher the likelihood that the same tact will be evoked, thus providing an opportunity for additional social reinforcement. In this way, children learn to generalize tacts to multiple items in the same stimulus class. In other words, the child learns that *dog* refers to many different dogs, not just the family pet. When an individual generalizes a tact to a novel item with similar properties, it is called an **extended tact**.

> When a tact is generalized to a novel item with similar properties, it is called an _____ _____.

Two special kinds of extension are **metaphorical extension** and **metonymical extension**. Metaphorical extension occurs when a tact is extended to an object in a different stimulus class with similar properties. An example of metaphorical extension might be when the tact *leg* that originally represented the four legs of an animal was extended to the legs on a table, which have similar functions and geometric qualities. If a metaphorical extension is reinforced by the verbal community, it may then become a generalized tact that is widely understood and accepted. Although the use of *legs* for the four structures holding up a table may have started as a metaphorical extension, today it would be considered a generalized tact.

Metonymical extension occurs when generalization of a tact accounts for a verbal operant that seems to have no controlling stimuli (Hegde, 2011; Skinner, 1957; Winokur, 1976). For example, when a person talks about an object that is not present, it may be difficult to determine what the discriminative stimulus is. When a child looks into a toy box and says, "No ball," it is tempting to think that the missing ball acted as the stimulus; however, a missing object cannot be a stimulus for a response, in the same way a missing cause does not produce an effect (Hegde, 2011). The child's response, *No ball*, was actually controlled by the stimuli that were currently present (i.e., the toys in the box along with the empty space) that previously coexisted with the missing ball. The response *ball* was likely reinforced in the past when the ball had been part of that group of toys; therefore, those toys are now the antecedent for the tact *No ball*. When groups of stimuli have common elements, a response conditioned to one of them may also be conditioned to all or some of the individual items in the group. Therefore, when the speaker confronts one or more of those same elements, the same response is likely to be emitted.

Reinforcement of a tact should be contingent on it having an appropriate relation or correspondence with the stimulus or event being tacted. If a child points to the neighborhood cat and says "dog," it would not be reinforced, thus decreasing the probability that the child would say "dog" the next time he or she sees a cat. When children are first developing their verbal repertoire, some leniency may be allowed. For example, an 18-month-old child who sees a helicopter and says "airplane" might still be reinforced. However, as the child's verbal repertoire increases, caregivers may require progressively better correspondence between the tact and the discriminative stimulus that evokes it. In this way, children learn to produce more differentiated tacts. It is through this process of appropriate social reinforcement that tacts are learned, generalized, and differentiated, thus expanding the child's verbal repertoire.

At times, it may difficult to tell if a young child is producing a tact or a mand. In order to make a determination, the entire interaction needs to be assessed. For example, if a young child is playing and suddenly points to a ball and says "ball," it may be difficult to tell if he wants the ball (mand) or if he is just labeling the toy he sees (tact). If the listener reinforces the child with a comment such as, "Yes, there's the ball" and the child says nothing further, his verbal behavior was a tact. If, however, the child continues to demand action by reaching or verbalizing, then it was most likely a mand. This example highlights the importance of considering the entire verbal episode when assessing verbal behavior.

Echoic Behavior

Skinner (1957) defined **echoic behavior** as verbal behavior that is under the control of another verbal stimulus and has a sound pattern similar to that of the stimulus. Stated simply, echoics are imitations of another's verbal behavior. The verbal behavior, acting as the stimulus for the imitation, is often called a **model**. The ability to imitate a model is important for language development. An earlier example demonstrated an echoic behavior when the child imitated his mother (the echoic) after she pointed to the family pet and said "dog" (the model). This resulted in positive social reinforcement from the mother, thus strengthening the response.

An _____ is a verbal behavior that is under the control of another verbal stimulus and has a sound pattern similar to that stimulus.

Echoics may be used as fill-ins while the listener is formulating a response. For instance, if a person is asked a question and needs a little time to answer, the person might repeat part of the question. For example, when asked, "Who was president of the United States in 1985?" a person might respond, "The person who was president in 1985 [speaking slowly and pausing slightly] . . . is Ronald Reagan." This echoic response would be self-reinforcing if it provides time for the speaker to compose an answer. An echoic response might also be used to indicate agreement, such as when one person says, "That's a beautiful sunset," and another person responds, "Beautiful sunset!" Echoic responses also might serve to confirm information received. For example, one person might say, "Let's meet at the park at 8:00" and another person repeats, "The park at 8:00," indicating both agreement and confirmation of the meeting place and time.

Applying the three-part contingency, antecedents for echoic behaviors are other persons' verbal behaviors (models). As with tacts, the consequence for echoic behavior is social reinforcement. This reinforcement is usually contingent on there being a good match between the model stimulus and the acoustic properties of the echoic response. A good match occurs when there is point-to-point correspondence and formal similarity with the antecedent stimulus. Point-to-point correspondence occurs when all components (i.e., the beginning, middle, and end) of the antecedent stimulus and behavior are the same. Formal similarity occurs when the antecedent and behavior are produced in the same sensory modality and resemble one another. In other words, positive reinforcement is more likely to occur if the echoic reproduces the antecedent stimulus or closely approximates it.

Although correspondence between the stimulus unit and the response unit is required, a certain degree of variability may be acceptable. Verbal echoic behaviors may differ somewhat from the stimulus or antecedent behavior. Vocal behaviors may differ in pitch, loudness, intonation, or other characteristics when compared to a vocal antecedent. With sign language, a sign may differ somewhat from the original signed behavior. Similarly, written echoics may differ somewhat in the way letters or shapes are formed when compared to the antecedent visual stimulus. If these differences fall within an acceptable range, the behavior will be reinforced. If not, reinforcement is unlikely. At times, an echoic may be reinforced because it is moving closer to an approximation than an earlier attempt. The label **partial echoic** is used when only a portion of what is heard is repeated. This may occur as a child is developing language or when someone echoes the last part of an utterance just heard in order to show agreement or to request clarification. Table 2–4 provides examples of echoic behaviors along with their antecedents and consequences.

Skinner (1957) also described self-reinforcing, self-echoic behaviors. Such behaviors may, as described later, occur during early language development in typically developing children. There are times, however, when self-echoics characterize a language problem. Verbal perseverations produced by individuals with neurological disorders may be described as self-echoics. When self-echoics are excessive, uncontrolled, or pathological in other ways, they may be labeled as **palilalia**.

Echoics have an important role in the development of verbal behavior. A baby's first vocalizations consist of unconditioned and indiscriminate babbling. This occurs naturally as air moves through the vocal folds, causing them to vibrate so random sounds are produced. A number of conditions can then occur to shape this unconditioned, nonoperant babbling into echoic behavior, which may then provide the foundation for the development of more complex verbal operants. First, before any kind of verbal behavior develops, including echoic behavior, it is possible that the babies are reinforced by hearing their own babbling. The sounds they hear themselves produce are immediately and automatically reinforced so babbling increases. This may explain why babies who are deaf begin to babble but then stop; they cannot hear their own

Table 2–4. Echoics

Antecedent	Behavior	Consequence
The child hears the word "ball"	Child says "ball"	The parent responds, "That's right!"
The child sees someone sign, "He has a blue shirt."	Child signs "blue shirt"	The parent responds, "Yes"
A parent says, "Mmmm . . . this pizza is yummy!"	Child says "Yummy!"	The parent smiles and nods, indicating he knows the child agrees

babbling, so this type of automatic reinforcement does not occur.

A second type of conditioning occurs because the parents experience a reinforcing effect when they hear their baby's nonoperant babbling. Parents take pleasure in hearing the sound of their baby's cooing and babbling. They tend to react by echo-babbling back to the baby or by repeating the sounds made by their baby while they are involved in other caregiver activities such as bathing or playing with the child. The parents' vocalizations then become associated with these pleasurable experiences, and ultimately these vocalizations become conditioned reinforcers for the child's vocalizations.

A third type of conditioning takes place as parents begin to socially reinforce their babies' babbling. Social reinforcement might include smiling, hugging, picking them up, or other similar reactions that strengthen the response and encourage more babbling. Several studies have shown that such contingent social reinforcers can increase babbling in babies (Bloom, Russell, & Wassenburg, 1987; Goldstein, King, & West, 2003; Goldstein & Schwade, 2008; Gros-Louis, West, Goldstein, & King, 2006; McLaughlin, 2006; Winokur, 1976).

Initially, parents reinforce any sounds made by their baby. Over time, parents begin to provide more refined reinforcement that is contingent upon hearing sounds that are used by their verbal community. For example, a baby who says "dada" for daddy is producing a partial echoic that parents are likely to reinforce, initially. Over time, however, the parents are likely to require progressively better approximations or a complete echoic. During this time when echoics are being reinforced, other environmental variables (e.g., events, objects, or persons) may become associated with the child's response and gain stimulus control over it (Hegde, 2011). This process of refined reinforcement gradually leads to the development of mands, tacts, and other verbal operants (McLaughlin, 2006; Pena-Brooks & Hegde, 2007).

Intraverbal Behavior

Like echoics, the controlling variables for **intraverbals** are prior verbal responses. However, unlike echoics, there is no point-to-point correspondence between intraverbal responses and their stimuli. Intraverbals may be generated by a speaker's own prior verbal behavior or by the verbal behavior of another person. Therefore, the antecedent for an intraverbal is an immediately preceding response that stimulates additional verbal responses. The consequence for intraverbals is social reinforcement that may be overt or subtle, as explained later in this section.

> Verbal operants that are generated by a speaker's own verbal behavior or by the verbal behavior of others, without point-to-point correspondence with the antecedent stimulus, are _____.

Intraverbals make up much of what people say throughout the day and explain how people can recite a long poem or go on talking in the absence of continuous physical stimuli. In essence, speech that is produced stimulates more speech in a chain-like fashion. When a speaker asks, "How are you?" the social response, "Fine, thank you" is likely intraverbal (Skinner, 1957). Responses to *wh*– questions may also be intraverbals; a response to a *why* question is likely going to start with *because*.

Some intraverbals are more obvious and consist of verbal behaviors that are somewhat routine because they were learned as a unit. If a speaker says "salt and . . . " a listener is likely to complete this phrase with the intraverbal *pepper*. Intraverbal control is often evident in common metaphors and literary allusions, such as when reciting *the early bird* prompts the intraverbal *gets the worm*. When an individual recites the alphabet, *A-B-C-D* becomes a stimulus that generates *E-F-G-H*, and so forth. Similarly, when reciting a long poem, each stanza becomes a stimulus for the next one. Children often learn mathematical, historical, or scientific facts as intraverbal responses. The verbal behavior *two plus two* stimulates the intraverbal response *equals four*, and *Columbus sailed the ocean blue* prompts the response *in fourteen hundred ninety-two*. Each of these examples demonstrates intraverbal control where one verbal response is the stimulus for the next verbal response, and so on. This type of intraverbal control likely contributes to the fluency of our speech, for without it, speech would contain more pauses, repetitions, and hesita-tions (Hegde, 1982). Table 2–5 provides examples of intraverbal behaviors along with their antecedents and consequences.

The consequence that reinforces intraverbal behavior is social reinforce-ment that may be overt or subtle. When a question is asked in the classroom, the correct answer is the one that is rein-forced. Therefore, it is likely to be repro-duced when the same or similar question is asked again. When reciting a poem or lengthy account of some historical event, each subsequent segment reinforces the preceding segment's accuracy. When a client with aphasia recites the phrase "salt and . . . " to stimulate the target word *pepper*, that client is using an intraverbal prompt to self-cue the response. This indi-vidual may be overtly reinforced by a cli-nician saying "that's right" or more subtly reinforced by an improved ability to com-municate. Thus, the client is more likely to use the same strategy in the future.

Intraverbals can take the form of chains or clusters (Winokur, 1976). When the response has a fixed order upon which the delivery of reinforcement is contingent, it is an **intraverbal chain**. Earlier examples of reciting the alphabet or a lengthy poem are intraverbal chains because one ver-

Table 2–5. Intraverbals

Antecedent	Behavior	Consequence
The listener says, "salt and . . ."	Speaker says "pepper"	The listener responds, "That's right!"
The child recites to himself, "Columbus sailed the ocean blue . . ."	Child continues, "in 1492"	The child is reinforced by completing the rhyme and remembering the fact accurately
A teacher asks, "Why are you late?"	The student says, "because I had car trouble"	The teacher responds, "I understand."

bal response stimulates the next. Skinner (1957) found it important to note that "any link in a chain of responses is not under exclusive control of the preceding link" (p. 72). In other words, just repeating the last letter in the alphabet or the last word in a poem is often not enough to stimulate the next verbal behavior. Instead, the speaker often needs to begin at the beginning of the chain in order to recite the entire sequence. A child who is interrupted while reciting the alphabet often needs to start back at the beginning in order to finish, or when asked, "What day is it?" a client with aphasia might need to recite the days of the week, "Monday, Tuesday . . . " until the correct day is stated.

Intraverbal clusters occur when groups of verbal operants evoke each other in the absence of a unidirectional relationship. Word associations or naming items in a category are examples of intraverbal clusters. The verbal stimulus *furniture* might evoke verbal responses such as *table, chair, couch,* and *bed.* In this example, one verbal stimulus evoked several intraverbal responses; therefore, it is an example of **divergent intraverbal control**. If the stimulus consisted of several verbal stimuli used to evoke a single response (e.g., the verbal stimuli *worn on the wrist* and *used to tell time* are used to evoke *watch*), it is an example of **convergent intraverbal control** (Michael, Palmer, & Sundberg, 2011).

Intraverbal clusters can be further described as **formal** or **thematic** (Michael et al., 2011; Winokur, 1976). In formal clusters, the stimuli and responses are linked together because they sound similar (e.g., *pie* may stimulate *my, try, high,* or *bye*). Therefore, rhyming skills are dependent on this type of intraverbal control. In thematic clusters, the stimuli and responses are linked together because they share a common meaning or have shared similar reinforcement contingencies. The cluster *chair, sofa, couch, bench* is an example of a thematic cluster.

In terms of language development, intraverbal relations are a higher level verbal behavior than the production of basic mands and tacts. Basic verbal operants such as pure echoics, mands, and tacts should be taught first (Hegde, 2011). This does not, however, diminish the importance of working on intraverbal relationships as the child's verbal repertoire develops. Children and adults with impaired intraverbal relations will often be described as having impaired word retrieval, poor conversational skills, poor sentence completion, difficulty with categories, difficulty generating antonyms and synonyms, poor topic maintenance, or limited continuous speech.

Textual Behavior

Skinner (1957) defined textual behavior as verbal behavior that "is under the control of a nonauditory verbal stimulus" (p. 66). The most common antecedent for textual behavior is written text; however, other forms of visual stimuli that evoke textuals might include the phonetic alphabet, hieroglyphs, musical notes, or other symbols. Braille, a tactile form of written text, could also be an antecedent for textual behavior. In other words, textual behavior is synonymous with reading. The consequence of textual behavior is social reinforcement contingent on there being good point-to-point correspondence between the stimulus (i.e., written text) and the textual behavior (i.e., reading). Without good point-to-point correspondence, a defective textual is produced and the stimulus is misread. Unlike echoics, formal similarity is not required as the antecedent, and the response involves different sensory modalities. Table 2–6 provides examples of textual behaviors along with their antecedents and consequences.

> A verbal behavior that is under the control of a nonauditory verbal stimulus such as written text, the phonetic alphabet, or musical notes is _____ behavior.

Initially, textual behavior is socially reinforced for purely educational reasons. A child beginning to read who says "dog" in the presence of the written stimulus *dog* is likely to be reinforced with overt social reinforcement such as "That's right" or "Good reading." As children get older, textual prompts can be used to establish other types of verbal operants. For example, the printed name may be placed next to a picture to teach a new verbal operant; picture dictionaries use this strategy. In this way, the child associates the written text with the picture and ultimately the actual object. This may result in the production of a tact when they later see that picture or object. Thus, textuals can contribute to the expansion of a child's verbal repertoire. As children get older and learn more textuals, reading becomes a primary mode for increasing their verbal repertoire and knowledge base. This explains why textbooks and libraries are important parts of most educational institutions.

Beginning readers are often reinforced by hearing themselves read (audible feedback) but later begin to read silently. It is also interesting to note that even experienced readers often resort to reading out loud when reading a particularly complex text or set of instructions, thus providing auditory feedback that is reinforcing. Most adult textual behavior, however, is covert (silent). Textual behavior is so strongly reinforced that individuals often find themselves reading such varied materials as books, letters, e-mails, newspapers, billboards, advertisements, and labels, to name just a few. Skinner (1957) stated that, "In the case of automatic self-reinforcement, the behavior may become so reduced in magnitude that it is no longer visible to [or observed by] others" (p. 141). Such is the case with silent reading. Textual behavior as silent reading may provide a type of automatic self-reinforcement and may continue to

Table 2–6. Textual Behavior

Antecedent	Behavior	Consequence
The written word C-A-T	Child says "cat"	The listener responds, "That's right!"
Musical text (musical notes and text)	The singer performs the song	The audience claps, and/or the singer is paid
A written poem	The reader reads the poem to himself	Reading the poem evokes a joyful emotional response

receive reinforcement by being useful to the reader in many ways (Skinner, 1957).

From a purely practical view, reading often results in completing a task more successfully or correctly. Reading directions or a map may result in finding a specific location. Reading a recipe may result in a delicious meal. Reading an advertisement might help save money. Reading instructions is important for properly taking medications or building something. A child whose textual behavior matches the instructions (pictures and text) for building a LEGO vehicle is reinforced with a new toy that he put together all by himself. As adults, the reinforcement for textual behavior may also be monetary. Such is the case when someone is paid to read during a public performance or when someone is paid to read a book for recording purposes.

In addition, reading, whether silent or overt, may evoke an emotional response because of a reader's past experience. This emotional response may be reinforcing in such a way that the reader wants to read more works by the same author or other similar texts. Readers may not be able to identify the exact stimulus or property of the stimulus that evoked the emotional response, but they know how it made them feel at the time. This emotional response occurred even though the reason for the response is not clear.

Transcription

Transcription is a nonvocal verbal behavior (i.e., writing) that requires support from the external environment. In order for this verbal behavior to occur, the writer must (a) obtain the necessary instruments (e.g., pen, pencil, paper), (b) make marks of differential form, and (c) transmit those marks to a reader. If no writing materials or reader are available, then the necessary environmental support is not available, and the behavior cannot occur.

Skinner (1957) described two types of transcription: copying written material or dictation. When a written response is controlled by a vocal stimulus, it is called **dictation**. With dictation, the antecedent is a verbal stimulus (auditory), and the consequence is social reinforcement based on point-to-point correspondence (i.e., accurate transcription). Formal similarity is not required as the antecedent (vocal behavior) and response (written text) involve different sense modalities.

If both the stimulus and response are written (i.e., copying text), the verbal behavior is actually echoic. Social reinforcement will require both point-to-point correspondence and formal similarity. Although correspondence between the stimulus unit and the response unit is required, a certain degree of variability may be acceptable as described earlier (see Echoic Behavior).

Social reinforcement for transcription may be educational (e.g., accurately transcribing notes from a textbook or from a teacher's lecture) or economic (getting paid to transcribe something). Accurate transcription may also result in a variety of other reinforcing consequences in everyday life. Accurately writing down a phone number that someone dictates to you might be reinforced by being able to talk to him or her later, accurately writing down a recipe that is being presented on the television might result in making a tasty dish, and accurately copying the directions to a friend's house might be reinforced when you get to visit him or her. If point-to-point correspondence does not occur in these examples, the results (e.g., dialing a wrong number, making a dish that tastes bad, or getting lost) might be disappointing and frustrating (i.e., punishing consequences).

It should be noted that spontaneous writing or composition is not considered a form of transcription. Unlike copying text or writing to dictation, spontaneous writing is a verbal response that does not have point-to-point correspondence with the antecedent event. Spontaneous writing is often under intraverbal control, which was discussed earlier (see Intraverbal Behavior), but could also have mand or tact properties. For example, when a teenager is talking on the phone, a mother may write down a note asking, "Who are you talking to?" This would most likely indicate mand behavior. Similarly, a child who writes a sentence about a picture engages in tact behavior.

Autoclitics: The Behavioral Explanation of Rules of Grammar

An **autoclitic** is supplementary verbal behavior that provides additional information about a speaker's response. Autoclitics are considered secondary verbal operants because their emission depends on the production of primary verbal operants (mands, tacts, echoics, intaverbals, and textuals) and an audience (Hegde, 2011). In essence, an autoclitic is the part of a verbal operant that tacts the controlling variable of the primary verbal operant.

Autoclitics include morphological structures and other elements of grammar, as well as any part of the verbal behavior that provides additional information about what the speaker has said and the circumstances under which a person is speaking (i.e., the controlling variables for the primary verbal operant). For example, if someone says, "I really want coffee," *I want coffee* is the primary verbal operant (i.e., a mand). The secondary verbal operant, *really*, adds strength to the statement that may result in the listener responding more readily. This secondary verbal operant is an autoclitic.

Secondary verbal operants that include morphologic structures and other elements of grammar, as well as any part of the verbal behavior that provides additional information about what the speaker has said and the circumstances under which a person is speaking, are _____.

The antecedent for autoclitics is the primary verbal behavior of the speaker, without which there would be no need for the autoclitic. The consequence is social reinforcement, typically in the form of listener agreement or some form of verbal or nonverbal behavior. Autoclitics are for the benefit of the listener who must discriminate whether to serve or not serve as the mediator of reinforcement for those verbal stimuli (Cooper et al., 2007). Speakers are already aware of the circumstances of their own verbal behavior, so autoclitics are not for their benefit. Listeners, on the other hand, may not have access to a speaker's controlling variables, so the speaker provides autoclitic information to clarify (a) why an utterance is made, (b) how strong that utterance is (operant strength), and (c) the spatial, temporal, quantitative, physical, and other properties of the stimuli that evoke that response (Hegde, 2011). This additional information may, however, influence the nature or precision of the listener's reaction, thus benefiting the speaker in return.

Descriptive Autoclitics

There are several types of autoclitics, each with a different function. Table 2–7 presents types and functions of autoclitics. Many autoclitics are descriptive. **Descriptive autoclitics** further describe the primary verbal operant; they tact the controlling variables of the verbal operant they accompany. The autoclitic *I said* . . . describes a speaker's previous verbal response, whereas the autoclitic *I will say*

. . . or *I was about to say* . . . describes an imminent response. Autoclitics may precede various tacts, such as *I declare* . . . , *I'm telling you* . . . , or *I remember* . . . . These autoclitics could be removed; however, their removal might change the effect that the verbal behavior has on the listener.

The statement *Mary has a fever of 102 degrees* might occur in several different scenarios. As it is, it could be a tact produced by her doctor where the controlling variables are Mary and the thermometer

Table 2–7. Autoclitics

Example	Function of the Autoclitic
I said the coffee is great. I *was about to say* the coffee is great.	Describes a prior verbal response or an imminent response, respectively
I *really* want some coffee.	Specifies the strength of the verbal behavior
I *don't* see the car.	Qualifies the verbal behavior (negation)
The cat *is* soft. The cat *was* soft.	Qualifies the verbal behavior (assertive) and provides temporal information
I *LOVE* taking out the trash.	Inflection reveals sarcasm
I see the ball*s*. I see *many* ball*s*.	Indicates plurality; the verbal behavior occurs in response to more than one ball (quantification)
I see *a* ball. (nonspecific) I see *the* ball. (indicates a specific ball)	Provides specificity and quantification; the verbal behavior occurs in response to a single stimulus
He walk*s* the dog. He walk*ed* the dog. He is walk*ing* the dog.	Indicates the temporal relationship between the controlling variables and when the verbal behavior occurs
The girl*'s* shoe.	Indicates a possessive relationship between two controlling variables (tacts).
The ball is *under* the chair.	Indicates the spatial relationship between controlling variables.

Note. The autoclitic in each example is indicated by italics.

the doctor is holding. If the same statement is preceded by the autoclitic *Cindy said* . . . , it implies that the controlling variable is a comment made by another person; if it preceded by the autoclitic *I see that* . . . in the context of a letter written by her mother, then a different controlling variable is identified. In each of these scenarios, the autoclitic acts upon the primary verbal operant, which then interacts with cues gathered from the environment and audience to provide additional information about the verbal behavior and the context in which it occurred.

Another group of autoclitics describe the relationship between a response and other verbal behavior of the speaker or listener, or other circumstances under which the behavior occurred. Examples include *I agree* . . . , *I disagree* . . . , *I confess* . . . , or *Between you and me* . . . . The information added by these autoclitics allows the listener to relate the verbal behavior that follows to other aspects of the current situation; thus, they may react to it more efficiently or successfully. Some common autoclitics indicate that what is said should have the same effect as the previous verbal behavior (e.g., *in other words* . . .), yet others reveal a subordinate relation to the previous verbal behavior (e.g., *for example* . . .).

Some autoclitics specify the strength of the verbal behaviors they are part of. Verbal behaviors that include autoclitics such as *I'm sure that* . . . , *I promise* . . . , or *Definitely* . . . indicate strong controlling variables. In contrast, autoclitics such as *I guess* . . . , *I hesitate to say* . . . , or *Possibly* . . . suggest a more tentative nature to the verbal behaviors that follow. Even though the verbal behavior that follows each of these autoclitic examples might be the same, the strength of the resulting statement is different; thus, it might have a different effect on the listener.

Quantifying Autoclitics

Quantifying autoclitics indicate the numerical properties of the controlling stimuli that prompted the primary verbal response (Hegde, 2011). These include autoclitics such as *many, some, all, few,* and others. In the statements *I want all blocks* and *I want few blocks,* the meaning of the primary operant *I want blocks* is changed by the quantitative autoclitic used. The articles *a* and *the* are two very common quantifying autoclitics that tact the numerical properties of the controlling variables while also indicating specificity. *The ball* implies a specific ball is the controlling stimulus as compared to *a ball,* which is more generic.

Qualifying Autoclitics

Qualifying autoclitics qualify the verbal behaviors they accompany in such a way that the intensity or direction of the listener's behavior is modified (Skinner, 1957). This is most often achieved through assertion or negation. **Assertive autoclitics** define the relationship between causal variables and responses in such a way that they move the listener in a positive direction or intensify behavior. **Negative autoclitics** qualify or cancel the verbal behavior they accompany and may signal the cessation or weakening of a behavior.

The verbal behavior *yes* is an assertive autoclitic that provides emphasis or encourages the continuation of a behavior (positive reinforcement). The verbal behavior *is* is the most common assertive autoclitic in the English language. It often serves the same function as *yes* as seen in the utterance, *Yes, it is!* A comparison of two statements, *I think it's Mary* versus *It IS Mary*, demonstrates the assertive power of *is* in that it turns a tentative statement into one with confidence and strength. It does this by clarifying the causal variables and the relationship between them. The autoclitic *is* in the second statement tells us with confidence that *it* and *Mary* are referring to the same discriminative stimulus. A second example, *The cat is soft*, is made up of two tacts (*the cat* and *soft*) plus the autoclitic *is*. Again, the autoclitic indicates that *the cat* and *soft* are controlled by the same discriminative stimulus. The autoclitic *was* has the same assertive power, but both *is* and *was* also serve another autoclitic function in that they describe temporal characteristics of the stimulus. *The cat is soft* implies currency, whereas *The cat was soft* describes something experienced in the past.

Just as "Yes!" may encourage the continuation of a behavior, so "No!" (emitted as a mand) may stop the nonverbal behavior of the listener (punishment). This is often a child's first exposure to *no*. Later, the behavior of *no* is extended to verbal responses. If a child describes a red car as *blue*, the parent may respond "no." The child may then self-correct by saying "red, no blue," and eventually this evolves into the autoclitic *no blue* or *not blue*. *No, not, never,* and *nothing* are examples of negative autoclitics. *No . . .* is also frequently used to indicate a stimulus that is absent (see the earlier description of *metonymical extension* in Tacts).

If the word *not* is added to a previous example, resulting in the utterance *The cat is not soft*, it provides an example of negation. In this case, the autoclitic *not* indicates that *soft* is not part of the tact *cat*. In other words, the controlling variables for the two tacts are not the same and have not been reinforced as a verbal operant. Similarly, other negative autoclitics can be used to qualify or cancel the verbal behaviors that they accompany, such as *I don't think . . . , I don't recall . . .* , or *I would not go as far as to say . . .*

Other types of qualifying autoclitics indicate the kind or degree of extension of a tact. Examples include *sort of* and *kind of* (e.g., *It's sort of heavy*). Earlier, responses such as *perhaps, probably, surely*, and *maybe* were presented as examples of descriptive autoclitics. At times, terms such as these actually function as qualifying autoclitics. If the effect on the listener is related to the speaker's inclination (the probability of the event described), it is qualifying. If the effect it has is related to the properties of the stimuli responsible for those inclinations (i.e., the strength of the speaker's verbal behavior), it is descriptive. For instance, the utterance *Surely, Bill is honest* might be interpreted to mean that it is highly likely the tact *honest* would be used to describe Bill (qualifying), or it might be interpreted to mean that the speaker is very sure Bill is honest (descriptive).

Autoclitic Mands

Cooper et al. (2007) describe **autoclitic mands** that are controlled by a specific motivating operation and are produced to mand the listener to react in some specific way to the primary verbal operant. For mands, the autoclitic functions to gain a specific reinforcer (Greer & Ross, 2008). Autoclitic mands frequently occur but are often difficult to recognize because the motivating operation is private. When a person says, "I want the *big* cookie" or "I want *a tall glass of* water," the autoclitics (indicated with italics) appear with the mand and indicate the size of the cookie or amount of water that will be reinforced.

Initially, the autoclitic functions for mands and tacts may need to be directly taught. Emitting a mand to request the *big* cookie is a different response than using the adjective *big* to tact a big dog. Autoclitics as mands and tacts are separate functions, and learning one does not generalize to the other (Twyman, 1996). Some children may confuse autoclitic mands and tacts. If a child says "juice please" to tact a bottle of juice, he or she has not learned the correct autoclitic function. A parent will respond by correcting the child or withholding reinforcement, and over time typically developing children learn to discriminate the different functions and use them correctly. Children with language disorders may require more specific training to teach these separate functions (Greer & Ross, 2008).

Grammatical Tags and Verbal Ordering

Some autoclitics appear as grammatical tags, bound morphemes, or inflections. These are called **fragmentary tacts** (Hegde, 2011). If someone says, "I LOVE taking out the trash," the inflection that puts emphasis on *love* reveals sarcasm, which changes the meaning of the verbal behavior. Grammatic tags like third-person singular present tense *–s*, regular past tense *–ed*, and present progressive *–ing* (e.g., walks, walked, and walking) tact the temporal relationship between the controlling variables and when the verbal behavior occurs. The plural *–s* (e.g., balls) informs the listener that the primary verbal operant, which tacts the stimulus *balls*, occurs in response to more than one ball.

> Autoclitics that appear as grammatical tags, bound morphemes, or inflections are called _____
> _____.

Several grammatic markers function as autoclitics that indicate various relationships between two or more controlling variables of verbal operants. The possessive marker *–'s* indicates a possessive relationship between two tacts in the same utterance (e.g., girl's shoe). The comparative *–er* and superlative *–est* markers specify attribute relationships between two or more controlling variables. Prepositions (e.g., *in, on, under, in back of*) generally indicate the spatial relationships between controlling variables, such as in *The ball is under the chair*.

The two conjunctions *and* and *or* indicate that more than one verbal operant is being controlled by the same discriminative stimulus. If the two operants are compatible in relation to a single stimulus, the autoclitic *and* is used (e.g., The dog is gentle and friendly). If two operants are not compatible, the autoclitic *or* is used (e.g., The dog is mean or friendly).

Skinner (1957) described an additional autoclitic function that explains the use of grammatical tags such as third-person singular present tense *–s*. It is to indicate agreement in number between the verb and the noun that serves as the subject. In the example *The girl runs*, the final *–s* in *runs* is a fragmentary tact under the control of specific features, which include (a) it identifies running as an activity rather than an object or property of an object, (b) it identifies the currency of the activity, and (c) it clarifies the singularity of what is running as well as the agreement in number between *runs* and *the girl*. This is opposed to *The girls run*, which denotes plurality (girls) and agreement in number between the verb (run) and the subject (girls).

This description does not contain examples of every possible grammatic feature identified and labeled by linguists; however, it demonstrates how grammatic features can be explained in terms of causal analysis as opposed to structural analysis. It also suggests that language does not emerge because of some innate knowledge or understanding; it is a learned behavior. Fragmentary tacts are learned because they serve a purpose and are reinforced by the community. They convey meaningful information to the listener and contribute to successful communication.

The same can be said for Skinner's explanation of verbal ordering. Proper sequencing is not the result of innate ability but occurs because it is an established pattern that is reinforced by the verbal community (Skinner, 1957). The verbal behaviors *top* and *pot* are different responses because one patterning of speech sounds is likely to evoke reinforcement in a given circumstance (e.g., tacting a pot), while the other is not. Likewise, *pancake* and *cake pan* are different responses. When a child looks at a car and says "red car," the words appear in that order because that is what has been modeled and reinforced by the verbal community; it is not an explicit act of composition.

Initially, children may learn phrases such as *thank you* or *how are you?* as a single functional unit; therefore, these types of verbal behaviors do not involve an ordering process. Most verbal behaviors, however, do require a specific ordering process to convey the proper message. At times, a first response may not be successful in communicating the desired message, and recasting may be required until

the verbal behavior is understood and reinforced. This is clearly seen in compositional freewriting, where a passage might be written and rewritten, manipulating the word order until the desired response is achieved.

Several processes can influence verbal ordering. The ordering of a verbal behavior may correspond to the sequence of relevant stimuli that generated it. When providing a personal history or narrating an event, verbal behaviors are usually temporally sequenced to coincide with the sequence of activities (stimuli) that occurred. Word order may also be influenced by the relative strength of verbal behaviors, with the strongest more likely to be emitted first and the weakest last (Skinner, 1957). With echoic responses, order is dictated by the antecedent stimuli. Likewise, intraverbal control may dictate word order, as seen when one verbal stimulus generates more verbal stimuli, such as with counting or reciting the alphabet.

In summary, autoclitics are classified as secondary verbal operants because their emission depends upon primary verbal operants (mands, tacts, intraverbals, echoics, textuals, and transcriptions). It is only when these other verbal operants have been established that the speaker finds himself subject to the contingencies that promote the development of autoclitic behavior. Autoclitics function to describe, qualify, negate, assert, quantify, or otherwise comment upon primary verbal operants in such a way as to clarify or alter their affects upon the listener. Autoclitics include fragmentary tacts (grammatic tags and bound morphemes) and, along with other processes, influence verbal ordering; they are Skinner's explanation as to how children acquire grammatical and syntactic structures.

Multiple Causation: Complex Verbal Operants

Skinner (1957) made a distinction between **pure verbal operants** and **impure verbal operants**. Pure verbal operants are those associated with a single controlling variable (antecedent) or consequence. Hegde (2011) described six kinds of stimulus control over the five types of verbal operants described thus far. These controlling variables include motivation (mands), environmental events (tacts), another speaker's speech (echoics), printed material or other visual stimuli (textuals), prior speech (intraverbals), and the audience that produces an effect on those verbal operants. Verbal operants do not occur in a vacuum, however, and verbal behavior is typically affected by multiple variables. When a verbal operant is under the control of multiple controlling relations (i.e., it results from a combination of multiple antecedents and/or consequences), it is an impure verbal operant.

If a child walks into a room, sees an orange on the table, and says "orange," it is likely a pure tact (if he is labeling the orange) or a pure mand (if he is requesting the orange). If a teacher holds up an orange and asks the child, "What is this?" and the child says "orange," the child's response is now both an intraverbal (controlled by the teacher's verbal behavior/question) and a tact (controlled by the object in the environment). These two controlling variables combined to evoke the response "orange"; therefore, the response is now an impure verbal operant or an intraverbal tact. In this way, multiple variables might evoke a single response, and different classes of verbal operants can be combined within a single utterance. In a different scenario, a child sees a box of cookies and says, "I really want a cookie." The listener responds, "Good asking" and hands the child a cookie. The child's mand also includes a tact (cookie) and several autoclitics (really, a). This verbal behavior was subsequently reinforced with both a primary reinforcer and a social reinforcer. Table 2–8 provides additional examples of complex verbal operants and controlling variables.

Multiple causation helps to explain why individuals produce certain verbal behaviors over others (i.e., their choice of words). The verbal behavior an individual produces is influenced by the number and strength of variables present in a given situation (Skinner, 1957). The probability that a specific response will be produced in a given situation is increased if there are multiple controlling variables currently available or if there are stronger variables with a longer history of reinforcement. The audience effect may also influence which verbal behaviors are used. For instance, a young adult may use a different set of verbal responses when speaking to a group of friends than when speaking to a parent. Each audience has become a controlling variable for a specific set of verbal behaviors.

It is also possible for a single variable to control more than one response. This explains how people can talk for an extended period of time without being exposed to a constant barrage of new stimuli. One controlling variable is enough to generate some speech, which in turn stimulates more speech through intraverbal control. The verbal behavior approach emphasizes the importance of identifying and assessing all the controlling variables for particular verbal operants so that teaching arrangements can be designed more effectively (Bondy, Tincani, & Frost, 2004).

Table 2–8. Complex Verbal Operants and Controlling Variables

Example (Verbal Episode)	Antecedent Conditions	Verbal Operants	Consequence Type(s)
A: The clinician says, "Say ball" B: Child says "ball" C: Clinician says, "good talking"	VB of clinician (mand) VB of clinician (model)	Intraverbal Echoic	Social/educational
A: Clinician holds up a ball and says "ball" B: Child says "ball" C: Clinician smiles and says, "That's right!"	VB of clinician (model) Aspect of current environment	Echoic Tact	Social/educational
A: A hungry child points to a cookie in view B: Child says "cookie" C: Parent gives child a cookie	Motivation (hunger) Aspect of current environment	Mand Tact	Primary (receives the cookie that was specified)
A: A child is hungry and mom says, "What do you want?" B: Child says "cookie" C: Parent gives child a cookie	VB of mother Motivation (hunger)	Intraverbal Mand	Primary (receives the cookie that was specified)
A: Clinician holds up a ball and says, "Say ball" B: Child says "ball" C: Clinician says, "That's right!"	VB of clinician (mand) VB of clinician (model) Aspect of current environment	Intraverbal Echoic Tact	Social/educational
A: Clinician holds up a glass of milk and says, "A glass of ___" B: Child says "milk" C: Clinician says, "That's right!" and gives the child the glass of milk.	VB of clinician Motivation (thirst) Aspect of current environment	Intraverbal Mand Tact	Social and primary (receives the milk that was specified)
A: Child is thirsty and mom says, "What do you want?" B: Child says, "Milk, please" C: Mother smiles and gives child some milk.	VB of mother Motivation (thirst)	Intraverbal Mand Autoclitic (please)	Social and primary (receives the milk that was specified)

Note. VB = verbal behavior.

Implications for Assessment and Treatment of Communicative Disorders

Historically, assessment in speech-language pathology has been concerned with the form or topography of responses, not with why speakers say what they say. Most traditional standardized language assessments designed for children result in establishing percentiles or age equivalencies by assessing receptive and expressive language abilities. This is typically done by assessing language that is under the control of discriminative stimuli such as pictures, objects, or questions. Sampling often focuses on naming (tacting), while verbal behaviors under the control of motivating operations (mands) are seldom sampled (Esch, LaLonde, & Esch, 2010). In addition, standardized tests may fail to adequately assess a child's intraverbal repertoire (Cooper et al., 2007). The information gathered may be helpful but will not distinguish between verbal operants or identify the delayed or absent language skills associated with motivating operations or intraverbal control often found in children with language disorders.

Viewing language as a learned behavior that involves a social interaction between speakers and listeners, with verbal operants as basic units, changes the way language needs to be assessed. As described throughout this chapter, verbal behavior is not classified or defined based on topography or form but on the controlling variables involved. Therefore, the assessment of verbal behaviors involves the identification and analysis of verbal operants.

Determining the strength and weakness of each of the verbal operants can result in a more complete understanding of a language deficit and a more effective intervention program (Sundberg & Partington, 1998). The assessment of verbal behavior is based on identifying (a) the verbal operants that are present, (b) their frequency, (c) the types of stimulus control under which they occur (both discriminative stimuli and motivating operations), and (d) what consequences seem to reinforce or maintain those verbal behaviors for the child being assessed (Bondy et al., 2004). This information is critical for designing an effective treatment plan, because it will help clinicians establish treatment targets (verbal operants that are weak or absent), design treatment circumstances that will increase the probability of a response occurring (antecedent events), establish a training sequence that is functional for the child (one that readily improves communication), and successfully reinforce the desired verbal behaviors that occur.

Most treatment methods used by speech-language pathologists today are based on behavioral principles in that they involve the manipulation of environmental events to teach specific response classes (Hegde, 1998, 2008; Hegde & Maul, 2006). A verbal behavior approach to teaching communication skills may be distinguished from more commonly used approaches in several ways. First, treatment targets are based on verbal operants rather than linguistically based topographical forms. Verbal operants are seen as the bases for building verbal behavior, so language intervention involves establishing each verbal operant repertoire, including impure verbal operants with multiple causation. Then more complex relations such as autoclitics are established.

Second, treatment targets should be functionally organized rather than topographically (Hegde, 2011). The same word can belong to different classes of verbal behaviors with different causes. When a child says "ball," is it to name the picture or object (tact), request the ball (mand), imitate a verbal model (echoic), read the written word (textual), or complete the phrase "throw the . . . " (intraverbal)? Topographically, the response did not change. Behaviorally and functionally, however, these are separate responses because the cause did change in each scenario.

This is important because a response produced in one context (i.e., as one type of verbal operant) may not occur in another. Different types of verbal operants, although topographically the same, may need to be taught separately (Drash, High, & Tudor, 1999; Duker, 1999; Hall & Sundberg, 1987; Kelley et al., 2007; Lamarre & Holland, 1985; Lerman et al., 2005; Michael, 1988; Oah & Dickenson, 1989; Oliver, Hall, & Nixon, 1999; Partington & Bailey, 1993; Sautter & LeBlanc, 2006; Twyman, 1996; Watkins, Pack-Teixeira, & Howard, 1989). Similarly, structures that have been linguistically considered the same class (irregular plurals, regular plural allomorph variations, and past tense morphemes) have been identified as separate response classes (Guess, Sailor, Rutherford, & Baer, 1968; Hegde & McConn, 1981; Hegde, Noll, & Pecora, 1979). On the other hand, structures that have been treated separately from a linguistic point of view (e.g., subject-noun and object-noun phrases) are functionally the same, and teaching one may be sufficient to generate the other (Hegde, 1980; Hegde & McConn, 1981; McReynolds & Engmann, 1974).

Finally, the verbal behavior approach places a unique emphasis on the listener, as well as the speaker; a verbal episode requires both. The listener plays an important role as the moderator for reinforce-ment of the speaker's behavior and can also become a discriminative stimulus for the behavior. In addition, from a verbal behavior standpoint, the traditional concepts of *understanding* or *receptive language* actually are referring to a type of listener behavior. The listener understands the speaker if he responds to the speaker's verbal behavior in an appropriate way. Viewing language as verbal behavior clearly affects the assessment and treatment procedures a speech-language pathologist might use. Additional considerations and specific procedures for the assessment and teaching of verbal behaviors are presented in subsequent chapters.

Chapter Summary

1. Skinner (1957) believed that language is a learned behavior that is effective only through the mediation of other people and called it verbal behavior.

2. Verbal behaviors include vocal behavior (speech), other audible behaviors such as clapping hands to get attention, gestures, and writing.

3. Verbal behaviors are analyzed in terms of (a) their antecedent stimuli, (b) the communication behaviors themselves, and (c) the consequences of those behaviors.

4. Skinner viewed verbal behavior acquisition as a process of operant conditioning in which a child is motivated to produce a response that is subsequently reinforced. Once a response is reinforced, that response is more likely to become part of the child's verbal repertoire. When many instances of a response are reinforced, that operant will increase in strength and is more likely to be repeated and maintained.

a. Motivating operations (MOs) are steps taken to increase the probability that a specific behavior will occur.

b. Successive approximation (reinforcement made contingent upon closer and closer approximations to the desired behavior) is used to shape complex verbal behaviors over time.

c. Stimulus and context variation facilitate generalization of a response.

5. A unit of verbal behavior functionally related to one or more independent variables is an operant.

a. Mands are motivated by a state of deprivation or aversive stimulus and typically specify the reinforcing consequence. Mands include verbal behaviors such as commands, requests, and questions.

b. Tacts are evoked by a particular object or event, or property of an object or event. Tacts often name, comment on, or describe objects or events in the environment.

c. Echoics are imitations of another person's verbal behavior.

d. Intraverbals are generated by a speaker's own verbal behavior or by the verbal behavior of others. Reciting a long poem, automatic responses, naming items in a category, sentence completion, and the learning of factual information are examples of verbal behaviors under intraverbal control.

e. Textual behavior (i.e., reading) is under the control of nonauditory verbal stimuli such as written text, phonetic transcription, or musical notes.

f. Transcription (i.e., writing) is a nonvocal verbal behavior.

6. Autoclitics are secondary verbal operants that include morphological structures and other elements of grammar, as well as any part of the verbal behavior that provides additional information about what the speaker has said and the circumstances under which the person is speaking.

a. Autoclitics function to describe, qualify, negate, assert, quantify, or otherwise comment upon primary verbal operants in such a way as to clarify or alter their affects upon the listener.

b. Fragmentary tacts are autoclitics that appear as grammatic tags, bound morphemes, or inflections. Traditional linguistic structures such as plural markers, tense markers, possessives, comparative and superlative forms, and prepositions are examples of fragmentary tact autoclitics.

7. The ordering of verbal behavior occurs because it is an established pattern reinforced by the verbal community. Verbal ordering can also be influenced by the sequence of stimuli that generated it, by the relative strength of the behaviors, or by intraverbal control.

8. Pure verbal operants are those associated with a single controlling variable (antecedent) or consequence. Much of the time, however, verbal behavior is affected by multiple controlling variables (i.e., multiple causation).

9. The assessment of verbal behavior is based on identifying (a) the verbal operants that are present, (b) their frequency, (c) the types of stimulus control under which they occur (both discriminative stimuli and motivating operations), and (d) what consequences seem to reinforce or maintain those verbal behaviors.

10. Verbal behavioral analysis is critical for designing an effective treatment plan because it helps clinicians (a) establish treatment targets (verbal operants that are weak or absent), (b) design treatment circumstances that will increase the probability of a response occurring (antecedent events), (c) establish a training sequence that is functional for the child (one that readily improves communication), and (d) successfully reinforce the desired verbal behaviors that occur.

11. A truly verbal behavior approach to teaching communication skills may be distinguished from more commonly used behavioral approaches in several ways:

    a. Treatment targets are based on verbal operants rather than linguistically based topographical forms.
    b. Treatment targets are functionally organized rather than topographically.
    c. The verbal behavior approach places a unique emphasis on the listener, as well as the speaker; a verbal episode requires both.

Application Exercises

1. Distinguish between the following types of primary verbal operants:
   a. Mand
   b. Tact
   c. Echoic behavior
   d. Intraverbal
   e. Textual behavior
   f. Transcription

2. For the verbal episodes given in Table 2–9, label the verbal behavior as a mand, tact, echoic, intraverbal, textual, or transcription.

3. Label the *complex verbal operants* for the italicized behaviors in the examples given in Table 2–10.

4. List several features that may contribute to the strength of a response.

5. Describe three examples where motivating operations are used to increase the probability that a desired response will occur.

6. How is successive approximation used to shape verbal behavior?

7. Once a verbal behavior is established, what steps can be taken to promote

Table 2–9. Verbal Episodes

Antecedent	Behavior	Consequence (Listener Response)
The child sees an airplane.	Child says "airplane"	"Yes, I see it!"
The teacher says, "one plus one . . . "	Child says "equals two"	"Yes, that's right!"
The child is hungry	Child signs, "I want apple"	Gives the child an apple
The written word D-O-G	Child says "dog"	"Yes, good reading!"
A parent says, "Bring me your coat?"	Child responds, "coat?"	"Yes, bring it to me."

Table 2–10. Complex Verbal Operants

Example (Verbal Episode)	Antecedent Conditions	Consequence Type(s)
A: The clinician says, "Say ball" **B:** *Child says "ball"* **C:** Clinician says, "Good talking"	VB of clinician (mand) VB of clinician (model)	Social/educational
A: A hungry child points to a cookie in view **B:** *Child says "cookie"* **C:** Parent gives child a cookie	Motivation (hunger) Object in environment (cookie)	Primary (receives cookie)
A: Clinician holds up a glass of milk and says, "A glass of ____" **B:** *Child says "milk"* **C:** Clinician says, "That's right!" and gives the child some milk	VB of clinician Motivation (thirst) Object in environment (milk)	Social and primary
A: Child is thirsty and mom says, "What do you want?" **B:** *Child says, "Milk, please"* **C:** Mother smiles and gives child some milk.	VB of mother Motivation (thirst)	Social and primary

generalization and maintenance of that response?

8. Identify the italicized autoclitics in the following utterances as descriptive, quantifying, or qualifying.
    a. *I said* the coffee is great.
    b. I *really* need some sleep.
    c. The music *is* loud.
    d. I see *many* cars.
    e. I see *the* car.
    f. *I think* that's the answer.
9. Identify the fragmentary tacts (autoclitics) in the following utterances and describe their function:
    a. He walked the dog.
    b. The girls are running.
    c. The shoes are in the closet.
    d. The truck is bigger than the car.

References

Bloom, K., Russell, A., & Wassenburg, K. (1987). Turn taking affects the quality of infant vocalizations. *Journal of Child Language, 14,* 211–227.

Bondy, A., Tincani, M., & Frost, L. (2004). Multiply controlled verbal operants: An analysis and extension to the Picture Exchange Communication System. *The Behavior Analyst, 27*(2), 247–261.

Cooper, J. O., Heron, T. E., & Heward, W. L. (2007). *Applied behavior analysis* (2nd ed.). Upper Saddle River, NJ: Pearson Education.

Drash, P. W., High, R. L., & Tudor, R. M. (1999). Using mand training to establish an echoic repertoire in young children with autism. *The Analysis of Verbal Behavior, 16,* 29–44.

Duker, P. C. (1999). The Verbal Behavior Assessment Scale (verBAS): Construct validity, and internal consistency. *Research in Developmental Disabilities, 20*(5), 347–353.

Esch, B. E., LaLonde, K. B., & Esch, J. W. (2010). Speech and language assessment: A verbal behavior analysis. *The Journal of Speech-Language Pathology and Applied Behavior Analysis, 5,* 166–191.

Goldstein, M. H., King, A. P., & West, M. J. (2003). Social interaction shapes babbling: Testing parallels between bird song and speech. *Proceedings of the National Academy of Sciences, USA, 100,* 8030–8035.

Goldstein, M. H., & Schwade, J. A. (2008). Social feedback to infants' babbling facilitates rapid phonological learning. *Psychological Sciences, 19,* 515–523.

Greer, R. D., & Ross, D. E. (2008). *Verbal behavior analysis.* Upper Saddle River, NJ: Pearson Education.

Gros-Louis, J. G., West, M. J., Goldstein, M. H., & King, A. P. (2006). Mothers provide differential feedback for infants' prelinguistic sounds. *International Journal of Behavior Development, 30,* 500–516.

Guess, D., Sailor, W., Rutherford, G., & Baer, D. M. (1968). An experimental analysis of linguistic development: The productive use of the plural morpheme. *Journal of Applied Behavior Analysis, 1,* 225–235.

Hall, G., & Sundberg, M. L. (1987). Teaching mands by manipulating conditioned establishing operations. *The Analysis of Verbal Behavior, 5,* 41–53.

Hart, B., & Risely, T. (1975). Incidental teaching of language in the preschool. *Journal of Applied Behavior Analysis, 8,* 411–420.

Hegde, M. N. (1980). An experimental-clinical analysis of grammatical and behavioral distinctions between verbal auxiliary and copula. *Journal of Speech and Hearing Research, 23,* 864–877.

Hegde, M. N. (1982). Antecedents of fluent and dysfluent oral reading: A descriptive analysis. *Journal of Fluency Disorders, 7,* 323–341.

Hegde, M. N. (1998). *Treatment procedures in communicative disorders* (3rd ed.). Austin, TX: Pro-Ed.

Hegde, M. N. (2008). *Hegde's pocketguide to treatment in speech-language pathology* (3rd ed.). Clifton Park, NY: Cengage Delmar.

Hegde, M. N. (2011). Language and grammar: A behavioral analysis. *Journal of Speech-Language Pathology and Applied Behavior Analysis, 5*(2), 90–113.

Hegde, M. N., & Maul, C. A. (2006). *Language disorders in children: An evidence-based approach to assessment and treatment.* Boston, MA: Allyn & Bacon.

Hegde, M. N., & McConn, J. (1981). Language training: Some data on response classes and generalization to an occupational setting. *Journal of Speech and Hearing Disorders, 44,* 301–320.

Hegde, M. N., Noll, M. J., & Pecora, R. (1979). A study of some factors effecting generalization of language training. *Journal of Speech and Hearing Disorders, 44*(3), 301–320.

Hegde, M. N., & Pomaville, F. (2013). *Assessment of communicative disorders in children: Resources and protocols* (2nd ed.). San Diego, CA: Plural.

Kelley, E. M., Shillingsburg, M. A., Castro, M. J., Addison, L. R., LaRue, R. H., Jr., & Martins, M. P. (2007). Assessment of the functions of vocal behaviors in children with developmental disabilities: A replication. *Journal of Applied Behavior Analysis, 40,* 571–576.

Lamarre, J., & Holland, J. G. (1985). The functional independence of mands and tacts. *Journal of the Experimental Analysis of Behavior, 43,* 5–19.

Laraway, S., Snycerski, S., Michael, J., & Poling, A. (2003). Motivating operations and terms to describe them: Some further refinements. *Journal of Applied Behavior Analysis, 36,* 407–414.

Lerman, D. C., Parten, M., Addison, L. R., Vorndran, C. M., Volkert, V. M., & Kodak, T. (2005). A methodology for assessing the functions of emergent speech in children with developmental disabilities. *Journal of Applied Behavior Analysis, 38,* 303–316.

McGee, G. G., Krantz, P. J., Mason, D. & McClannahan, L. E. (1983). A modified incidental-teaching procedure for autistic youth: Acquisition and generalization of receptive object labels. *Journal of Applied Behavior Analysis, 16*(3), 329–338.

McLaughlin, S. (2006). *Introduction to language development* (2nd ed.). Clifton Park, NY: Thomson Delmar Learning.

McReynolds, L. V., & Engmann, D. L. (1974). An experimental analysis of the relationship between subject and object noun phrases (ASHA Monograph 18). In L. V. McReynolds (Ed.), *Developing systematic procedures for train-*

ing children's language (pp. 30–46). Rockville, MD: American Speech-Language-Hearing Association.

Michael, J. (1982). Skinner's elementary verbal relations: Some new categories. *The Analysis of Verbal Behavior*, *1*, 1–3.

Michael, J. (1988). Establishing operations and the mand. *The Analysis of Verbal Behavior*, *6*, 3–9.

Michael, J., Palmer, D., & Sundberg, M. (2011). The multiple control of verbal behavior. *The Analysis of Verbal Behavior*, *27*(1), 3–22.

Oah, S., & Dickenson, A. (1989). A review of empirical studies of verbal behavior. *The Analysis of Verbal Behavior*, *7*, 53–68.

Oliver, C., Hall, S., & Nixon, J. (1999). A molecular to molar analysis of communicative and problem behaviors. *Research in Developmental Disabilities*, *20*(3), 197–213.

Partington, J. W., & Bailey, J. S. (1993). Teaching intraverbal behavior to preschool children. *The Analysis of Verbal Behavior*, *11*, 9–18.

Pena-Brooks, A., & Hegde M. N. (2007). *Assessment and treatment of articulation and phonological disorders in children* (2nd ed.). Austin, TX: Pro-Ed.

Sautter, R. A., & LeBlanc, L. A. (2006). Empirical applications of Skinner's analysis of verbal behavior with humans. *The Analysis of Verbal Behavior*, *22*(1), 35–48.

Skinner, B. F. (1957). *Verbal behavior*. New York, NY: Appleton-Century-Crofts.

Sundberg, M. L., & Partington, J. W. (1998). *Teaching language to children with autism or other developmental disabilities*. Danville, CA: Behavior Analyst.

Twyman, J. S. (1996). The functional independence of impure mands and tacts of abstract stimulus properties. *The Analysis of Verbal Behavior*, *13*, 1–19.

Watkins, C. L., Pack-Teixeira, L., & Howard, J. S. (1989). Teaching intraverbal behaviors to severely retarded children. *The Analysis of Verbal Behavior*, *7*, 69–81.

Williams, G., & Greer, R. D. (1993). A comparison of verbal-behavior and linguistic communication curricula for training developmentally delayed adolescents to acquire and maintain vocal speech. *Behaviorology*, *1*, 31–46.

Winokur, S. (1976). *A primer of verbal behavior: An operant view*. Englewood Cliffs, NJ: Prentice-Hall.

CHAPTER 3

Defining and Measuring Behaviors

This text emphasizes the speech-language pathologist's (SLP's) role in helping clients develop desirable communicative behaviors that will support their overall quality of life. That being said, the question often arises regarding how improvement will be measured and determined. Subjective statements such as, "You have come so far" and "He is doing so well" are typically meaningful to clients and their significant others and may support the **social validity** of treatment given. Social validity is established when treatment goals, procedures, and results are subjectively determined to be successful by the client, therapist, and significant others (Foster & Mash, 1999). However, clinicians should not solely rely on subjective criteria to judge improvement in their clients' communicative skills. Objective techniques are needed to measure behavioral change.

> _____ _____ is established when treatment goals, procedures, and results are subjectively determined to be successful by the client, therapist, and/or significant others.

When utilizing a behavioral approach to treatment, clinicians determine the effectiveness of the selected treatment methods by developing objective goals that can be measured over time. Through the process of data collection, SLPs determine the baseline levels of a given behavior, develop a treatment plan to address that skill, make any needed changes based on the data obtained, sequence treatment in a way that promotes the client's progress, and ascertain if the goal has been generalized and maintained. Data collection allows clinicians to make therapeutic deci-

sions that are objective in nature. Methods for defining and measuring behavior are discussed in detail in this chapter.

Defining Behaviors

Within the field of speech-language pathology, target behavior selection is a key component of both the assessment and treatment processes. Although traditional treatment methods often involve collecting assessment data and then developing target behaviors based on the obtained information, it can be beneficial to draft definitions of priority target behaviors prior to initiating assessments with the client. During initial interviews with the client and/or significant others, SLPs should have a candid discussion regarding areas of concern. This information can be used to develop working definitions of the target behaviors to facilitate observations and informal assessment trials. These definitions can be used to collect data and determine possible maintaining antecedent and consequence stimuli. This topic is discussed in further detail in Chapter 4.

Topography (Form) Versus Function

When defining target behaviors, whether it be for assessment or treatment, clinicians consider both the topography and function of the response. **Topography** refers to the form and structure of a given response. Topographically written target behaviors will specify, in detail, what the behavior looks like, sounds like, or both. For example, a clinician may write a goal that a child will point to common objects in a field of two within 5 seconds of a verbal stimulus. Similarly, an articulation client may be expected to produce an acoustically and visually correct initial /s/ while reading a short passage. In these examples, the form of the target behavior is clearly and objectively defined. In most cases, SLPs write goals based on topography to facilitate the data collection process.

In some cases, clinicians may elect to write treatment goals based on function rather than topography. **Response function** refers to the consequence an individual receives for engaging in a response. In a general sense, it is the reason a client is exhibiting a specific behavior. In order to gain the attention of his mother, a child may wave, call out, or pull on her hand. In this case, all of the listed behaviors have the same function, namely, getting the mother's attention. When writing function-based objectives, clinicians typically develop target behaviors that specify one of the verbal operants discussed in Chapter 2. For example, a clinician may write a goal that states a child will engage in tact behavior a minimum of five times during the school day. A target behavior for a high school student who has experienced a traumatic brain injury may be to mand for information (i.e., ask clarifying questions) at least three times a week during biology class. When writing such target behaviors, clinicians do not specifically define the structure of a given response. Rather, they indicate the effect engaging in the behavior will have on the client's environment.

> _____ refers to the structure or form of a behavior, whereas _____ is related to the reason the client engages in a behavior.

Response Classes

Function-based definitions of behavior are built on the concept of response classes. **Response classes** refer to sets of behaviors that occur under highly similar or identical antecedent and consequence conditions. Therefore, each behavior within the response class serves the same function for the client. In the previously discussed example, waving, calling, and pulling on his mother's hand were all part of the same response class for the little boy who was trying to get his mother's attention. Because each response resulted in the same consequence, the behaviors can be said to have served the same function.

Although there is often a reliance on topographically based target behaviors within our field, it is beneficial to address response classes during treatment when possible. Targeting response classes can make treatment more efficient, because it increases the likelihood that generalization to other behaviors within the class will occur (see Chapter 7 for additional information regarding generalization). For example, addressing intraverbal behavior by teaching a child to respond to a set of 10 "where" questions may result in generalization to new, untaught "where" questions as well. Similarly, studies have shown that auxiliary and copula verb forms may also belong to the same response class (Hegde, 1980; Hegde & McConn, 1981). Although they are separate grammatical structures, teaching use of auxiliary *is* (e.g., *She is walking*) may generalize to copula *is* (e.g., *She is funny*) without the need for direct teaching.

While addressing response classes can make the treatment process more efficient, there is still much research that needs to be done on this topic within the field of speech-language pathology.

Clinicians are cautioned against stating that behaviors constitute a response class without empirical evidence to support this assumption. Over time, functions of behavior can change, resulting in changes to the response class as well. For example, the child who called to his mother to get her attention may start exhibiting this behavior in order to gain access to a preferred item instead. Furthermore, although a set of behaviors may serve as a response class for one client, the same behaviors may serve different functions for other individuals. Accordingly, whether utilizing a topographical or functional approach to defining responses, SLPs should allow their clients' individual needs and characteristics to guide the development of observable, measureable target behaviors.

Observable and Measureable

Prior to providing behaviorally based treatment services, SLPs ensure that the selected target behaviors are defined in a way that will promote accurate data collection. In order to facilitate this process, **operational definitions** of target behaviors are constructed. Operational definitions describe behaviors that can be both observed and measured. Therefore, anyone who reads the operational definition should be able to observe the client engaging in the target behavior and measure it accurately. When target behaviors are not written operationally, a clinician is unable to determine if progress has been attained. As a result, the clinician would be unable to determine when to start, continue, change, or cease treatment services for a given behavior or client. Table 3–1 provides examples of nonoperationally defined target behaviors and how they

can be revised in order to make them observable and measurable).

Developing operationally written target behaviors can be a challenging process. In many cases, the clinician must thoughtfully consider how the target behavior can be most clearly defined. Although this process may take time, every speech-language skill can be written in observable and measurable terms. Considering the following five components is beneficial when developing operational definitions of target behaviors (adapted from Hegde, 1998):

1. Response topography (RT): As previously discussed, topography refers to the form and structure of a given response. SLPs describe the observable qualities of a behavior rather than presumed, mentalistic constructs. For example, instead of listing that a client will "process" or "understand" commands, operationally written target behaviors state that a client will follow directions. Several examples of topographically defined responses include:
   a. Point to objects (RT)
   b. Answer "why" questions (RT)
   c. Produce present progressive –*ing* (RT)
   d. Produce initial and final /t/ (RT)
   e. Imitate (RT) syllables
   f. Maintain eye contact (RT)
   g. Produce fluent syllables (RT)
   h. Make requests (RT)
2. Level (L): Clinicians specify the level at which treatment will be provided. This component refers to the level of difficulty at which the behavior will be taught. For receptive language goals, level descriptors typically express the complexity of the antecedent stimuli used to evoke the target behavior

Table 3–1. Writing Observable and Measurable Goals

Nonobservable and/or Measurable Target Behavior	Reason	Observable and Measurable Target Behavior
Improve his receptive language skills with 80% accuracy.	• Response topography not specified. • Stimuli are not specified. • Setting is not specified.	Follow one-step directions (e.g., sit down, stand up, give me _____) with 80% accuracy in 20 trials in response to verbal stimuli in the clinical setting.
Use sign language to communicate with 90% accuracy.	• Response topography is not specified. • Stimuli are not specified. • Setting is not specified. • Use of sign language would be more appropriately measured using frequency data.	Use the sign "help" to request assistance during independent work in the classroom at a minimum rate of two times during the school day.
Production of initial and final /m/ with 80% accuracy in 50 trials in response to pictured stimuli in the clinic setting.	• Level of treatment is not specified.	Production of initial and final /m/ with 80% accuracy in 50 trials at the word level in response to pictured stimuli in the clinic setting.
Drink without aspirating.	• Level of treatment is not specified. • Stimuli are not specified. • Setting is not specified.	Tolerate an 8-oz. glass of thin liquids with no audible or visible signs of aspiration while using a chin tuck posture with 100% accuracy during lunchtime in the hospital room.
Require fewer than two cues to sustain eye contact with the clinician for at least 5 minutes in the clinic room.	• In this example, the SLP would be measuring her own behavior (i.e., number of cues provided) rather than the client's.	Sustain eye contact throughout 80% of the 5-second intervals during a 5-minute conversation with the clinician in the clinic room.

(e.g., two-step directions, a field of four, etc.). When writing expressive language and articulation objectives, the length of the client's response is specified (e.g., word level, two to four word phrases, conversation, etc.). For other goals, the level may indicate the amount of time the client has to engage in a behavior. Level descriptors have been added to the target behaviors listed below:

a. Point to objects (RT) in a field of two (L)
b. Answer "why" questions (RT) in sentences of at least five words (L)
c. Produce present progressive –*ing* (RT) in sentences of at least three words (L)
d. Produce initial and final /t/ (RT) in conversational speech (L)
e. Imitate (RT) CV and VC (L) syllables
f. Maintain eye contact (RT) for a total duration per session of at least 4 minutes (L)
g. Produce fluent syllables (RT) during a 10-minute conversation (L)
h. Make requests (RT) in three to five word phrases (e.g., I need _____., Can I have _____?, etc.) (L)

3. Accuracy criterion (AC): Accuracy criteria indicate when the target behavior will be considered met. They are a measure of the precision with which the client uses the target behavior. The accuracy criterion should be directly tied to the data collection method used to measure progress toward acquisition of the target behavior. For example, if the target behavior specifies an accuracy criterion of 80%, percentage data should be taken during treatment to measure progress. In most cases, it is beneficial

to specify the number of consecutive trials and/or length of time in which the criterion must be maintained (e.g., across three sessions, in 20 consecutive trials, etc.). Data collection methods will be discussed in greater detail later in this chapter. Accuracy criterion examples include:

a. Point to objects (RT) in a field of two (L) with 80% accuracy in 20 consecutive trials (AC)
b. Answer "why" questions (RT) in sentences of at least five words (L) with 90% accuracy in 20 consecutive trials (AC)
c. Produce present progressive –*ing* (RT) in sentences of at least three words (L) with 80% accuracy in 20 trials (AC)
d. Produce initial and final /t/ (RT) in conversational speech (L) with 80% accuracy during a 10-minute conversation (AC)
e. Imitate (RT) CV and VC (L) syllables with 90% accuracy in 50 trials (AC)
f. Maintain eye contact (RT) for a total duration per session of at least 4 minutes (L) during a 10-minute conversation (AC)
g. Produce 95% (AC) fluent syllables (RT) during a 10-minute conversation (L)
h. Make requests (RT) in three to five word phrases (e.g., I need _____., Can I have _____?, etc.) (L) at a minimum rate of three times in two of three consecutive center rotations (AC)

4. Stimuli (ST): This component refers to the antecedent stimuli that will be used to evoke the target behavior. Antecedent stimuli should be carefully selected based on the nature of target behavior. For example, tacting

skills should be taught with visual stimuli (e.g., pictures, objects, etc.) rather than verbal stimuli (e.g., questions posed by the clinician). Similarly, pictured stimuli could not be used when teaching a client to follow directions. Instead, the antecedent stimuli would be verbal in nature. Examples of stimuli include:

a. Point to objects (RT) in a field of two (L) with 80% accuracy in 20 consecutive trials (AC) in response to toys (ST)

b. Answer "why" questions (RT) in sentences of at least five words (L) with 90% accuracy in 20 consecutive trials (AC) in response to questions posed by the clinician (ST)

c. Produce present progressive *–ing* (RT) in sentences of at least three words (L) with 80% accuracy in 20 trials (AC) in response to pictured stimuli (ST)

d. Produce initial and final /t/ (RT) in conversational speech (L) with 80% accuracy during a 10-minute conversation (AC) with the clinician (ST)

e. Imitate (RT) CV and VC (L) syllables with 90% accuracy in 50 trials (AC) in response to verbal stimuli (e.g., *Say* _____) (ST)

f. Maintain eye contact (RT) for a total duration per session of at least 4 minutes (L) during a 10-minute conversation (AC) with a peer (ST)

g. Produce 95% (AC) fluent syllables (RT) during a 10-minute conversation (L) with a teacher (ST)

h. Make requests (RT) in three to five word phrases (e.g., I need _____., Can I have _____?, etc.) (L) at a minimum rate of three

times in two of three consecutive center rotations (AC) in response to not having materials needed to complete an activity (e.g., a pencil, scissors, etc.) (ST)

5. Setting (SE): The setting indicates the environment in which the target behavior will be learned and/or maintained. In the initial stages of treatment, contrived settings such as clinic or treatment rooms are typically listed. As the client acquires the target behavior, more naturalistic settings, such as the home, classroom, playground, or job site, may be specified. With the addition of the target settings, the below listed examples present target behaviors that are both observable and measurable in nature:

a. Point to objects (RT) in a field of two (L) with 80% accuracy in 20 consecutive trials (AC) in response to toys (ST) in the home setting (SE)

b. Answer "why" questions (RT) in sentences of at least five words (L) with 90% accuracy in 20 consecutive trials (AC) in response to questions posed by the clinician (ST) in the clinical setting (SE)

c. Produce present progressive *–ing* (RT) in sentences of at least three words (L) with 80% accuracy in 20 trials (AC) in response to pictured stimuli (ST) in the speech room (SE)

d. Produce initial and final /t/ (RT) in conversational speech (L) with 80% accuracy during a 10-minute conversation (AC) with the clinician (ST) in the clinical setting (SE)

e. Imitate (RT) CV and VC (L) syllables with 90% accuracy in 50 trials (AC) in response to verbal stimuli (e.g., say _____) (ST) in the treatment room (SE)

f. Maintain eye contact (RT) for a total duration per session of at least 4 minutes (L) during a 10-minute conversation (AC) with a peer (ST) in the cafeteria (SE)

g. Produce 95% (AC) fluent syllables (RT) during a 10-minute conversation (L) with a teacher (ST) in the classroom (SE)

h. Make requests (RT) in three- to five-word phrases (e.g., I need _____., Can I have _____?, etc.) (L) at a minimum rate of three times in two of three consecutive center rotations (AC) in response to not having materials needed to complete an activity (e.g., a pencil, scissors, etc.) (ST) in the classroom (SE)

In order to develop operational definitions of behavior, SLPs consider (1) _____ _____, (2) _____, (3) _____ _____, (4) _____, and (5) _____.

Requirements of Various Settings

By describing response topographies, levels, accuracy criteria, stimuli, and settings, SLPs increase the likelihood that the target behaviors they develop will be operational in nature. Although these components can help develop observable, measurable definitions of behavior, clinicians may be expected to include additional information in the goals they develop. Additional goal writing requirements in the school and medical settings are discussed below.

Schools

School-based SLPs are typically expected to develop annual goals and related objectives that are time bound. Therefore, school-based clinicians write goals that include dates by which the student can be reasonably expected to acquire the skill. For example, an articulation goal for a third-grade student may state that, "By April 10, 2016, Emma will use initial, medial, and final /s/ during conversational speech with 80% accuracy in a 10-minute conversation with the clinician in the speech room." Although this is a common practice, it poses some ethical dilemmas for SLPs. Specifying the date by which the student will acquire a skill implies a guarantee that the child will make progress and meet the established accuracy criterion. Although SLPs can make a "reasonable statement of prognosis" (American Speech-Language-Hearing Association [ASHA], 2010, p. 2), they are ethically cautioned against promising that treatment will be effective. For this reason, the previously listed examples do not include dates by which the objectives are attained.

An additional requirement in the school setting is that speech-language goals must be educationally relevant. Therefore, the goals targeted during speech-language treatment should allow the child to make some measure of progress within the school setting. Aligning speech-language goals with grade-level standards can help facilitate this requirement. In most states, this entails writing target behaviors that address the Common Core State Standards (Common Core State Standards Initiative, 2010). Table 3–2 provides examples of speech-language goals written to address specific Common Core State Standards).

Table 3–2. Speech-Language Goals Tied to Common Core State Standards (2010)

Speech-Language Target Behavior	Common Core Standard Addressed
By January 22, 2016, Jose will produce initial, medial, and final /k/ at the phrase level in response to pictured stimuli with 80% accuracy in 20 consecutive trials in the speech room.	CCSS.ELA-Literacy.SL.K.6: Speak audibly and express thoughts, feelings, and ideas clearly.
By December 16, 2016, Sophie will label items by category at the sentence level in response to object stimuli with 80% accuracy in 20 trials in the speech room. Target items will include cat, horse, dog, fish, shoe, shirt, pants, socks, pencil, paper, crayons, scissors, car, bus, plane, train, apple, sandwich, ice cream, and chips.	CCSS.ELA-Literacy.L.1.5.B: Define words by category and by one or more key attributes (e.g., a duck is a bird that swims; a tiger is a large cat with stripes).
By August 28, 2016, Max will produce at least 95% fluent syllables during a conversation with a peer in the cafeteria as measured by a 10-minute conversational speech sample.	CCSS.ELA-Literacy.SL.2.4: Tell a story or recount an experience with appropriate facts and relevant, descriptive details, speaking audibly in coherent sentences.
By May 6, 2016, Jenny will use the below listed irregular plural nouns at the sentence level in response to pictured stimuli with 80% accuracy in 20 consecutive trials in the speech room. Target irregular plural nouns will include men, women, people, children, mice, feet, teeth, geese, deer, and sheep.	CCSS.ELA-Literacy.L.3.1.B: Form and use regular and irregular plural nouns.
By November 10, 2016, William will ask a minimum of five questions during a 10-minute conversation with the speech-language pathologist in the speech room.	CCSS.ELA-Literacy.SL.4.1.C: Pose and respond to specific questions to clarify or follow up on information, and make comments that contribute to the discussion and link to the remarks of others.
By February 8, 2016, Rene will answer intermixed "Who" and "Where" questions regarding a fifth-grade reading selection of at least one page with 80% accuracy in 20 trials in the classroom.	CCSS.ELA-Literacy.RF.5.4.A: Read grade-level text with purpose and understanding.
By March 9, 2016, Ana will compare/contrast common objects by providing one similarity and one difference between the two items in sentences with 80% accuracy in 20 trials in the speech room.	CCSS.ELA-Literacy.RI.6.9: Compare and contrast one author's presentation of events with that of another (e.g., a memoir written by and a biography on the same person).

Although writing treatment goals that address academic progress is stressed within educational systems, school-based SLPs should ensure that the student's areas of need drive goal development rather than specific standards. For example, although kindergarten standards state that a student is expected to sort common items by category (Common Core State Standards Initiative, 2010), this should not be written as a goal unless it is truly an area of need for the individual student. School-based SLPs should identify areas of need, cross-reference those areas of need with grade-level standards, and then select specific skills that may be targeted as treatment goals. In some cases, the standard must be shaped down to ensure that treatment is provided in a way that facilitates the child's success. Too many times, clinicians are called upon to write goals that may not be appropriate for their students due to pressure to align treatment with classroom curriculum. Holding the child's needs paramount and using clinical discretion is necessary. In almost all cases, it is possible to perform a child-specific assessment and then examine the curricular standards, which are quite extensive, when selecting treatment goals.

Medical Facilities

Medical facilities also expect SLPs to develop observable, measurable goals that will be addressed in therapy. According to the ASHA (2011) Medical Review Guidelines for Speech-Language Pathology Services, clinicians are expected to be able to take objective measurements of their clients' progress. Specifying response topographies, levels, accuracy criteria, stimuli, and settings when writing target behaviors can help facilitate this.

SLPs in medical settings also write goals that allow their patients to function more independently in their everyday lives. Therefore, SLPs develop goals that help individuals make progress toward their premorbid status. When drafting goals in the medical setting, clinicians take input from clients and significant others in order to develop appropriate goals. For example, a clinician working in an outpatient setting may recognize that a client who recently experienced a stroke has difficulty using morphological markers such as regular past tense *–ed* or third-person singular *–s*. Upon further discussion with the client and his wife, the clinician may learn that, secondary to learning English later in life, the client had difficultly using these bound morphemes prior to his stroke. As a result, the clinician would be unlikely to target these skills, as they would not allow the client to make progress toward his premorbid level of functioning.

Similarly to school-based SLPs, clinicians working in medical settings may also be expected to write goals that are time bound. In order to receive funding for services rendered, SLPs may need to provide an estimation of the amount of time needed to attain treatment goals (ASHA, 2004). This poses the same ethical concern faced by SLPs working in the school setting. Clinicians should be careful to clarify that any acquisition dates discussed with clients do not indicate a promise of improvement. Rather, they are goals that the clinician hopes the client will be able to meet based on current prognostic indicators. Furthermore, if the clinician can document through data collection that a patient is making reasonable progress toward meeting identified goals, third-party payers (e.g., insurance companies) often authorize a further time period for continued therapeutic intervention.

Measuring Behaviors

In addition to ensuring that target behaviors are observable, SLPs make certain that the client's progress can be reliably measured throughout treatment. According to Cooper, Heron, and Heward (2007), measuring behavior entails "describing and comparing behavior with a set of labels that convey a common meaning" (p. 73). Therefore, **measurement** typically involves assigning numerical values to observed phenomena. If the selected target behavior is written in an operational manner, measuring a client's progress should be an objective, unambiguous process.

Measurement is important to both practitioners and researchers within the field of speech-language pathology. Clinical practitioners repeatedly measure their client's progress toward acquisition of a given target behavior in order to make sound clinical decisions and determine the effectiveness of treatment (ASHA, 2007). Accordingly, data collection helps clinicians know when to continue an effective treatment method or discontinue an ineffective procedure. For example, a clinician who elects to provide verbal praise each time a client correctly follows one-step directions will take data to determine the success of using verbal praise as a consequence procedure. If the client demonstrates progress, the clinician would continue providing verbal praise as positive reinforcement for the client's behavior. If the data indicate no improvement, the clinician can determine that verbal praise is not serving as a positive reinforcer for the client, and therefore changes need to be made to the treatment plan.

Objective measurement of communicative behaviors is also important for researchers. Measurement allows researchers to accurately describe their observations. Without data collection, research would be based on conjecture. Researchers also use data to identify relationships between behaviors and antecedent and consequence events. Therefore, data collection is the process by which researchers determine if a given treatment method is effective or not. As a result, measurement is helpful in identifying treatments that are evidence based in nature. There are a variety of methods that practitioners and researchers use for measuring communicative behavior. The following sections discuss several of the most commonly utilized data collection methods employed by SLPs.

Accurate measurement techniques are important to both _____ and _____.

Frequency Measures

Frequency measures involve taking a tally of the number of times a client exhibits a target behavior during a specific time frame. Frequency measures are often used when determining a client's use of a specific verbal operant (see Chapter 2 for additional information). For example, a clinician may measure the number of times a preschool-aged student engages in tact behavior during a 10-minute center rotation. Table 3–3 shows an example of a completed data sheet for this goal. When

Table 3–3. Data Collection Sheet: Frequency Measures

Client's Name: Harper Smith   DOB: 05/16/2012

Clinician: James Reid   Preschool Teacher: Mrs. Sandoval

Target Behavior: Production of tacts that are two to three words in length in response to visual stimuli at a minimum rate of nine times in two of three consecutive 10-minute center rotations across 3 consecutive days in the preschool classroom.

Date	Center	Length of Observation	Tally of Instances of the Target Behavior	Total Frequency of the Target Behavior
9/1/15	Mathematics	10 minutes	HHH	5
9/1/15	Language Arts	10 minutes	HHH III	8
9/1/15	Art	10 minutes	HHH I	6
9/2/15	Language Arts	10 minutes	HHH IIII	9
9/2/15	Mathematics	10 minutes	HHH I	6
9/2/15	Structured Free Play	10 minutes	HHH HHH	10
9/3/15	Structured Free Play	10 minutes	HHH IIII	9
9/3/15	Art	10 minutes	HHH HHH I	11
9/3/15	Mathematics	10 minutes	HHH II	7

working with an individual who exhibits pragmatic language concerns, an SLP may take frequency data on the number of questions the client asks the clinician (i.e., mands for information) during a 5-minute conversation.

When utilizing frequency measures, the clinician should always reference the time frame in which the data were collected (e.g., in a 30-minute session, during the school day, etc.). If the unit of time is not referenced, the clinician will be unable to compare frequency data collected across sessions. Cooper et al. (2007) also cautioned against using frequency data to measure behaviors that occur

within the context of discrete trials. They stated that discrete trials present the client with opportunities to engage in a target behavior that they may not encounter in naturalistic settings. Therefore, using frequency data within discrete trials can run the risk of inflating the client's actual response rate. Finally, frequency data are not appropriate for behaviors that occur for long periods of time. For example, it would not be recommended to use frequency data when measuring out-of-seat behavior. Knowing the number of times (i.e., frequency data) the client was out of his seat is less meaningful than knowing the amount of time the child was not sitting in his chair. Behaviors of this nature are better measured by taking duration data.

Durational Measures

Durational measures are used to quantify the amount of time a client engages in a target behavior. There are two types of durational measures that clinicians typically use: total duration per session or duration per occurrence (Cooper et al., 2007). If an SLP is interested in the total amount of time a client engages in a behavior during a set time period, total duration per session should be used. For example, a clinician may use total duration per session recording to measure the amount of time a client engages in eye contact during a 30-minute session. In order to measure this, the clinician would start a stopwatch when the client first establishes eye contact. Once the client looks away, the stopwatch would be stopped but not reset. Upon subsequent instances of eye contact, the stopwatch would be restarted, and this procedure would be repeated until the end of the session. The SLP would then be left with the total amount of time the client made eye contact during the 30-minute session. If the clinician were concerned about the amount of time for each occurrence of eye contact made during the session, duration per occurrence data would be taken. When using this procedure, the SLP would measure the length of each instance of eye contact and write it down. The clinician could then calculate the range and/or mean amount of time the client maintained eye contact per occurrence of the target behavior.

Durational measures are particularly well suited for pragmatic language target behaviors. Because behaviors such as eye contact, topic maintenance, and proximity are continuous in nature, duration data can be used to measure their occurrence. Durational measures can also be used with various cognitive rehabilitation goals. A clinician may measure the amount of time a client who has experienced a traumatic brain injury can sustain attention to a specific task. Similarly, duration data may be collected for home health clients who are working on completing activities of daily living (ADLs) such as cooking, cleaning, and managing a checkbook in a more time-efficient manner.

Latency Measures

Like duration data, latency measures also include a reference to time. **Latency** refers to the amount of time between an antecedent stimulus and the client's response. Reducing clients' response latencies can help improve the fluency with which they exhibit the target behavior. As a result, latency measures are best suited for skills that need to be exhibited within a certain time frame (e.g., word finding, following directions, etc.). Clients who exhibit aphasia may demonstrate word-finding difficulties that result in long latencies between the presentation of antecedent stimuli and their responses. In such cases, clinicians may write a goal stating that the client will label pictures of common objects with an average response latency of less than 3 seconds in 20 consecutive trials in the clinic room. During treatment, the clinician would measure the amount of time between the presentation of the antecedent stimulus and the client's response during each trial. Using these data, the SLP could then calculate average response latency across 20 trials to measure the client's progress toward the goal.

Interval Measures

A third technique that incorporates time is interval measurement. When using **interval measures**, the clinician first divides the assessment or treatment session into a series of short intervals. In order to obtain the most reliable data, these intervals should be relatively short in duration (e.g., 5–15 seconds). The clinician then takes data on whether or not the client engages in the target behavior during each of the established intervals. Table 3–4 shows an example of a data collection sheet for interval data. As with durational measures, it is most appropriate to use interval recording when the target behavior addressed during treatment is continuous in nature. Therefore, this technique can be used with pragmatic language or cognitive rehabilitation targets as well.

The two primary types of interval measurement used by SLPs are whole- and partial-interval recording. When using **whole-interval recording**, the clinician only gives the client credit for engaging in the target behavior if it is exhibited throughout the entire interval. For example, a clinician using 10-second, whole-interval recording to measure a client's eye contact would chart that eye contact occurred only if it was maintained throughout the entire 10-second interval. Even if eye contact were maintained for part of the interval, the clinician would not document that the target behavior occurred unless it was present for the entire 10 seconds. Conversely, **partial-interval recording** gives the client credit for engaging in the behavior if it occurs at any time during the interval. Therefore, in the previous example, the clinician would document that eye contact occurred if it was exhibited at any time during the interval. Whether using whole- or partial-

interval recording, the obtained data are converted into a percentage of intervals in which the behavior was exhibited during the session (e.g., 80% of 10-second intervals during a 30-minute session).

Although interval measurement can be used to collect data on some speech-language target behaviors, there are several problems associated with interval recording. Because whole-interval recording documents behaviors that are exhibited throughout an interval, some instances of the behavior will go unrecorded if they only occur for part of the interval. Therefore, whole-interval recording may result in underestimating the client's actual use of the target behavior. On the other hand, partial-interval recording can overestimate the prevalence of a target behavior. This occurs because the client receives credit for engaging in the target behavior whether it is exhibited for a split second or throughout the entire interval. SLPs should keep these limitations in mind when interpreting interval data.

Derivative Measures

Derivative measures involve combining two sets of data obtained during an observation session. Undoubtedly, the most commonly encountered derivative measure within the field of speech-language pathology is percentage data. When collecting percentage data, clinicians chart clients' correct (typically with a "+") and incorrect (typically with a "−") responses during a session. This information is then used to derive a ratio of correct responses compared to the total number of response opportunities. For example, a child working on production of irregular past tense forms may respond correctly in 12 of 20 consecutive trials. The clinician could

Table 3–4. Data Collection Sheet: Interval Measures

Client's Name: <u>Samuel Brown</u>   DOB: <u>06/03/2000</u>

Clinician: <u>Jamie Davis</u>   Date: <u>12/05/2015</u>

Length of Observation: <u>9:00 AM to 9:20 AM, 20 minutes</u>

Target Behavior: <u>Sustain eye contact throughout 65% of the 10-second intervals</u>
<u>during a 20-minute conversation with the clinician in the clinic room.</u>

Type of Interval Data Being Collected: _____ Partial Interval   __X__ Whole Interval

Length of Intervals: <u>10 seconds</u>

Number of Minutes	Interval #						Total
	1	2	3	4	5	6	
1	+	+	−	−	−	+	3
2	−	−	+	+	+	+	4
3	+	−	−	−	+	−	2
4	+	+	+	−	+	+	5
5	−	−	+	−	+	−	2
6	−	+	+	+	−	−	3
7	−	−	+	+	+	+	4
8	+	+	−	−	−	+	4
9	+	+	−	+	−	−	3
10	−	+	−	+	−	−	2
11	+	−	+	+	+	+	5
12	−	−	−	−	+	+	2
13	+	+	−	−	−	+	3
14	−	+	+	+	−	−	3
15	+	+	+	−	+	+	4
16	−	−	+	+	−	−	2
17	−	+	+	−	−	+	3
18	+	−	+	−	+	+	4
19	+	−	−	+	+	−	3
20	−	+	−	−	+	−	2
Total % of intervals in which the target behavior was present: 63/120 = 52.5%							

then divide 12 by 20 and multiply by 100 in order to obtain a percentage of correct responses (e.g., $12/20 = 0.6 \times 100 = 60\%$).

Percentage data have broad applicability to a variety of articulation, language, voice, and fluency goals. Furthermore, it is frequently used to measure client progress when using a discrete trial teaching (DTT) approach during treatment. Chapter 5 provides additional information regarding this topic (also, see Table 5–5 for an example of a data sheet for collecting percentage data). Although percentage data are widely used, they may result in an inaccurate description of a client's performance if there are an inadequate number of response opportunities. Cooper et al. (2007) stated that percentage data are most reliable when there are at least 100 opportunities for the client to engage in the target behavior. They cited Guilford (1965), who cautioned against using percentage data if there will be fewer than 20 response opportunities within the observation session. Clinicians should consider these guidelines when determining whether or not to use derivative measures during treatment.

Verbal Interaction Sampling

Verbal interaction sampling (Hegde, 2003) is a specific measurement technique that can be used with any of the previously discussed data collection methods. When utilizing verbal interaction sampling, clinicians collect data on the communicative behavior of at least two individuals during a social interaction. For example, a school-based SLP may use verbal interaction sampling when observing how a preschool teacher works with students at center time. Frequency data could then be

taken on the number of questions posed by the teacher and the number of utterances produced by the students. If the data indicate that minimal communicative behavior is being evoked during center time, the SLP can collaborate with the teacher to help increase opportunities for speech-language development in the classroom. Similarly, durational measures could be used to determine the amount of time the teacher spends introducing certain concepts or how long students are able to attend to instruction. This information can be used to tailor teaching to the students' individual needs. Note that verbal interaction sampling is not a specific data collection procedure. Rather, it is a method for observing the communicative behaviors of clients and their significant others during typical social situations using the data collection methods discussed previously.

Graphing and Interpreting Measurement Data

The importance of accurate data collection has been stressed in the preceding sections of this chapter. Although data collection is important, it has minimal functional value if clinicians do not refer to the collected data in order to guide clinical decision making. Therefore, it is crucial that SLPs understand how to interpret data in order to determine whether or not treatment is resulting in improved use of the selected target behaviors. Analyzing graphed data will enable clinicians to determine when to initiate, continue, change, or cease treatment for a target behavior.

SLPs typically construct line graphs to help visualize their clients' progress (or lack of progress). Line graphs help clinicians interpret data taken over the course of treatment. Figure 3–1 shows an example of a line graph displaying data taken over a number of treatment sessions. Important components of line graphs include the following:

1. X-axis: The *x*-axis, also referred to as the horizontal axis, symbolizes the passage of time. In Figure 3–1, the *x*-axis is labeled with the word "Sessions."
2. Y-axis: The *y*-axis, also referred to as the vertical axis, is a measure of the client's use of the target behavior. The *y*-axis should be tied directly to the data collection method used to measure the target behavior. In Figure 3–1, the *y*-axis is labeled as the "Number of Mands per School Day" because frequency data were taken.

3. Condition Labels: Condition labels are used to separate phases (i.e., baseline, treatment, or probe). Figure 3–1 uses condition labels to separate the "Baseline" and "Treatment" phases.
4. Data Points: Data points represent a measurement of the client's correct production of a target behavior during each session.
5. Data Path: Connecting consecutive data points with straight lines creates the data path.

Once a graph has been developed, SLPs can then use the graphed data to analyze their client's performance. According to Cooper et al. (2007), graphs are used to "organize, store, interpret, and communicate the results" (p. 127) of treatment. Clinicians who use a behavioral approach to speech-language treatment determine their clients' progress through visual

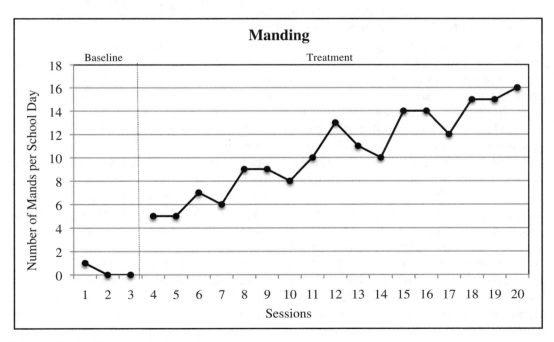

Figure 3–1. Line graph: Manding.

inspection of graphed data. This is accomplished through examining the variability, level, and trend of the data path.

> Progress on target behaviors is determined through _____ _____ of graphed data.

Data **variability** refers to the distance between data points on the y-axis. Describing the variability present in a data set indicates how much the behavior varies from session to session. Data points that are fairly close together on the y-axis can be described as stable or steady in nature. Steady states of performance are particularly important in applied behavior analysis because they permit comparisons between treatment phases. For example, if a low, steady state is observed during a baseline phase and a high, steady state is observed posttreatment, the clinician can be fairly confident that the treatment method was appropriate for addressing the defined target behavior. In most cases, three consecutive stable data points are needed to demonstrate a steady state. Significant variability between treatment data points could indicate that the selected procedure is not establishing control over the target behavior. Therefore, the clinician may need to make changes to the treatment plan in order to obtain more stability. Figure 3–2 illustrates the difference between steady and variable responding during a baseline phase.

The **level** of a data point is a reference to its placement on the y-axis. The level of a data point can be described as low, moderate, or high in nature. Figure 3–3 demonstrates different levels of performance data on a graph. For most communicative behaviors, data points that have high levels indicate improved use of the target behavior. Conversely, lower levels of performance may suggest that the client is making minimal growth.

Finally, **trend** refers to the direction of the data set. In most cases, data paths that demonstrate increasing trends suggest that the client is making progress toward the target behavior. Alternatively, data paths with decreasing trends indicate that the client's use of the target behavior is deteriorating. If the data points remain fairly stable, the clinician may state that the data set shows a zero trend. A zero trend suggests that the client is neither progressing nor regressing. Instead, the client is maintaining a relatively steady level of performance over time. Figure 3–4 provides a graphic representation of zero, increasing, and decreasing trends in a data path.

Determining Baseline Measures

The first data points that a clinician obtains for a target behavior are baseline levels of performance. **Baselines** are measures of the target behavior in the absence of treatment. Baseline data points provide a numerical value of the client's performance prior to initiating treatment. Therefore, they are conducted immediately after operational definitions of target behaviors have been developed. Baseline measures should be taken only of those target behaviors that will immediately be treated. Taking baseline measures of target behaviors that will not be treated for a while will be a waste of valuable clinical time. By the time the clinician gets around to treating those behaviors, the baseline measures will not be valid, and baseline procedures will have to be repeated.

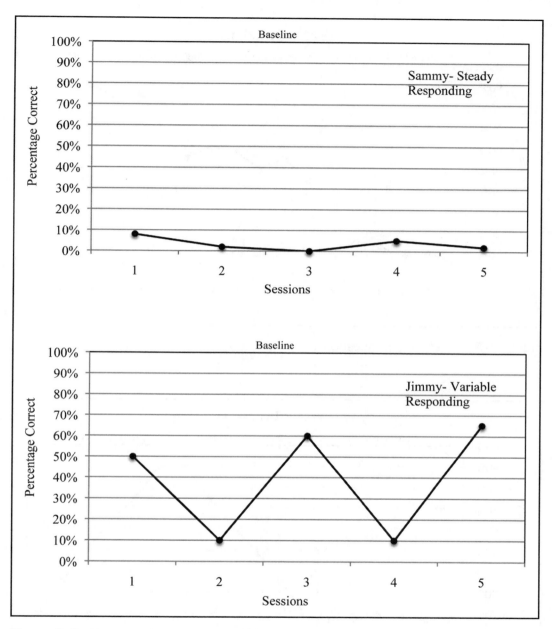

Figure 3–2. Variability: Production of initial /s/.

Any of the previously discussed data collection methods can be used to obtain baseline data; however, the utilized measurement technique must be consistent across baseline and treatment trials. It is important to conduct baselines because they serve as a valid measure to compare with the client's level of performance

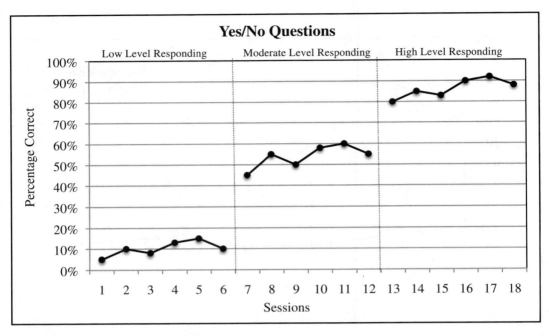

Figure 3–3. Level: yes/no questions.

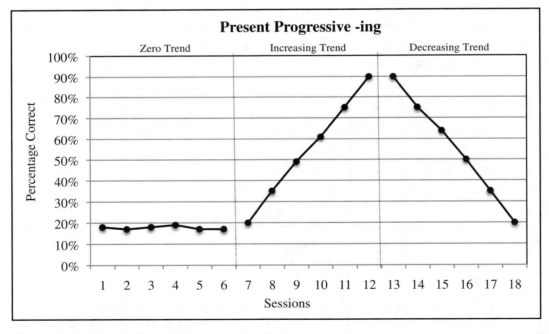

Figure 3–4. Trend: Present progressive –*ing*.

during treatment. If baseline measures are not well established before treatment is provided, there will be no way of determining whether or not the client is improving. Documenting client improvement is necessary to establish clinician accountability; in other words, because the client can be shown to improve after treatment is instated, clinicians can demonstrate that they have done their job.

Characteristics of Baseline Measures

Regardless of the data collection method being utilized, baseline measures have several distinct characteristics (Hegde, 1998). Baseline measures should (a) be stable and reliable over time, (b) adequately sample the target behavior, and (c) be taken in all relevant settings. Therefore, prior to initiating treatment for a target behavior, SLPs should establish stable and reliable baseline measures. In order to accomplish this, it is recommended that at least three stable baseline data points be obtained before providing treatment. If the target behavior is an appropriate one, baseline data should reflect low levels of performance. If baseline data indicate an increasing trend, it may suggest that a client is obtaining the target behavior without the need for instruction. If therapy were initiated after baseline measures that indicate an increasing trend, the clinician would be unable to determine whether the client was responding to the selected treatment method or some other variable. Therefore, if repeated baseline measures reveal high or improving levels of performance, another target behavior should be selected for treatment.

Although taking multiple baseline measures is best practice, it may not always be feasible in some settings. Therefore, many SLPs elect to conduct baselines once and then initiate treatment. Although this can complicate accurate interpretation of data, it is preferable to take one baseline measure rather than none at all. Also, an exception to taking multiple measures is when repeated data collection indicates a sharp decreasing trend within the baseline phase. For example, baseline data may indicate that a client's overall conversational fluency is decreasing. In such a case, the clinician would be ethically called upon to initiate treatment in an attempt to help combat the decreasing data trend.

A second characteristic of baseline measures is that they adequately sample the target behavior. When conducting baselines, clinicians provide clients with enough opportunities to engage in the target behavior so that a reliable measure is obtained. A common problem with standardized tests is that they often only provide the client with one or two opportunities to exhibit the assessed communicative behavior. Baseline measures avoid this issue by providing the client with multiple opportunities to engage in the target behavior (typically at least 20). This helps ensure that the target behavior is adequately sampled.

A final characteristic of baselines is that they should be conducted in all relevant settings whenever possible. Frequently, baselines are only conducted within the clinical setting. In order to measure generalization of the target behavior later in treatment, the clinician may accompany the client to other settings such as the home, school, or job site in order to establish baselines in these locations as well. When trips to extra-clinical settings are not feasible, the client or significant others may be instructed to audio or video record conversations in natural settings that the clinician can then analyze to determine baseline levels of performance. Furthermore, clinicians may find significant differences in baseline rates of behavior across various settings. The settings in which the response is being used most consistently can then be analyzed to provide suggestions for structuring future treatment sessions.

Procedures for Taking Baseline Data

Depending on the nature of the target behavior, the clinician may use several different procedures in order to take baseline data. A method used frequently by SLPs is to conduct baselines within the context of discrete trials. When using this technique, clinicians start by preparing their antecedent stimuli and a data recording sheet. Table 3–5 provides an example. Once these items have been prepared, the clinician administers discrete evoked baseline trials. First, the clinician presents the evoking antecedent stimuli (e.g., a picture, question, etc.) and waits a few seconds for the client's response. After a response is provided, the clinician documents the client's performance, removes the antecedent stimuli, and pauses briefly before presenting the next trial. This procedure is then repeated until all of the selected antecedent stimuli have been presented. The clinician can then use the collected data to calculate baseline levels of performance.

In some cases, clinicians may elect to conduct discrete modeled baseline trials as well. This procedure would look very similar to that of discrete evoked baseline trials; however, the clinician would model production of the target behavior immediately after presenting the antecedent stimuli. Results of modeled baseline trials can help indicate the client's prognosis for improvement with treatment. If the client responds better to modeled than to evoked baseline trials, the clinician can assume that it will be beneficial to use this antecedent manipulation during treatment (see Chapter 6 for more information regarding treatment techniques).

Baseline levels of performance can also be determined through analysis of spontaneous speech-language samples. By analyzing such samples, clinicians are typically able to determine baselines in a more naturalistic context. In order to facilitate the collection of baseline data, the clinician may gather antecedent stimuli that are likely to evoke the target behaviors of interest. For example, when taking baseline measures of regular plural –s, the clinician may have duplicates of several toys available (e.g., blocks, balls, dinosaurs, etc.) that the child can play with. Using the measurement method specified by the target behavior, the clinician could then take data on the client's use of regular plural –s during conversation.

Noncontingent Reinforcement During Baseline Procedures

When conducting baselines within the context of discrete trials or spontaneous conversation, clinicians do not provide contingent consequences for clients' responses. For example, a clinician would not provide verbal praise to a client who answered a yes/no question correctly during baseline trials. Similarly, corrective feedback would not be provided following incorrect responses. Contingent consequences are avoided in order to ensure that valid baseline levels of performance

Table 3–5. Baseline Recording Sheet

Client's Name: _____   Date: _____

DOB: _____   Clinician: _____

Target Behavior: _____

Physical Stimuli: _____

Verbal Stimuli: _____

Target Response	Trials	
	Evoked	Modeled
1.		
2.		
3.		
4.		
5.		
6.		
7.		
8.		
9.		
10.		
11.		
12.		
13.		
14.		
15.		
16.		
17.		
18.		
19.		
20.		
Percentage correct		

are obtained in the absence of treatment. Although contingent consequences are prohibited, noncontingent reinforcement can be provided during baseline trials. This procedure involves providing time-based reinforcement that is unrelated to the client's use of the target behavior. Statements such as, "You're working so hard," "Thank you for paying attention," or "You are doing just what I need to have you do" can be provided noncontingently while maintaining the reliability of baseline measures.

After stable, reliable baseline measures of the target behaviors to be immediately addressed have been obtained, treatment can begin. Chapter 5 outlines the discrete trial procedure, which has broad applicability to the treatment of communicative disorders, and Chapter 6 offers a broad array of specific techniques to increase desirable behaviors. However, before addressing treatment procedures, the application of behavioral principles to assessment procedures is discussed in Chapter 4, which addresses functional behavior assessment and its application to communicative behaviors.

Chapter Summary

1. SLPs rely on objective data collection rather than social validity to determine the effectiveness of the treatment they provide.

2. Clinicians consider both response topography and function when developing target behaviors to be addressed during treatment.

3. Response topography refers to the form and structure of a given response. Therefore, definitions of this nature specify what the behavior looks and/or sounds like.

4. Response function refers to the consequence the client receives for engaging in a response. It is essentially what a person gets as a result of performing a certain behavior.

5. Function-based definitions of behavior are built on the concept of response classes, which specify a group of behaviors that are exhibited for the same function.

6. Although topography-based definitions of behavior are more frequently used in the field of speech-language pathology, addressing response classes can promote generalization to untaught skills.

7. SLPs develop operational definitions of communicative behavior to help ensure that treatment goals are observable and measureable in nature.

8. It is recommended that clinicians consider the following components when writing operational definitions of target behaviors: (a) response topography, (b) level, (c) accuracy criterion, (d) stimuli, and (e) setting.

9. Clinicians may encounter additional requirements when writing goals in school and medical settings (e.g., making goals time bound, etc.).

10. Measurement is the process of assigning numerical values to observed phenomena; accurate measurement procedures facilitate objective data collection.

11. Measurement is important to both practitioners and researchers.

12. There are a variety of data collection methods employed by SLPs. They include (a) frequency measures, (b) durational measures, (c) latency measures, (d) interval measures, (e) deriv-

ative measures, and (f) verbal interaction sampling.

13. Percentage data are frequently collected by SLPs.

14. SLPs determine client progress through visual inspection of graphed data.

15. Visual inspection of graphed data includes examining the variability, level, and trend of the data path.

16. Baseline data are a measurement of the target behavior in the absence of treatment.

17. By comparing baseline performance with treatment data, clinicians are able to determine how much the client is improving.

18. Baseline measures should be stable and reliable prior to implementing treatment.

19. Baseline procedures can be conducted using discrete evoked and modeled trials.

20. Baseline data can also be obtained via analysis of spontaneous speech-language samples.

21. Because baselines are a measure of the behavior in the absence of treatment, contingent reinforcement should not be provided during these trials.

Application Exercises

1. How could you write a goal to address mand behavior based on response topography? Would this definition need to be revised if focusing on response function?

2. Write operational definitions of the behaviors listed below. What measurement techniques would you use to collect data on the following speech-language skills?

   a. Topic initiation
   b. Orientation to person, place, and time
   c. Use of irregular plural nouns
   d. Production of final consonants
   e. Following two-step directions

3. The data set below reflects a client's use of present progressive *–ing* during baseline and treatment sessions. Compose a line graph and chart the client's progress. Describe the data path in terms of variability, level, and trend. Based on the graph, what would you recommend that the clinician's next steps be?

   a. Session 1 (Baseline): 0%
   b. Session 2 (Baseline): 0%
   c. Session 3 (Baseline): 0%
   d. Session 4 (Treatment): 20%
   e. Session 5 (Treatment): 35%
   f. Session 6 (Treatment): 25%
   g. Session 7 (Treatment): 45%
   h. Session 8 (Treatment): 60%
   i. Session 9 (Treatment): 65%
   j. Session 10 (Treatment): 75%

4. Describe how you will take baselines for the target behaviors listed below:

   a. Describe common nouns by category, color, and size at the word level with 80% accuracy in 20 consecutive trials in response to pictured stimuli paired with a question posed by the clinician (e.g., *What category does it belong to? What color is it? What size is it?*) in the clinic room.

   b. Produce initial, medial, and final /l/ at the phrase level with 80% accuracy in 50 consecutive trials in response to pictured stimuli in the clinic room.

   c. Use the sentence frame, "I want _____" to request food items at a minimum rate of four times during snack time in the classroom across 3 consecutive days.

d. Answer yes/no questions at the word level with 90% accuracy in 20 consecutive trials in response to questions posed by the clinician and/or fellow clients during aphasia group activities.

References

American Speech-Language-Hearing Association. (2004). *Medical review guidelines for speech-language pathology services.* Retrieved from http://www.asha.org/uploadedFiles/practice/reimbursement/medicare/DynCorpSLPHCEC.pdf

American Speech-Language-Hearing Association. (2007). *Scope of practice in speech-language pathology* [Scope of practice]. Retrieved from http://www.asha.org/policy

American Speech-Language-Hearing Association. (2010). *Roles and responsibilities of speech-language pathologists in schools* [Professional issues statement]. Retrieved from http://www.asha.org/policy

American Speech-Language-Hearing Association. (2011). *Speech-language pathology medical review guidelines.* Retrieved from http://www.asha.org/practice/reimbursement/SLP-medical-review-guidelines/

Common Core State Standards Initiative. (2010). *Common core state standards for English language arts & literacy in history/social studies, science, and technical subjects.* Retrieved from http://www.corestandards.org/wp-content/uploads/ELA_Standards.pdf

Cooper, J. O., Heron, T. E., & Heward, W. L. (2007). *Applied behavior analysis* (2nd ed.). Upper Saddle River, NJ: Pearson Education.

Foster, S., & Mash, E. (1999). Assessing social validity in clinical treatment research: Issues and procedures. *Journal of Consulting and Clinical Psychology, 67*(3), 308–319.

Guilford, J. P. (1965). *Fundamental statistics in psychology and education.* New York, NY: McGraw-Hill.

Hegde, M. N. (1980). An experimental-clinical analysis of grammatical and behavioral distinctions between verbal auxiliary and copula. *Journal of Speech and Hearing Research, 23*(4), 864–877.

Hegde, M. N. (1998). *Treatment procedures in communicative disorders* (3rd ed.). Austin, TX: Pro-Ed.

Hegde, M. N. (2003). *Clinical research in communicative disorders: Principles and strategies.* Austin, TX: Pro-Ed.

Hegde, M., & McConn, J. (1981). Language training: Some data on response classes and generalization to an occupational setting. *Journal of Speech and Hearing Disorders, 46*(4), 353–358.

CHAPTER 4

Functional Behavior Assessment and Applications to Communicative Disorders

Chapter Outline

- Definition of Contingencies
- A-B-C Contingencies
- Definition and Purpose of Functional Behavior Assessment (FBA)
- Questions FBA Seeks to Answer
  - What Is the Behavior of Concern?
  - What Antecedent Variables Precipitate the Behavior?
    - Where Does the Behavior Occur?
    - When Does the Behavior Occur?
    - Who Is Present When the Behavior Occurs?
  - How Is the Behavior Reinforced?
    - Positive Reinforcement
    - Negative Reinforcement
    - Automatic Reinforcement
- Gathering Data
  - Indirect Methods
  - Direct Observation
  - Functional Analysis
- FBA: Applications to Verbal Behavior
- Assessment of Verbal Operants

One of the primary clinical activities speech-language pathologists (SLPs) engage in is providing assessment services (American Speech-Language-Hearing Association [ASHA], 2007). Conducting comprehensive assessments allows clinicians to identify clients who may require therapy and develop treatment plans to address the documented areas of need. Traditionally, speech-language assessments have focused on the topographical aspects of communication (Esch, LaLonde, & Esch, 2010). Although clinicians frequently examine response form (e.g., production of speech sounds, morphology, syntax, etc.), analyses of verbal behavior are often less robust in speech-language assessments. Diagnostic tools that fail to examine the functional bases of a client's verbal responses overlook a crucial component of the evaluation process. As a result, clinicians must supplement traditional assessment measures with techniques used to describe the functions of communicative responses as well. The following sections discuss a variety of assessment procedures and how they can be applied to communicative behaviors.

Definition of Contingencies

Behaviorally based assessments are built on the concept of contingencies. **Contingencies** refer to the correlation between a behavior and various other environmental stimuli. Therefore, the presence or absence of such stimuli affects the occurrence of the behavior. Hegde (1998) describes two primary types of contingencies that may affect speech-language development: neurophysiologic contingencies and environmental contingencies.

Neurophysiologic contingencies refer to the medical variables that may underlie an observed behavior. For example, a child who has an unrepaired cleft palate will exhibit a hypernasal vocal quality. A patient who has experienced a stroke may display significant word-finding difficulties due to the associated brain damage. Although SLPs must be aware of the neurophysiologic contingencies that affect a client's performance, there is very little clinicians can do to manipulate variables of this nature. Such contingencies are best addressed by the medical community.

A _____ occurs when there is a correlation between a behavior and various other environmental stimuli.

SLPs are involved in manipulating environmental contingencies to affect the frequency of verbal behavior. An **environmental contingency** is present when there is a consistent relationship between environmental stimuli and a behavior. Chapter 2 discussed how verbal behavior is a product of specific antecedent and consequence stimuli. Therefore, there are certain environmental events that occur before (i.e., antecedents) and after (i.e., consequences) communicative behaviors that make them more or less likely to occur. For example, a clinician may provide verbal praise when a child labels pictures of various animals. If the child's performance increases over time, the clinician created an environmental contingency between showing the child a picture (i.e., the antecedent), the child's response (i.e., the tact behavior), and providing verbal praise (i.e., the consequence). By establishing new environmental contingencies, SLPs help their clients develop more appropriate forms of verbal behavior.

A-B-C Contingencies

A-B-C contingencies are the primary contingencies manipulated by SLPs during treatment. **A-B-C contingencies** describe the relationship between antecedent stimuli (the "A" in A-B-C contingencies), behaviors (the "B" in A-B-C contingencies), and consequence stimuli (the "C" in A-B-C contingencies). These are often referred to as three-term or S-R-C (i.e., stimulus-response-consequence) contingencies as well. It is important that SLPs have a solid understanding of A-B-C contingencies because they help clinicians understand the specific environmental stimuli that need to be either added or

removed in order to affect the frequency of verbal behavior. Refer to Table 4–1 for examples of A-B-C contingencies related to speech-language pathology.

Understanding A-B-C contingencies helps clinicians identify environmental stimuli that need to be _____ or _____ in order to affect the frequency of verbal behavior.

As discussed in previous chapters, antecedents refer to the environmental stimuli that occur prior to a behavior. Antecedent stimuli can serve to evoke a variety of behaviors within the natural environment. Seeing boxes of cereal on a grocery store shelf may serve as an antecedent stimulus for a child to request a specific type of cereal that he wants. Similarly, seeing an overly talkative coworker

Table 4–1. Examples of A-B-C Contingencies

Antecedent	Behavior	Consequence
A woman is thirsty.	She says, "Can you get me a glass of water?"	Her husband pours her a glass of water.
A child sees a ball.	The child says, "Look, ball!"	His mother says, "You're right! I see it too."
An individual asks, "What day is it?"	You respond by saying, "Wednesday."	The individual thanks you.
An SLP says, "Say snake."	The child repeats the word *snake* correctly.	The clinician provides verbal praise for the child's correct production.
Per a sound level meter, the client's vocal intensity is too high.	The client reduces his overall volume.	The dB level on the sound level meter goes down and the clinician praises the client.

may cause an individual to walk out of the lunchroom while at work. Within treatment sessions, antecedent stimuli such as picture cards, storybooks, toys, functional objects, written materials, verbal questions, and so forth are frequently used to evoke speech-language target behaviors. For example, a clinician may show a child pictures of various items that start with /s/ (i.e., sink, sock, soup, etc.) when evoking production of this phoneme in the initial word position. A client who exhibits aphasia may be shown common household objects (e.g., a spoon, toothbrush, remote control, etc.) in order to address confrontational naming skills.

The next component of A-B-C contingencies is the behavior itself. A behavior is any observable activity that a person engages in (Cooper, Heron, & Heward, 2007). Behavior can be either overt or covert in nature (Chance, 2006). Overt behavior can be observed by the people in the client's environment. Examples of overt behavior include production of speech sounds, following directions, answering questions, asking for help, pointing, signing, hitting, gesturing, yelling, and so forth. In most cases, clinicians assess and treat overt forms of behavior exhibited by their clients. Covert behavior can only be observed by the individual who is engaging in the response. Covert behavior is typically not targeted during speech-language treatment; however, SLPs may teach their clients specific types of covert behavior to improve their performance of target speech-language skills. For example, an SLP may teach a client with short-term memory deficits to engage in silent rehearsal, a technique that may help the client to remember previously presented information.

Consequences are the final component of A-B-C contingencies. Consequences refer to the environmental stimuli that occur after a behavior. These stimuli affect the probability that an individual will engage in a behavior again in the future. Consequence stimuli that increase the likelihood that a behavior will be exhibited are called reinforcers. There are a wide variety of stimuli that may serve as reinforcers for clients (see Chapter 6 for detailed information regarding reinforcement). Consequence stimuli that decrease the probability of a behavior being exhibited in the future are called punishers. Refer to Chapter 8 regarding the clinical use of punishment to decrease undesirable behaviors.

Definition and Purpose of Functional Behavior Assessment (FBA)

As discussed at the beginning of this chapter, most standardized speech-language assessments are primarily concerned with response topography. Evaluation tools of this nature often fail to describe the functions of verbal responses. Without knowledge of this information, clinicians may have difficulty selecting and treating speech-language target behaviors. Therefore, traditional assessment measures must be supplemented with additional procedures to examine the use of verbal operants. The field of applied behavior analysis (ABA) has described a variety of such techniques.

Functional behavior assessments (FBA) are the primary set of procedures used by board certified behavior analysts (BCBAs) in the field of ABA to determine potential functions of behaviors. The overall purpose of FBAs is to identify possible contingencies between a behavior and its maintaining antecedent and consequence stimuli. Therefore, FBAs are used to help clinicians develop hypotheses about A-B-C contingencies that are present in a client's environment. Although some FBA techniques can be used by SLPs (e.g., interviews, checklists, etc.), clinicians must be cognizant of their level of training. SLPs should refer to BCBAs when an FBA is deemed necessary. Although conducting a formal FBA is outside of an SLP's scope of practice, clinicians may be called upon to collaborate with BCBAs during the assessment process. Also, knowing about FBA techniques is helpful when devising a plan to address behavior problems that may interfere with therapy. Therefore, SLPs should be knowledgeable about what the FBA process entails.

> Functional behavior assessments help identify potential relationships between a behavior and its maintaining _____ and _____ stimuli.

Questions FBA Seeks to Answer

FBAs strive to answer a series of questions in order to identify potential relationships between behaviors and environmental stimuli. These questions help clinicians define the undesirable behavior, identify antecedent variables that precipitate the behavior, and make assumptions about how the behavior is being reinforced. The following sections describe these questions in greater detail.

What Is the Behavior of Concern?

The first step in conducting an FBA is to identify the behavior(s) of concern. Clinicians initially identify potential behaviors for assessment through interviewing clients and their significant others. The interview process should yield specific, topographical information regarding the behavior of concern. For example, if an interviewee states that a child is aggressive, the clinician should ask follow-up questions to obtain clarification regarding the specific form the behavior takes (e.g., "What constitutes aggression?" "What does he do when he is aggressive?" etc.). Once clinicians identify the undesirable behavior, an observable and measurable definition should be developed (see Chapter 3 for additional information). It is important to develop a definition that is operational in nature in order to facilitate direct observation of the behavior later on in the FBA process.

What Antecedent Variables Precipitate the Behavior?

Once the behavior has been operationally defined, clinicians attempt to identify the antecedent variables present in the environment prior to the client engaging in the response. Antecedent variables are identified through consideration of the following questions.

Where Does the Behavior Occur?

Clinicians initially attempt to determine if there are specific locations where the behavior is more or less likely to be evoked. This is the first step in identifying potential antecedent stimuli associated with undesirable responses. Answering this question allows clinicians to determine where direct observations will need to be conducted. For example, a clinician may learn that a client engages in an undesirable behavior frequently at home but not at school. Similarly, an informant may report that a patient exhibits undesirable verbal responses in her hospital room but not in the day room, gym, and so forth. In such cases, information of this nature would lead clinicians to conduct additional assessment sessions in the locations where the behavior was reportedly being demonstrated in order to determine possible maintaining variables in these settings.

When Does the Behavior Occur?

After the locations where the behavior typically occurs have been determined, clinicians identify specific times when the client is likely to exhibit the undesirable response. This is accomplished by identifying the **discriminative stimuli** and **motivating operations** associated with the undesirable behavior. Discriminative stimuli are antecedent variables that serve as signals to the client that reinforcement may be available for engaging in a behavior. Therefore, antecedent conditions in which discriminative stimuli are present increase the probability that the client will engage in the undesirable behavior. Specific tasks or activities may serve as discriminative stimuli for the undesirable behavior. A student who has difficultly learning science may exhibit noncompliance during instruction of this subject. A patient with dementia who lives in a skilled nursing facility may engage in aggression during dressing or bathing activities. Clinicians may often find that

transitions between activities can evoke undesirable behavior as well. Many clients have difficulty switching from a preferred to a nonpreferred task. Similarly, unanticipated schedule changes may serve to evoke undesirable behavior. Identifying the immediate antecedent stimuli associated with undesirable behaviors is a key component of conducting FBAs.

Clinicians also attempt to identify potential motivating operations that precipitate undesirable behaviors. For example, a clinician may find that aggressive behavior such as hitting or biting may be associated with a child not eating breakfast. Increased elopement from the classroom may occur when a student did not receive adequate sleep the night before. Changing doses of medication may also serve as a motivating operation for undesirable behavior. Such motivating operations may make it more likely that an undesirable behavior will be displayed. Therefore, motivating operations must be identified during the FBA process so they can be adequately addressed during treatment.

Who Is Present When the Behavior Occurs?

Clinicians also identify the individuals present when the undesirable behavior is exhibited. It is likely that certain people will be serving as discriminative stimuli for engaging in the undesirable behavior. Therefore, clinicians use the interview and direct observation process to identify who is present in the client's environment when the behavior occurs. A clinician who works in the hospital setting may find that a patient's agitation is correlated with the presence of a specific nurse or therapist. An SLP who works on a high school campus could observe that a student's behavior is related to certain teachers or classmates in the educational setting. Clinicians may also find that the absence of certain people may be associated with the undesirable behavior. While working in the school setting, this author has observed on many occasions that students can demonstrate increased behavioral concerns when their teachers or classroom instructional assistants are out sick for the day. The number of people present in the client's environment can also result in increased instances of the undesirable behavior. More people can result in greater crowding, noise, and general confusion (O'Neill et al., 1997). This is true in both the educational and medical communities. If this is the case, clinicians may advocate for their clients to have access to smaller class sizes or private hospital rooms in an attempt to decrease the undesirable behavior.

Determining who is present when the behavior occurs signals to the clinician the people who may be reinforcing the client's responses. For example, a student may be disruptive in the classroom when his peers are present but stay on task during one-on-one treatment sessions. This could indicate that attention from peers is reinforcing the student's disruptive behavior. Likewise, a child may throw tantrums when told to make his bed by his father while complying with similar directions provided by his mother. This suggests that the father may be allowing the child to escape the nonpreferred task of making his bed. Understanding who is present in the client's environment when the undesirable behavior is exhibited leads us to the next question that clinicians must answer while conducting FBAs: How is the behavior reinforced?

How Is the Behavior Reinforced?

As previously discussed in this chapter, consequences that follow a behavior that serve to increase its future frequency are known as reinforcers. The concept of reinforcement is applicable to both desirable and undesirable forms of behavior. For example, a clinician may provide verbal praise, which helps increase correct production of the /r/ phoneme. While at home, the child may also receive verbal praise for incorrect production of this sound because the parent thinks that it is cute or charming. Providing verbal praise contingent upon incorrect productions may increase the use of this typically undesirable behavior. In some cases, individuals may be reinforcing an undesirable behavior even though they have no intention of doing so. A child may be able to terminate participation in an aversive classroom activity by engaging in an aggressive behavior. In this example, the people in the child's environment would be strengthening the aggressive behavior, although this may not have been their intention.

> The concept of reinforcement is applicable to both _____ and _____ forms of behavior.

According to Hegde (1998), it is up to society to differentiate between appropriate and undesirable responses in order to provide reinforcement suitably. In order to facilitate the development of appropriate behaviors, clinicians must first identify how the undesirable behavior is being reinforced. There are three types of reinforcement that may maintain undesirable behaviors: (a) **positive reinforcement**,

(b) **negative reinforcement**, and (c) **automatic reinforcement** (Figure 4–1).

Positive Reinforcement

Positive reinforcement is the process of providing a consequence contingent upon a behavior, resulting in the increase of that behavior in the future (this concept is discussed in greater detail in Chapter 6). Therefore, a reinforcer is *added* to the environment in order to *increase* the frequency of a behavior. Many undesirable behaviors are maintained through positive reinforcement. A child's screaming behavior that is displayed while at the grocery store may be positively reinforced if her parent buys her the candy she wants in order to calm her down. In this example, the parent is adding a stimulus (i.e., the candy) that maintains the undesirable behavior (i.e., the screaming). Therefore, the child's screaming serves as a mand that provides her access to a specific reinforcer that she wants.

A variety of undesirable behaviors may be maintained through attention as well. Undesirable classroom behaviors such as refusing to complete a task, running around the classroom, being loud, or making inappropriate comments can result in attention from peers or classroom staff. If providing this attention results in an increase in the undesirable behavior, it is likely that the response is being maintained through positive reinforcement. If the clinician determines that an undesirable behavior results in positive reinforcement, the treatment plan should include procedures to ensure that the response no longer results in the maintaining consequence. This topic is discussed in greater detail in Chapter 8.

Negative Reinforcement

Negative reinforcement is the process of taking away a stimulus contingent upon a behavior, resulting in an increase in the future frequency of the behavior (this topic is also discussed in greater detail in Chapter 6). Whereas positive reinforcement involves adding a stimulus to increase the frequency of a response, negative reinforcement accomplishes this task through stimulus *removal*. As was the case with positive reinforcement, a variety of

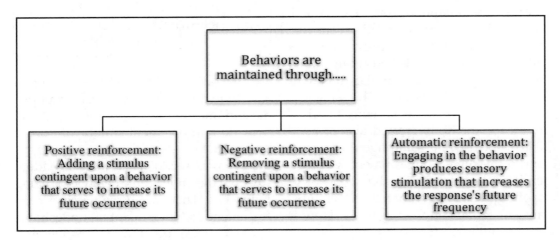

Figure 4–1. How behaviors are maintained.

undesirable behaviors can be maintained through negative reinforcement. Some clients engage in undesirable behaviors in order to avoid an aversive stimulus. People who stutter may avoid certain situations (e.g., talking on the phone, giving presentations, having conversations with specific people, etc.) in which they have demonstrated increased stuttering in the past. Students who view school as an aversive setting may refuse to enter the classroom or feign being sick in order to avoid the educational environment.

Additionally, behaviors that are negatively reinforced may allow clients to escape aversive stimuli that they have already come in contact with. An adult client who asks off-topic questions receives negative reinforcement if the behavior results in avoidance of difficult treatment activities. In such cases, the clinician is removing a stimulus (i.e., the difficult treatment activity) contingent upon the client's off-topic questions (i.e., the undesirable behavior). Allowing a child to take a "sensory break" can serve as a negative reinforcer if made contingent upon instances of aggression during nonpreferred activities. This example also includes removal of an aversive stimulus (i.e., cessation of the nonpreferred activity) that increases an undesirable response (i.e., aggression). When assessment results indicate that an undesirable behavior is being maintained by negative reinforcement, the treatment plan includes procedures to ensure that the response no longer results in termination of the aversive stimulus (see Chapter 8 for additional information regarding extinction).

Automatic Reinforcement

It is sometimes difficult to identify specific positive or negative reinforcers associ-ated with undesirable behaviors. In these cases, the behavior could be maintained by automatic reinforcement. Automatic reinforcement is not dependent upon the mediation of another person. Therefore, instances of the undesirable response typically do not result in attention or access to a preferred item (i.e., positive reinforcement). Likewise, engaging in the behavior does not result in avoiding or terminating an aversive stimulus (i.e., negative reinforcement). Instead, the behavior itself produces sensory stimulation that automatically reinforces the undesirable response.

Responses that are automatically reinforced are often referred to as self-stimulatory behaviors. The sensation obtained by engaging in the behavior may come from any of the major sensory systems. Infants who display babbling behavior may do so to obtain automatic auditory reinforcement. Similarly, immediate or delayed echolalia can result in auditory stimulation that is reinforcing in nature. A client who spins in circles or rocks back and forth may do so in order to obtain vestibular feedback. Finger shadowing can be maintained by automatic visual reinforcement. Furthermore, a client may show an affinity for certain food textures (e.g., soft, crunchy, etc.) based on a history of automatic tactile reinforcement. Some automatically reinforced behaviors may be self-injurious in nature. Behaviors such as head banging, skin picking, eye gouging, scratching, hair pulling, or hand biting can result in sensory stimulation that is automatically reinforcing for some clients. Treatment techniques for automatically reinforced undesirable responses involve dampening the sensory feedback the client receives as a result of engaging the behavior (refer to Chapter 8 for more detailed information).

Gathering Data

Hypotheses about the contingencies between undesirable behaviors and antecedent and consequence stimuli should not be made based on conjecture. Instead, clinicians use specific techniques to answer the previously discussed questions. These questions are addressed through several widely used data collection methods. These procedures represent a continuum of FBA techniques that are used to identify potential relationships between environmental stimuli and undesirable behaviors. This continuum of techniques includes indirect methods, direction observations, and functional analyses (Figure 4–2).

Indirect Methods

Indirect FBA methods do not include observation of the client engaging in the undesirable behavior. Instead, they involve asking clients and their significant others a series of questions to evoke information about the behavior. Examples of indirect assessment techniques include clinical interviews, checklists, questionnaires, and so forth.

Most traditional speech-language assessments include the use of indirect methods. Clinical interviews allow SLPs to clarify information documented in the client's case history (Hegde & Pomaville, 2013). Clinicians also use this opportunity to solicit additional information pertinent to the client's potential participation in therapy, including primary areas of concern, medical and developmental history, educational exposure, and so forth. In addition to this information, interviews conducted as part of an FBA provide further insight into the undesirable behavior itself. BCBAs who conduct FBAs ask clients and their significant others interview questions regarding the nature of

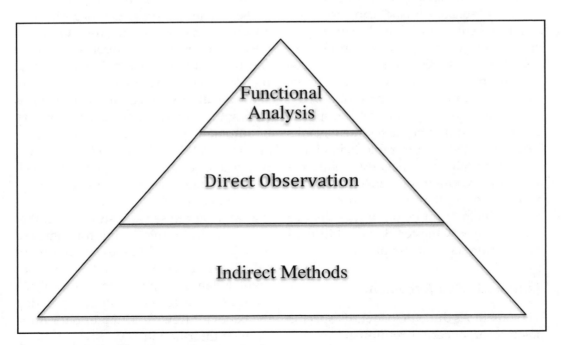

Figure 4–2. Continuum of FBA methods.

the undesirable behavior, the antecedent stimuli present before the response, and the consequences provided by the individuals in the environment after the behavior has been exhibited. This information can then be used to schedule direct observations of the client's behavior more efficiently. The SLP can also collect this type of data regarding undesirable communicative behaviors a client may display. Display Box 4–1 provides examples of questions clinicians can ask during the interview process to identify potential functions of undesirable behaviors.

After conducting a clinical interview that indicates the presence of an undesirable behavior, additional indirect methods such as checklists or questionnaires can be administered. Checklists and questionnaires are conducted to provide extra clarification regarding the antecedent and consequence stimuli maintaining the client's use of the undesirable behavior. A second reason clinicians use these indirect assessment techniques is to verify information obtained during the interview process. If informants report similar information during both the clinical interview and administration of a checklist or questionnaire, there is a greater probability that their responses are reliable. When the results across indirect assessment measures vary, the clinician should help explain any ambiguous terms to ensure

---

Display Box 4–1. Sample Interview Questions

The following questions may be asked during a clinical interview to clarify information regarding potential functions of the behavior:

1. What are the primary areas of concern?
2. What do the concerning behaviors look and sound like?
3. Have you noticed anything that seems to trigger the behavior?
4. What could you do to ensure that he or she engages in the behavior?
5. What could you do to ensure that he or she does not engage in the behavior?
6. What does his or her daily routine look like?
7. Are there certain times of day when the behavior is exhibited more often?
8. Are there certain places where the behavior occurs more frequently?
9. Who is typically in the environment when the behavior occurs?
10. How do you respond when he or she engages in the behavior?
11. How do others respond when he or she engages in the behavior?

that all questions are salient and accurately answered. Display Box 4–2 gives an example of a checklist that can be used during an FBA.

There are a variety of advantages to using indirect FBA assessment measures. As previously discussed, these techniques help clinicians schedule their direct observation sessions. Planning efficient observation sessions saves clinicians time and results in reduced cost to the client and financing agencies. These techniques are also convenient in that they can be completed fairly quickly and often yield useful information. Although indirect methods are a core component of the FBA process, there are several disadvantages associated with their use. Most significantly, informants may provide inaccurate information. This may occur due to the informant having incorrect recollections regarding the behavior and its associated environmental events. Occasionally, the informant may have preconceived notions about the undesirable behavior that result in a reporting bias. In addition to informant concerns, there is minimal efficacy research that has been conducted on the reliability of indirect assessment methods. Although there are drawbacks related to the use of these techniques, they are typically helpful and widely used within the field of ABA.

Direct Observation

It is best practice for clinicians to follow up on the results of indirect assessment methods with the use of direct observations. Observing clients as they engage in the behavior allows clinicians to confirm or rebuff the information obtained during clinical interviews, checklists, or questionnaires. When conducting direct observations, clinicians attempt to examine the client's use of the undesirable response

as it naturally occurs within the environment. For this reason, specific environmental conditions are not contrived to evoke the behavior. Instead, the clinician simply watches the client in situations where the behavior has occurred in the past and attempts to identify stimuli associated with the response. Therefore, the purpose of conducting direct observations is to describe the antecedent and consequence stimuli that affect the behavior and use this information to develop hypotheses about potential functions the response serves for the client.

> Direct observations involve examining the client's use of the undesirable response as it _____ occurs within the environment.

As is the case with all behaviorally based assessment and treatment procedures, data collection plays a key role in direct observations. Behaviorists use direct observations as an opportunity to develop hypotheses about the functions of behaviors that are backed by data. **ABC recording** is one way data can be collected during direct observations conducted within FBAs. As one might expect, the "A-B-C" in ABC data collection refers to antecedents, behaviors, and consequences. Therefore, this technique involves observing the client and documenting the antecedent stimuli present prior to the behavior, the nature of the behavior itself, and the consequences provided as a result of engaging in the behavior. Table 4–2 provides an example of a data collection sheet for ABC recording.

> When using ABC recording, clinicians document (a) _____ stimuli, (b) the _____, and (c) _____ stimuli.

Display Box 4–2. Sample Checklist

Instructions: Read each of the items below. Place check marks next to the items that accurately describe the nature of the undesirable behavior.

Antecedents:

_____ The behavior occurs at home.

_____ The behavior occurs at school.

_____ The behavior occurs at work.

_____ The behavior occurs across many different people.

_____ The behavior occurs across settings.

_____ The behavior occurs at certain times during the day.

_____ The behavior occurs in cycles.

Behavior:

_____ The behavior is exhibited for long periods of time.

_____ The behavior is exhibited with great intensity.

_____ The behavior occurs frequently.

_____ Engaging in the behavior results in physical harm to self.

_____ Engaging in the behavior causes physical harm to others.

_____ Engaging in the behavior results in property damage.

Consequences:

_____ People provide attention following the behavior.

_____ Engaging in the behavior allows the client to escape or avoid nonpreferred activities.

_____ The client is allowed to take a break after engaging in the behavior.

_____ The client is provided access to a preferred item following the behavior.

_____ People try to console the client after engaging in the behavior.

_____ The client engages in the behavior when alone.

Table 4–2. Data Collection Sheet: ABC Data

Client's Name: _____ DOB: _____

Clinician: _____ Date: _____

Setting: _____

Time of Observation: _____

Instructions: Each time the behavior is observed, document when it occurred, what happened just prior to the behavior, what the behavior looked like, and what happened immediately after the behavior. Document perceived functions of the behavior in the final column.

Time	Antecedents	Behavior	Consequences	Perceived Function

Scatterplots are another data collection method that may be used to collect information during direct observation sessions. This technique involves determining the times of the day when the behavior is most likely to occur. The clinician first divides the day into a series of intervals during which the client will be observed. For example, when conducting an assessment for a high school student, the clinician may divide the day according to the client's typical academic schedule (e.g., homeroom, English language arts, algebra, physical education, lunch, etc.). For a child who receives services in the home, the day may be divided into a series of 30-minute segments in which data will be collected. During each time interval, the clinician documents whether or not the client engages in the undesirable response. Table 4–3 provides an example of a scatterplot data collection sheet).

Frequently, BCBAs will rely on individuals in the client's environment (e.g., teachers, parents, care workers, etc.) to collect scatterplot data rather than directly observe the client themselves. In such cases, SLPs may be called upon to take scatterplot data regarding whether or not the behavior occurred while the client participated in speech-language services. Once scatterplot data have been obtained, the BCBA analyzes the information to determine any temporal patterns related to the undesirable response. Contexts during which the behavior occurred more frequently are further analyzed to identify antecedent and consequence stimuli associated with the behavior.

After indirect methods and direct observations have been completed, the BCBA aggregates the obtained data to make a hypothesis regarding the function of the undesirable behavior. The BCBA clearly defines this hypothesis by developing a summary statement (O'Neill et al., 1997). Summary statements describe the potential A-B-C contingency between the

Table 4–3. Data Collection Sheet: Scatterplot

Client's Name: _____ DOB: _____

Clinician: _____ Date: _____

Setting: _____

Instructions: At the end of each interval, fill in the box completely if the behavior was observed. If the client did not engage in the behavior during the interval, place an "x" in the box to document no occurrence of the response.

Time		Dates												
From	To													
8:00	8:30													
8:30	9:00													
9:00	9:30													
9:30	10:00													
10:00	10:30													
10:30	11:00													
11:00	11:30													
11:30	12:00													
12:00	12:30													
12:30	1:00													

undesirable behavior and its antecedent and consequence events. These statements are the clinician's best guess regarding the function of the behavior based on the available data. The following are examples of summary statements:

1. Upon being presented with picture cards (i.e., the antecedent), Ayden hits his head with a closed fist (i.e., the behavior), which results in attention from the clinician and avoidance of treatment tasks (i.e., the consequences).
2. When prompted to initiate daily hygiene activities (e.g., brushing teeth, washing hair, etc.) (i.e., the antecedent), Mr. Johnson hits (i.e., the behavior) caregivers, which postpones the activity (i.e., the consequence).
3. While walking by the candy aisle in the grocery store (i.e., the antecedent), Sally yells (i.e., the behavior) so that her mother will put the candy in the shopping cart (i.e., the consequence).
4. When presented with a math worksheet (i.e., the antecedent), Christopher crawls under his desk (i.e., the behavior) in order to escape (i.e., the consequence) completing the activity.

Functional Analysis

In most cases, indirect methods and direct observations provide BCBAs with clear patterns regarding the environmental events that affect the frequency of a behavior. However, when potential contingencies are not identified, additional assessment techniques may be warranted. Although the previously discussed techniques help BCBAs develop hypotheses about the functions of behaviors, BCBAs cannot make firm statements regarding

functional relationships based on indirect methods and direct observations as experimental control is not established. The process of experimentally testing hypotheses about the functions of undesirable behaviors is known as a **functional analysis**.

> A _____ _____
> is the process of testing hypotheses about the functions of undesirable behaviors.

Multiple functional analysis methods have been described (see Repp & Horner, 1999, for an in-depth review of various procedures). Iwata and his colleagues developed what is arguably the most widely used functional analysis technique (Iwata, Dorsey, Slifer, Bauman, & Richman, 1994). Based on the results of this study, four conditions were developed to experimentally examine the functions of behavior. These four conditions are described in greater detail below (Figure 4–3):

1. Contingent attention: This condition involves providing attention as a consequence each time the client engages in the undesirable behavior. If clients demonstrate increased responding during this condition, it is likely that the undesirable behavior is maintained as a result of positive reinforcement in the form of social attention.
2. Contingent escape: When conducting the contingent escape condition, the clinician first presents a nonpreferred task (e.g., an academic activity) to the client. The nonpreferred task is terminated contingent upon the undesirable behavior, thus allowing the client to escape the activity. Increased responding in this condition sug-

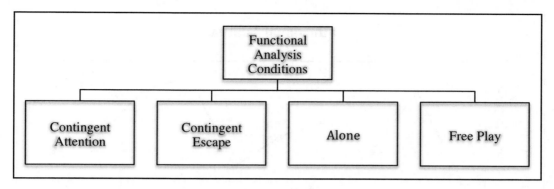

Figure 4–3. Conditions included in functional analyses of behavior.

gests that the behavior is maintained through negative reinforcement in the form of escape.

3. Alone: The alone condition helps the clinician determine if the client engages in the behavior as a result of automatic reinforcement. Clients are left by themselves in a setting with minimal stimuli. The clinician monitors the client (often through a two-way mirror) to ensure their safety and measure instances of the undesirable behavior. Clients who demonstrate increased responding in this condition likely do so in order to obtain the self-stimulation available through automatic reinforcement.

4. Free play: The free play condition serves as a control for the other conditions. The client is provided free access to a variety of preferred items. No demands are placed upon clients in this condition, and attention is provided noncontingently. As a result of free access to a variety of favored stimuli, it is unlikely that the client will engage in the undesirable behavior during this condition. If responding is observed during this condition, it is likely due to the automatic reinforcement that can only be obtained

through engaging in the undesirable behavior itself.

The clinician repeats these four conditions repeatedly, collecting data regarding the frequency of the undesirable behavior throughout. The data collected during each condition are graphed to determine the function of the undesirable behavior. The function of the response is represented by the condition in which the undesirable behavior is exhibited most frequently. Figure 4–4 shows data graphed from a functional analysis that suggest the client engaged in yelling in order to get attention. Often, a behavior may serve several functions for a client. For example, a child may crawl under the table to escape treatment tasks and gain the clinician's attention. In such cases, graphed functional analysis data will indicate elevated response rates in more than one experimental condition. If this is the case, the clinician must ensure that treatment is developed to address all functions of the undesirable behavior.

There are several distinct advantages to conducting functional analyses. Most significantly, functional analyses are the only FBA method that results in an experimentally validated definition of the function

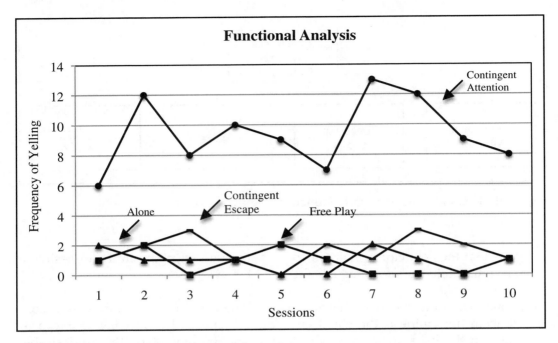

Figure 4–4. Graphed functional analysis data.

of a behavior. Therefore, functional analyses tend to provide the clearest description of the antecedent and consequence stimuli that maintain undesirable responses. BCBAs and SLPs collaborating with BCBAs can use the information garnered from functional analyses to design more effective treatment plans that address the undesirable behavior appropriately.

A primary drawback to functional analyses is that they must be conducted by trained, knowledgeable clinicians with experience in the area of behavior. As a result, it is not within a SLP's scope of practice to administer functional analyses. Furthermore, many individuals may view functional analyses unfavorably because they require clinicians to set up conditions that evoke the undesirable behavior. BCBAs who conduct functional analyses must consider the risks involved in evok-

ing the undesirable behavior and take any necessary precautions to maintain the client's safety during the assessment process.

FBA: Applications to Verbal Behavior

As previously discussed, SLPs frequently utilize indirect methods and direct observations to assess communicative behaviors. The use of functional analyses is less frequently used in the field of speech-language pathology. Although this may be the case, behavioral researchers have developed functional analysis techniques to determine the maintaining variables of verbal behaviors (Ewing, Magee, & Ellis, 2002; LaFrance, Wilder, Normand, & Squires, 2009; Lerman et al., 2005; Normand, Machado, Hustyi, & Morley, 2011; Normand, Severtson, & Beavers, 2008; Plavnick & Normand, 2013). The conditions included in such studies vary from those previously discussed. Instead, these methods are used to determine which verbal operant a communicative behavior represents.

Studies examining the function of verbal responses involve the manipulation of motivating operations, discriminative stimuli, and consequences to determine the nature of the verbal response. Data are collected in a series of conditions where the clinician attempts to evoke verbal operants according to their controlling antecedent and consequence stimuli (see Chapter 2 for additional information). For example, when conducting a mand condition, a clinician might set up a situation where the client had not eaten breakfast and was hungry (i.e., the motivating operation). Instances of the word *eat* would then be reinforced contingently by access to food. To set up a tact condition for the same verbal utterance, the clinician might show the client pictures of a person eating (i.e., the discriminative stimulus) and provide social attention contingent upon describing the scene using the word *eat*. The condition in which the client used the communicative response most frequently would indicate the function of the behavior and the verbal operant the response reflected.

Assessment of Verbal Operants

Although speech-language assessments do not include formal functional analyses of verbal behavior, SLPs do thoroughly examine their clients' use of the various

verbal operants. This is a key component of the assessment process that provides valuable information regarding a client's functional communication skills (Baker, LeBlanc, & Raetz, 2008; Gross, Fuqua, & Merritt, 2013; Hegde & Pomaville, 2013; Tager-Flusberg et al., 2009). Assessments should yield findings that describe how clients make requests and protests (i.e., mands), comment about things in their environment (i.e., tacts), repeat the behaviors of others (i.e., echoics), respond to questions and statements posed by communicative partners (i.e., intraverbals), and use grammar skills (i.e., autoclitics). For clients who have experienced neurogenic language disorders, an assessment of textual and transcription behavior may be needed as well.

Speech-language assessments include an analysis of clients' use of the various _____ _____.

Similar to the assessment procedures conducted by behaviorists, SLPs set up specific environmental conditions to evoke the client's use of the verbal operants. To assess a child's mand behavior, a clinician may place preferred toys on a high shelf to see how the child requests additional play time. Similarly, the SLP could present a nonpreferred activity to see how the child engages in protest behavior. To assess the client's tact repertoire, the clinician would present a variety of novel items and take note of how the client responds. Echoic behavior could be assessed by evaluating the client's ability to imitate gross motor movements (e.g., clapping), vowels, simple syllable shapes, single words, and utterances of increasing length and complexity. Intraverbal behavior can be examined by documenting the client's responses to questions, sentence completion prompts, or other verbal stimuli. Autoclitic behavior is best assessed by conducting a thorough conversational language sample. Reading and writing tasks may be used to evoke textual and transcription behavior.

Regardless of the specific conditions that the SLP decides to include in the assessment, it is important to ensure that objective data are collected on the verbal operants of interest. It is not enough to simply provide a subjective assessment of the client's communication skills. Clinicians must also support general descriptions of verbal behavior with objective data. This is frequently accomplished by taking either frequency or percentage data on the client's current communicative methods. Table 4–4 provides an example of a data collection sheet that can be used during assessments of verbal operants. Using Table 4–4, the clinician would tally the number of times the client engaged in the various topographical forms of the listed verbal operants. This information could then be used to document baseline levels of performance and select goals that would be addressed during treatment.

Chapter Summary

1. Standardized speech-language assessment measures tend to focus on response topography rather than function.
2. Clinicians must supplement traditional assessment tools with additional procedures to analyze response function.
3. Assessments that analyze response function are based on the concept of contingencies. Although neurophysiologic contingencies may affect a cli-

ent's performance during treatment, SLPs are primarily concerned with manipulating environmental contingencies to affect the frequency of communicative behavior.
4. A-B-C contingencies describe the relationship between antecedent stimuli, behaviors, and consequence stimuli.
5. Antecedents refer to the stimuli that occur prior to a behavior.
6. Behaviors may be overt or covert in nature.
7. Consequences can increase (i.e., reinforcers) or decrease (i.e., punishers) the likelihood of a behavior occurring again in the future.
8. Functional behavior assessments (FBAs) are a set of procedures used to identify relationships between antecedents, behaviors, and consequences. FBAs should be conducted by individuals who have experience assessing and analyzing behavior.
9. There is a continuum of FBA techniques, including indirect methods, direct observation, and functional analysis.
10. Examples of indirect FBA methods include interviews, checklists, and questionnaires.
11. Direct observation techniques include ABC data collection and scatterplots.
12. Functional analyses are experimental assessments of the functions of behaviors. They are the most intrusive form of FBA and typically used only if other FBA techniques fail to identify predictors of behavior.
13. The typical conditions included during functional analyses include contingent attention, contingent escape, alone, and free play.
14. Functional analyses have been adapted to assess a variety of undesirable verbal behaviors.

Table 4–4. Assessment of Verbal Operants

Client's Name: _____ DOB: _____

Clinician: _____ Date: _____

Setting: _____

Time of Observation: _____

		Verbal Operants				
		Mand	**Tact**	**Echoic**	**Intraverbal**	**Autoclitic**
Nonvocal Verbal Behavior	Hand Leading					
	Grabbing					
	Giving Item					
	Pointing					
	Gesturing					
	Eye Contact					
	Aggressive Behavior					**Refer to attached conversational language sample**
	Crying					
	Signing					
Vocal Verbal Behavior	Vocalization					
	Word Approximations					
	Single Words					
	Rote phrases/ sentences					
	Novel phrases/ sentences					
	Other: _____					

15. SLPs should evaluate their client's use of the various verbal operants during the assessment process.
16. Clinicians must collect objective data when assessing their clients' use of the various verbal operants.

Application Exercises

1. Search for videos online related to children engaging with peers in a preschool classroom. Attempt to describe A-B-C contingencies present in the child's environment. You may choose to describe contingencies related to communication, socialization, play skills, behavior, and so on.
2. Jason is a 4-year-old boy who has autism. He has been referred to the clinic where you work secondary to concerns regarding self-injurious behavior and difficulty expressing his wants and needs appropriately. Given the following information from clinical interviews, how should the clinician plan subsequent direct observation sessions?

   Jason's parents' primary concern is that he repeatedly hits his head with a closed fist. They report that he tends to engage in the behavior during challenging academic tasks and transitions between activities while at school. His preschool teacher states that he hits his head rather forcefully between three and five times during each occurrence. She reports that the classroom staff typically addresses the behavior by telling him to stop, attempting to block the self-injury, or redirecting him to the academic task. Jason seems to engage in the behavior most often when moving from floor to tabletop activities in the classroom. The behavior has not been observed during recess, snack time, or art.

3. Given the ABC data in Table 4–5, develop a summary statement that represents your hypothesis regarding the function of the client's behavior.
4. Based on the functional analysis data graphed in Figure 4–5, describe the function of the client's biting.
5. Search online journal databases (e.g., *The Analysis of Verbal Behavior*, *The Journal of Applied Behavior Analysis*, etc.) for research articles related to the application of FBA principles to verbal behavior. What types of conditions did the experimenters develop to test the functions of the subjects' communicative responses?
6. You are planning a speech-language assessment for a 3-year-old child who is a nonvocal communicator. How would you plan an assessment session to evaluate the child's use of the various verbal operants?

Table 4–5. Data Collection Sheet: ABC Data

Client's Name: <u>Kailey Smith</u>   DOB: <u>03/21/2010</u>

Clinician: <u>Denise Jones</u>   Date: <u>02/02/2016</u>

Setting: <u>Classroom</u>

Time of Observation: <u>8:00 AM to 12:15 PM</u>

Instructions: Each time the behavior is observed, document when it occurred, what happened just prior to the behavior, what the behavior looked like, and what happened immediately after the behavior. Document perceived functions of the behavior in the final column.

Time	Antecedents	Behavior	Consequences	Perceived Function
8:34 AM	Kailey is presented with a math worksheet	Kailey crawls under her desk and says no	Kailey is able to escape doing the math worksheet	Escape
9:27 AM	Kailey is given a coloring activity	Kailey crawls under her desk and refuses to make eye contact with the teacher	Kailey is able to escape the coloring activity	Escape
10:15 AM	Kailey is asked to cut and paste during an art project	Kailey gets out of her seat and crawls behind a table	Kailey is able to escape the art project Kailey's teacher provides a redirection to sit back down	Escape and Attention
11:51 AM	Kailey is asked to copy letters on a piece of paper	Kailey runs away from the teacher and hides under another student's desk	Kailey is able to escape having to copy letters	Escape

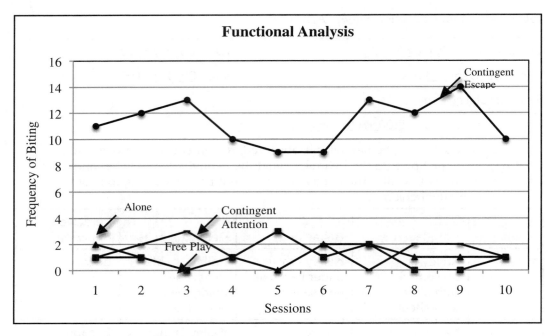

Figure 4–5. Functional analysis.

References

American Speech-Language-Hearing Association. (2007). *Scope of practice in speech-language pathology* [Scope of practice]. Retrieved from http://www.asha.org/policy

Baker, J. C., LeBlanc, L. A., & Raetz, P. B. (2008). A behavioral conceptualization of aphasia. *The Analysis of Verbal Behavior, 24,* 147–158.

Chance, P. (2006). *First course in applied behavior analysis.* Long Grove, IL: Waveland Press.

Cooper, J. O., Heron, T. E., & Heward, W. L. (2007). *Applied behavior analysis* (2nd ed.). Upper Saddle River, NJ: Pearson Education.

Esch, B. E., LaLonde, K. B., & Esch, J. W. (2010). Speech and language assessment: A verbal behavior analysis. *The Journal of Speech and Language Pathology and Applied Behavior Analysis, 5*(2), 166–191.

Ewing, C. B., Magee, S. K., & Ellis, J. (2002). The functional analysis of problematic verbal behavior. *The Analysis of Verbal Behavior, 18,* 51–60.

Gross, A. C., Fuqua, R. W., & Merritt, T. A. (2013). Evaluation of verbal behavior in older adults. *The Analysis of Verbal Behavior, 29*(1), 85–99.

Hegde, M. N. (1998). *Treatment procedures in communicative disorders* (3rd ed.). Austin, TX: Pro-Ed.

Hegde, M. N., & Pomaville, F. (2013). *Assessment of communicative disorders in children: Resources and protocols* (2nd ed.). San Diego, CA: Plural.

Iwata, B. A., Dorsey, M. F., Slifer, K. J., Bauman, K. E., & Richman, G. S. (1994). Toward a functional-analysis of self-injury. *Journal of Applied Behavior Analysis, 27*(2), 197–209.

LaFrance, D., Wilder, D. A., Normand, M. P., & Squires, J. L. (2009). Extending the assessment of functions of vocalizations in children with limited verbal repertoires. *The Analysis of Verbal Behavior, 25*(1), 19–32.

Lerman, D. C., Parten, M., Addison, L. R., Vorndran, C. M., Volkert, V. M., & Kodak, T. (2005). A methodology for assessing the functions of emerging speech in children with developmental disabilities. *Journal of Applied Behavior Analysis, 38*(3), 303–316.

Normand, M. P., Machado, M. A., Hustyi, K. M., & Morley, A. J. (2011). Infant sign training and functional analysis. *Journal of Applied Behavior Analysis*, 44(2), 305–314.

Normand, M. P., Severtson, E. S., & Beavers, G. A. (2008). A functional analysis of nonvocal verbal behavior of a young child with autism. *The Analysis of Verbal Behavior*, 24(1), 63–67.

O'Neill, R. E., Horner, R. H., Albin, R. W., Sprague, J. R., Storey, K., & Newton, J. S. (1997). *Functional assessment and program development for problem behavior: A practical handbook* (2nd ed.). Pacific Grove, CA: Brooks/Cole.

Plavnick, J. B., & Normand, M. P. (2013). Functional analysis of verbal behavior: A brief review. *Journal of Applied Behavior Analysis*, 46(1), 349–353.

Repp, A. C., & Horner, R. H. (1999). *Functional analysis of problem behavior: From effective assessment to effective support*. Belmont, CA: Wadsworth.

Tager-Flusberg, H., Rogers, S., Cooper, J., Landa, R., Lord, C., Paul, R., Rice, M., Stoel-Gammon, C., Wetherby, A., & Yoder, P. (2009). Defining spoken language benchmarks and selecting measures of expressive language development for young children with autism spectrum disorders. *Journal of Speech, Language, and Hearing Research*, 52, 643–652.

CHAPTER 5

Discrete Trial Teaching (DTT): A Framework

Discrete trial teaching (DTT) is an intensive behavioral approach to teaching specific skills. This method of teaching was originally named discrete trial training and is currently sometimes referred to as discrete trial instruction, but those terms are synonymous with discrete trial teaching. Lovaas and his colleagues developed DTT as a method of instruction to teach children with autism (Lovaas, 1987; McEachin, Smith, & Lovaas, 1993). Lovaas (1987) reported remarkable results in this initial study. Between two groups of young children with autism, 47% of the 19 participants in the experimental group receiving intensive DTT therapy for 40 hours a week achieved "normal intellectual and educational functioning in contrast to only 2% of the control group" consisting of 19 participants receiving only 10 hours of DTT a week (p. 7). A follow-up study 4 years later revealed maintenance of the gains made by children in the experimental group (McEachin et al., 1993).

_____ is an intensive behavioral approach to teaching specific skills.

Although modern-day home-based applied behavior analysis (ABA) therapy for children with autism incorporates DTT procedures, ABA should not be confused with DTT. In fact, the term *discrete trial* is mentioned only once in the major textbook on ABA (Cooper, Heron, & Heward, 2007, p. 78). Furthermore, in the behavior analyst task list, published by the Behavior Analyst Certification Board (BACB), the use of "discrete-trial . . . arrangements" is only one of 21 "fundamental elements of behavior change" that a person seeking to become a board certified behavior analyst (BCBA) must master (BACB, 2012, p. 4).

Yet, of all the procedures based on behavioral principles, DTT is possibly the most relevant to what speech-language pathologists (SLPs) seek to do—effectuate improvement in clients' communicative behaviors in the relatively short period of therapy time typically allotted in school and medical settings. Although first developed to teach children with autism, the DTT procedure is also an efficient, effective way to teach children and adults diagnosed with a wide variety of communicative disorders (Maul & Ambler, 2014; Pomaville & Kladopoulos, 2013; Skelton & Hagopian, 2014). Hegde (1998) developed a framework for delivering speech and language therapy using DTT (Display Box 5–1), and his description of the course of treatment is frequently referred to throughout this chapter.

What Is a Discrete Trial?

A **discrete trial** is an instructional unit designed to teach a specific skill. Discrete trials are brief, often lasting no more than 5 to 20 seconds, and potentially offering hundreds of learning opportunities during a one-on-one therapy session (Smith, 2001). Discrete trials are particularly well suited for teaching behaviors that are short-lived, with a clearly identified beginning and end (e.g., correct production of a phoneme or a specified language structure, identification of a common object, following two-step directions, answering *wh–* questions, etc.). Behaviors that are more complex can be broken down through task analysis (see Chap-

---

> ## Display Box 5–1. A Treatment Framework
>
> 1. Write target behaviors.
> 2. Take baseline measures of target behaviors to be treated first.
> 3. Begin DTT treatment, using modeling.
> 4. After five consecutively correctly imitated modeled responses, drop modeling.
> 5. After two incorrect evoked responses, reinstate modeling.
> 6. When the client reaches the criterion level for evoked trials over at least two consecutive sessions, conduct an intermixed probe.
> 7. When the client reaches the criterion level for the intermixed probe, conduct a pure probe.
> 8. When the client reaches the criterion level for the pure probe, conduct a final conversational probe in natural settings.
> 9. When the client reaches criterion level during repeated final conversational probes in natural settings, consider dismissal or move on to another target behavior.
> 10. Address issues of generalization and maintenance throughout the treatment framework.
>
> *Source:* Adapted from Hegde (1998).

ter 6), and each small step can then be taught with DTT procedures.

A _____ _____
is an instructional unit designed to teach a specific skill.

Preparing to Administer DTT

Before beginning DTT, there are several steps that must be taken, including:

1. Conducting a full assessment of the client's speech and language skills
2. Determining and writing appropriate client-specific target behaviors; these are the specific skills to be taught with DTT
3. Preparing the physical and verbal stimuli to evoke the target behavior; these constitute the antecedent component of a discrete trial
4. Preparing data sheets for baseline and treatment trials
5. Determining baseline measures of target behaviors to be treated first

After these steps have been completed, the clinician is ready to begin treatment, using the DTT procedure.

Components of the Discrete Trial

Discrete trials are highly structured, consisting of components that have been described in different ways by different authors. According to Smith (2001), a discrete trial consists of the following five parts: (1) the *cue,* (2) the *prompt,* (3) the *response,* (4) the *consequence,* and (5) the *intertrial interval.* Smith's use of the term *cue* will be replaced in this discussion with *antecedent,* a currently used term

that describes more succinctly what takes place to begin a discrete trial. A clinician can plan a therapy session, using these components as a framework for each discrete trial to be conducted. Tables 5–1, 5–2, 5–3, and 5–4 provide examples of a protocol for planning a DTT session.

The Antecedent

The antecedent component of a discrete trial consists of a **discriminative stimulus,** annotated S^D and pronounced "ess-dee."

Table 5–1. Protocol for Planning a DTT Session

Client's Name: _____   DOB: _____

Clinician's Name: _____   Session Date: _____

Target Behavior: _____

_____

Antecedent	Physical:
	Verbal:
Prompt	Type:
	Criterion for moving to independent:
	Criterion for reinstating prompt:
Response	
Consequence	For a correct response:
	For an incorrect response:

The S^D is "a stimulus in the presence of which a particular response will be reinforced" (Malott, 2007, p. 202; see Chapter 1 for further information regarding S^D). It is a stimulus that is carefully chosen to evoke a correct response that can then be reinforced by the clinician. In short, it is a stimulus that signals to the client that reinforcement is available for engaging in a response, thus increasing the likelihood of the client producing the target behavior. Everyday life is replete with examples of people responding with learned behaviors to discriminative stimuli. We stop the car when the light is red, go when the light is green, and slow down (when we are wise!) when the light is yellow. We answer the phone when it rings, smile when others smile at us, dance when we hear music, and stand when a bride walks down the aisle.

> In DTT, the antecedent consists of a _____ _____, annotated S^D.

In discrete trial therapy, the S^D is designed to evoke a verbal behavior from a client that has not been established by

Table 5–2. Example of a Completed Protocol for an Articulation Target Behavior

Client's Name: <u>John Doe</u>   DOB: <u>3/5/07</u>

Clinician's Name: <u>Mary Speechly</u>   Session Date: <u>9/22/14</u>

Target Behavior: <u>Production of /s/ in initial word position in response to picture stimuli with 90% accuracy in the clinic setting</u>

Antecedent	Physical: Picture cards depicting objects beginning with /s/
	Verbal: The clinician will say, "What is this?"
Prompt	Type: Full model
	Criterion for moving to independent: The model will be dropped after five consecutive correct imitative responses
	Criterion for reinstating prompt: The model will be reinstated after two incorrect independent responses
Response	John will verbally name the object in the picture
Consequence	For a correct response: Praise and a token for every correct response (FRI)
	For an incorrect response: Corrective feedback coupled with a demonstration of the correct production

Table 5–3. Example of a Completed Protocol for an Expressive Language Target Behavior

Client's Name: Sally Smart   DOB: 4/5/08

Clinician's Name: Mary Speechly   Session Date: 10/3/14

Target Behavior: Production of plural –s at the phrase level in response to picture stimuli with 90% accuracy in the clinic setting

Antecedent	Physical: Pairs of picture cards with one object on one and more than one object on the other (e.g., a picture of one ball paired with a picture of three balls). The clinician will place a set of paired cards on the table, in front of John for each discrete trial.
	Verbal: The clinician will say, "Here is one ball" while pointing to the picture of one ball; then the clinician will point to the picture of three balls and say, "Here are _____."
Prompt	Type: Visual cue; an index card with an *s* will be placed in front of John
	Criterion for moving to independent: The visual cue will be withdrawn after five consecutive correct responses
	Criterion for reinstating prompt: The visual cue will be reinstated after two incorrect independent responses
Response	John will produce phrases, such as "three balls"
Consequence	For a correct response: Praise and a token for every correct response (FRI)
	For an incorrect response: Corrective feedback; for example, "Oh-oh! I didn't hear the –s on the end of that word. Let's try again."

discriminative stimuli encountered in the natural environment that usually serve to shape verbal behavior in people who do not have a communicative disorder. People request help from SLPs because they are seeking control over their verbal behavior that can be established by special stimuli provided by clinicians during therapy sessions. Clinicians provide these special stimuli by fashioning appropriate physical and verbal antecedents that are

likely to evoke a correct response, which can then be reinforced.

In preparing the antecedent S^D for DTT, clinicians need to carefully consider physical and verbal stimuli that increase the likelihood of the client producing a correct response that can then be reinforced. Sometimes, this is a relatively easy task. For example, for articulation or phonological target behaviors, the physical stimulus is typically a picture of an object

Table 5–4. Example of a Completed Protocol for a Receptive Language Target Behavior

Client's Name: <u>Mike Elderly</u>   DOB: <u>4/15/1940</u>

Clinician's Name: <u>Jerry Garcia</u>   Session Date: <u>5/10/2014</u>

Target Behavior: <u>Identification of common objects by function in a field of four with</u> <u>80% accuracy in the clinic setting</u>

Antecedent	Physical: Several common functional objects (e.g., a toothbrush, a comb, a fork, a washcloth, a key, a cell phone, etc.); four objects will be placed on the table in front of Mike
	Verbal: The clinician will say, "Give me what you _____" (e.g., "open your door with," "fix your hair with," "talk to your friends with," etc.)
Prompt	Type: Positional; the object asked for will be placed closer to Mike than the others
	Criterion for moving to independent: The positional prompt will be dropped after five correct responses
	Criterion for reinstating prompt: The positional prompt will be reinstated after two incorrect independent responses
Response	Mike will give the clinician the requested object
Consequence	For a correct response: Verbal praise and informative feedback (e.g., "Yes, that's right! You open your door with a key!")
	For an incorrect response: Corrective feedback coupled with pointing to the correct object; "No. You open your door with a key. This is a key."

and the verbal stimulus is, "What is this?" to evoke production of a word, phrase, or sentence containing the targeted phoneme or phonological structure (e.g., consonant clusters, final consonants, etc.). For language target behaviors, however, constructing physical and verbal stimuli can be more complex (e.g., see Table 5–3 for antecedent stimuli for plural *–s*). Clinicians must ensure that the physical and verbal stimuli they are presenting are a

good S^D for the correct response they hope to evoke.

Sometimes, the antecedent stimuli may include irrelevant, or distractor, stimuli in the presence of which a response will *not* be reinforced, annotated S$^\Delta$ and pronounced "ess-delta." A response involving these stimuli is incorrect and therefore will not be reinforced. For example, a client may have a receptive language target behavior for identification of common objects in a field of three. The clinician would present three objects, such as a comb, a fork, and a key, and then say, "Give me the fork." The S^D for that verbal stimulus is the fork, and if the client selects the fork to give to the clinician, that response will be reinforced. If the client responds by identifying one of the S^Δs, either the comb or the key, that response will not be reinforced.

The Prompt

In the initial stages of treatment, the client is not likely to correctly respond just to the presentation of the antecedent stimuli. Therefore, the clinician often must provide a hint to the client, in addition to the special antecedent stimuli. The hints that a clinician gives a client to increase the probability of a correct response are called **prompts**. There are many different categories of prompts, with many specific procedures corresponding to those categories, and these are more fully explained in Chapter 6.

> Hints clinicians give to clients to increase the probability of a correct response are called _____.

Prior to beginning DTT, clinicians should explore possible prompting techniques that may be of benefit to the client during therapy. Pretreatment assessment sessions often end with **stimulability testing**, during which clinicians attempt to evoke correct productions of identified possible target behaviors through any necessary prompt. The most common check of stimulability tests how well the client responds to the clinician providing a **model** of a correct response. If the client does not adequately imitate a model, the clinician might try other verbal, visual, or tactile-kinesthetic prompts to evoke a correct or more appropriate response. When a prompt results in a better response, the clinician then has a good indication of the possible effectiveness of that prompt during treatment. The clinician may also elect to run a baseline measure of the target behavior in the presence of a selected prompt, to see to what extent baseline correct production might increase. This must be done *after* all evoked baseline measures and all modeled baseline measures have been taken. In the initial stages of treatment, it is best to deliver just a model or one type of some other prompt, while taking data on the correct response rate. If the correct response rate increases, the clinician can be more confident that the specific prompt being used is affecting behavior change. If the clinician bombards the client with different types of prompts, and the correct rate increases, there will be no way of determining which specific prompt was effective.

Although prompts often assist the client to produce correct responses, they should be **faded** as soon as possible. Fading refers to the gradual reduction of the special stimuli provided by the clinician, so that the response is maintained in the presence of more natural stimuli. To state this more plainly, the clinician should pull back on prompting until the response is produced in the absence of prompts (see Chapter 6 for further information regarding fading). This is done so that the client does not become **prompt dependent**, meaning that the client overdiscriminates and produces the correct response only in the presence of the special S^D presented during DTT. To prompt effectively, in a manner that leads to fading:

1. Prompt more in the initial stages of treatment
2. Deliver prompts immediately after presentation of the antecedent stimuli
3. Use subtle or short prompts, rather than loud and lengthy prompts
4. Use, whenever possible, silent or gestural prompts, rather than verbal prompts
5. Fade prompts as soon as possible, referring to data collected on the correct response rate as a guide (adapted from Hegde, 1998)

> Clients who overdiscriminate and produce correct responses only in the presence of the special stimuli presented by the clinician during treatment may have become _____ _____.

The Response

If the clinician has carefully prepared antecedent stimuli and used an effective prompt, the client will usually give a response. At times, the client may produce a response that appears to be irrelevant to the antecedent stimuli. When this occurs, the clinician should carefully consider whether or not the antecedent stimuli presented are appropriate for evoking the targeted response. For example, for the expressive language target behavior of production of third-person singular present tense –s, a clinician might show a client a picture of a man walking and mistakenly ask, "What is he doing?" In this case, there is a mismatch between the target behavior and the verbal stimulus given, which is appropriate for evoking present progressive –ing but not third-person singular present tense –s. Hopefully, the clinician will soon realize this and change the verbal stimulus to, "What does he do?"

At other times, the client may not give any response at all. When this happens, the clinician should consider whether or not the client understands what is expected. Further instructions, with or without a demonstration, may be necessary. Also, sometimes picture cards are ambiguous, represent a concept that is not easily understood, or represent a word that is not in the client's vocabulary. The clinician might find it necessary to take some time to teach the client what word or phrase the pictures represent. Other times, clinicians may decide to abandon certain picture stimuli altogether and find those that are less problematic for the client.

For most discrete trials, however, the client will produce some kind of a response. The correctness or incorrectness of that response will determine the next step in the discrete trial procedure—delivery of a consequence.

The Consequence

In treatment, the clinician delivers a consequence contingent upon the correctness or incorrectness of a client's response. If the response is correct, the clinician immediately reinforces the response, using one or a combination of the types of reinforcers described more fully in Chapter 6, and records the response as correct on the data sheet. If the response is incorrect, the clinician immediately delivers a consequence designed to discourage the incorrect response and records the response as incorrect on the data sheet. As a consequence for an incorrect response, the clinician can:

1. Give corrective feedback or some other type of punishment (see Chapter 8)
2. Give a prompt to evoke a correct or more correct response; if the response is correct, reinforce and record the correct response and, if incorrect, record the incorrect response and move on to the next trial
3. Ignore the incorrect response and move on to the next discrete trial

(Adapted from the National Professional Development Center on Autism Spectrum Disorders, 2010)

Sometimes, beginning clinicians may be tempted to pause after receiving a response from a client to reflect on whether or not it was a correct response. This is not recommended. To be effective, the consequence, either reinforcement or corrective feedback, should be delivered *immediately* after the response, as described in the following sections.

Reinforcement as a Consequence

During DTT, reinforcement is delivered immediately after a correct response. It should be delivered warmly, with a delighted facial expression. However, subjective feelings do not determine whether or not a technique is a true reinforcer. A clinician may "feel good" about delivering warm, enthusiastic verbal praise, and a client may appear to be enjoying the procedure; however, if the correct response rate is not increasing, then there is no reinforcement going on, and the clinician

must explore other possible reinforcers. Reinforcing effects can only be demonstrated through data collection indicating an increase in the correct response rate.

> Reinforcing effects can only be demonstrated through the collection of
> _____.

Also, a technique that proves to be reinforcing to one client cannot be assumed to also be reinforcing to another. A child, for example, who loves art may work hard to gain access to the high probability behavior of painting, while a child who loves physical movement may work hard for the privilege of jumping on a small trampoline for a while. The clinician must also be prepared for the fact that a reinforcer that has been effective for a client during one session may lose its effectiveness in subsequent sessions. For example, a clinician might spend some time constructing a milk carton "monster" for a child to "feed" upon production of a correct response and see the correct response rate improve impressively during the first session that technique is used. If that activity is repeated the next session, the response rate might decrease, because the child has grown tired of feeding that silly monster. Clinicians, therefore, should have several alternative methods on hand to reinforce correct responses during any one clinic session.

Punishment as a Consequence

One of the options a clinician has during DTT is to deliver punishment immediately after an incorrect response. The word **punishment** falls ill on the ears of many, but recall from Chapter 1 that punishment simply means that some contingency placed on a behavior has resulted in a *decrease* of a specified behavior. There are a number of punishment techniques that are applicable to DTT delivered during speech and language therapy; those techniques are described more fully in Chapter 8.

Punishment during DTT should be delivered firmly, but not harshly, and with a neutral facial expression and tone of voice. In other words, there should be a definite contrast between a clinician's facial expression and tone of voice when delivering punishment and when delivering reinforcement. A common mistake that beginning clinicians make is to deliver punishment with a bright smile, a cheery attitude, and verbal stimuli (e.g., "Nice try!") that are incompatible with the goal of punishment—namely, to decrease an undesirable behavior. Also, clients with receptive language disorders or cognitive or intellectual disabilities may find it confusing to see a contradiction between a clinician's facial expression and the words being said.

Recall that there are two types of punishment: positive punishment and negative punishment (see Chapters 1 and 8). Positive punishment involves the presentation of a stimulus immediately after an undesirable behavior. Negative punishment involves the withdrawal of a desired stimulus directly after an undesirable behavior. Both positive and negative punishment result in a decrease in the behavior. Just as in reinforcement, the effects of punishment are not determined by subjective feelings. For example, a parent might feel that harshly scolding a child for hitting a sibling is a suitable punishment. However, if the hitting behavior does not decrease, then scolding the child is not serving as a punishment. Punishing

effects can only be demonstrated through data indicating a decrease in the occurrence of the undesirable behavior or, during DTT, a decrease in the rate of incorrect responses.

Corrective feedback is the most commonly used form of positive punishment to decrease incorrect responses during DTT for speech and language therapy. It is especially valuable because the client receives specific information about what must be done to improve the response. For example, a client working on correct production of the phoneme /s/ may produce a full frontal lisp, responding with /θop/, when presented with antecedent stimuli to evoke the word /sop/. Using corrective feedback, the clinician would say, "No, that's not it. I saw your tongue come out between your teeth. Tuck your tongue back, lightly touching the bumps right behind your upper front teeth." The clinician might also use a further tactile-kinesthetic prompt, touching the alveolar ridge with an orange stick, to further illustrate tongue placement.

> The most commonly used technique to reduce incorrect responses during DTT for speech and language therapy is _____ _____.

Response cost is a negative punishment technique that can also be employed during DTT. As discussed in Chapter 8, response cost is best used in combination with a token economy, or generalized conditioned reinforcement. A client earns tokens for correct responses (generalized conditioned reinforcement) and loses tokens for incorrect responses (response cost). Display Box 5–2 presents a slight variation on this technique.

Display Box 5–2. A Slight Variation on Response Cost

Sometimes, even the most evidence-based clinicians may find a technique to be aversive, not only to the client but also to themselves. It has been the experience of this author that some small children have emotional reactions to the well-established technique of response cost. A variation that I have employed seems to cut down on this upset and encourages correct response rates. The steps I use in combining a token economy as reinforcement with response cost as punishment are as follows:

1. Start with a generous amount of tokens (I usually use poker chips) in a plastic cup.
2. For every correct response, add a token to the cup.
3. For an incorrect response, withdraw a token from the cup, but hold it over the cup, looking at the child with an expectant look.
4. Deliver the next discrete trial; if the child responds correctly, the token gets plopped right back into the cup.
5. If the child responds incorrectly, the token is withdrawn, as is consistent with the procedure.

The good news is—very rarely do I get to Step 5!

Christine A. Maul, PhD, CCC-SLP

The Intertrial Interval

The **intertrial interval** refers to a brief pause, between 1 and 5 seconds, after one discrete trial has been presented and before another begins. Although brief, the intertrial interval is a vital component to DTT. Remember that a discrete trial represents *one* opportunity and *only* one opportunity for the client to produce a response. Discrete trials are discrete because they are separated from each other. The intertrial interval clearly indicates the end of one discrete trial and the beginning of another, giving integrity to DTT and facilitating data collection. Clinicians who do not understand the importance of the intertrial interval may make errors in terms of data collection that will weaken the validity of their calculation of correct response rates. Display Box 5–3 is an illustration of a poor application of the intertrial interval.

Display Box 5–3. Misapplication of the Intertrial Interval

Sometimes beginning clinicians may disregard the importance of the intertrial interval. When this happens, data collection may be skewed, resulting in invalid calculations of correct response rates. For example, consider the following dialogue between a clinician and a client during DTT:

Clinician: [showing a picture of a boy eating] What is he doing?

Client: No response [clinician does not record data]

Clinician: Come on, now, tell me, what is he doing?

Client: He. . . . [clinician does not record data]

Clinician: Almost! Try again! He _____.

Client: He is walking.

Clinician: Good! You got it! [records a + for a correct response]

The clinician actually gave not one but three opportunities for the client to produce a correct response. However, because data were not recorded for each opportunity presented, the data so far reflect a 100% correct response rate, instead of a 33% correct response rate. Clinicians using DTT effectively adhere to predetermined physical and verbal stimuli, remember to separate each discrete trial by an intertrial interval, and record data for each opportunity presented.

Data Collection and Criterion Levels

Data collection is an integral part of DTT. As discussed in Chapter 3, there are various ways to measure target behaviors. In DTT, the most commonly used method is a derivative measure, usually expressed in terms of a percentage of correct response rates. Table 5–5 provides an example of a data collection sheet for DTT. Careful data collection helps a clinician to make certain necessary judgments during the course of DTT. For example, if a client's correct response rate is increasing, then the clinician can be assured that the selected reinforcement technique is an effective one. Conversely, if the correct response rate is not improving at all or even decreasing,

Table 5–5. Treatment Recording Sheet

Client's Name: _____ Date: _____

DOB: _____ Clinician: _____

Target Behavior: _____
_____

Correct Response: +   Incorrect Response: –   No Response: N/R
Correct Response (Modeled) +M   Incorrect Response (Modeled): –M
Correct Response (Prompted) +P   Incorrect Response (Prompted) –P

Target Response	Treatment Trials																								

Percentage correct evoked: _____

Percentage correct evoked plus modeled: _____

Percentage correct evoked plus modeled plus prompted: _____

the clinician knows it is necessary to find another reinforcer.

The clinician also refers to data collected during treatment to determine when modeling or prompting should be dropped or reinstated. This is a matter of clinical judgment; however, Hegde (1998) has suggested that DTT should begin with modeled trials (see Display Box 5–1). After five correct imitative responses, modeling should be dropped, and evoked trials should continue. After discontinuing modeling (or whatever prompt the clinician decides to use) and moving to evoked trials, the client should not be allowed to produce too many incorrect responses before reinstating modeling or prompting. The suggested criterion is no more than two incorrect responses during evoked trials before the clinician switches back to either modeled or prompted trials (Hegde, 1998).

The most important criterion level involved in DTT is the one that is set for the target behavior—the criterion level that indicates that the target behavior has been met. As treatment progresses, the correct response rate should be carefully calculated to determine when the client has reached that criterion level and the target behavior is ready to be probed for generalization. The following sections outline procedures for a number of different generalization probes that should be conducted to determine progress toward meeting the criterion level set for the target behavior.

uli—in other words, if the target behavior is showing **generalization**, a concept that is discussed in detail in Chapter 7. In treatment, the clinician begins by presenting a predetermined number of stimulus items as the antecedent; as few as four to six stimulus items may suffice to establish a target behavior (Hegde, 1998). As DTT progresses, the client may reach the criterion level set by the target behavior in response to those stimulus items. However, before a target behavior can be considered to have been met, the behavior should generalize and be maintained across stimuli, settings, and audiences. Therefore, during treatment, clinicians should periodically probe to check for generalization of the target behavior in response to new, untrained stimuli. Probe procedures are usually conducted after the client has met the criterion level as stated in the target behavior over at least three consecutive treatment sessions. There are three types of probe procedures that are particularly useful during DTT: an **intermixed probe**, a **pure probe**, and a **conversational probe**. Hegde (1998) has suggested a particular sequence for conducting these probe procedures and methods of analyzing probe data to determine the course of treatment; much of the following discussion is based on those suggestions.

> Probe procedures are conducted to see if the target behavior has _____ to untaught stimuli.

Probe Procedures

Probe procedures are conducted to determine if correct response rates are maintained in the presence of untrained stim-

The Intermixed Probe Procedure

The intermixed probe procedure can also be called the initial probe, because it is the first probe procedure that should be conducted after the client has met the criterion level for a target behavior over at least three consecutive sessions. The intermixed probe consists of two sets of stimulus items: a set that has been used during treatment (the "taught" items) and a set consisting of new stimulus items the client has not previously seen (the "untaught" items). During the intermixed probe procedure, the clinician alternates between taught and untaught stimulus items. When presenting a taught stimulus item, the clinician delivers either reinforcement for a correct answer or corrective feedback for an incorrect answer, just as for any discrete trial given during treatment. However, when presenting an untaught stimulus item, no reinforcement or corrective feedback is given. The response is simply recorded, and the clinician switches back to a taught stimulus item. Display Box 5–4 is a list of steps to take when conducting an intermixed probe.

> During an intermixed probe, the clinician presents _____ and _____ stimuli in an alternating fashion.

Data are collected and a percentage correct is calculated only for responses to untaught stimuli. Table 5–6 shows an intermixed probe data recording sheet and Tables 5–7 and 5–8 are examples of intermixed probe data recording sheets filled out for an articulation and for a language target behavior. The percentage correct for untaught stimuli should then be considered to determine next steps in treatment. If the percentage correct is low, say only 70% or less, the clinician should continue to treat using the same stimulus items previously used but also introducing a few new stimulus items. On the other hand, the percentage correct may be high but not high enough to reach

---

Display Box 5–4. Conducting an Intermixed Probe

1. Present a taught stimulus item.
2. Ask the predetermined question.
3. Wait a few seconds (e.g., 1–5 seconds) for the client to respond.
4. Reinforce the response contingently or provide corrective feedback for incorrect responses.
5. Record the response.
6. Wait a few seconds to establish an intertrial interval.
7. Present an untaught stimulus item.
8. Ask the predetermined question.
9. Allow a few seconds for the client to respond.
10. Record the response.
11. Provide no reinforcement or corrective feedback.
12. Repeat, starting with Step 1.

Table 5–6. Data Recording Sheet for an Intermixed Probe

Client's Name: _____   Date: _____

DOB: _____   Clinician: _____

Target Behavior: _____

Physical Stimuli: _____

Verbal Stimuli: _____

Target Response: Taught	Response	Target Response: Untaught	Response
1.			
		2.	
3.			
		4.	
5.			
		6.	
7.			
		8.	
9.			
		10.	
11.			
		12.	
Percentage correct for **untaught** stimuli: _____			

the criterion level required by the target behavior. For example, a target behavior might specify a criterion level of 90%, and the client may have an 80% correct response rate for untaught stimuli during an intermixed probe. If that is the case, the clinician should simply continue to treat, because treatment is going well, and the client may just need a little more time to generalize the target behavior to untaught stimuli. Finally, if the client reaches the criterion level during the intermixed probe procedure, the next step is to administer a pure probe.

For the intermixed probe procedure, the percentage correct is calculated only for responses given in the presence of _____ stimuli.

Table 5–7. Example of a Data Recording Sheet for an Intermixed Probe: Articulation

Client's Name: <u>Johnny Smith</u>   Date: <u>April 5, 2015</u>

DOB: <u>February 20, 2007</u>   Clinician: <u>Sally Speechly</u>

Target Behavior: <u>Production of /l/ in initial word position with 90% accuracy</u>

Physical Stimuli: <u>Picture cards of objects beginning with /l/</u>

Verbal Stimuli: <u>"What is this?"</u>

Target Response: Taught	Response	Target Response: Untaught	Response
1. lime			
		2. light	
3. lion			
		4. lamp	
5. lips			
		6. lemon	
7. lamb			
		8. leg	
9. lip			
		10. lock	
11. log			
		12. lunch	
Percentage correct for **untaught** stimuli: _____			

The Pure Probe Procedure

The pure probe procedure is conducted to determine if the correct response is produced in the presence of only new, untaught stimuli. The clinician presents a series of discrete trials, using nothing but untaught stimuli. No reinforcement for correct responses or corrective feedback for incorrect responses is given during a pure probe, and data are collected and analyzed based on all responses given.

There is no set number of stimulus items to use, but the clinician should administer a sufficient number of discrete trials to determine generalization of the response to untaught stimulus items in the absence of reinforcement. As a general rule, at least 20 trials should be conducted; Cooper et al. (2007) have recommended administering 100 trials when collecting percentage data. The pure probe procedure should be administered only when it is likely that the response has generalized,

Table 5–8. Example of a Data Recording Sheet for an Intermixed Probe: Language

Client's Name: <u>Mary Sunshine</u>   Date: <u>April 4, 2015</u>

DOB: <u>February 20, 2007</u>   Clinician: <u>Dudley Doright</u>

Target Behavior: <u>Production of plural –s and –z at the word level with 90% accuracy</u>

Physical Stimuli: <u>Pairs of picture cards of common objects; one object on one; two</u>
<u>objects on the other</u>

Verbal Stimuli: <u>e.g., "Here is one duck; here are two _____."</u>

Target Response: Taught	Response	Target Response: Untaught	Response
1. balls			
		2. ducks	
3. cars			
		4. apples	
5. babies			
		6. socks	
7. blocks			
		8. dogs	
9. chairs			
		10. pots	
11. pens			
		12. forks	

Percentage correct for **untaught** stimuli: _____

as indicated by the results of the intermixed probe. If the client reaches the criterion level during a pure probe, a final conversational probe should be administered in natural settings.

Conversational Probes

A target behavior cannot be considered to have been mastered until it has been determined that the client produces the behavior at criterion level in natural settings. Therefore, the final probe to be conducted is a series of conversational probes in the client's natural environment. Clinicians gather speech and language samples from clients while observing them at home, in school, on the job, or in the community. When direct observations are not possible, alternative procedures include audio or video recordings. In some cases, these procedures can be a more valid measure of generalization, because the clinician is not present and possibly serving as an S^D for the target behavior.

The collected samples are then analyzed to determine if the criterion level for the target behavior is sustained in the natural environment. If the client reaches the criterion level set for the target behavior, as indicated by analysis of speech and language samples in natural settings, it is an indication that (a) the client is ready to move on to a new level of the same target behavior, (b) the client is ready to move on to a different target behavior, or (c) the client is ready to be dismissed from treatment.

Variations on Probe Procedures

The sequence of probe procedures that has been described is appropriate for many target behaviors, particularly those having to do with articulation, phonological, and language disorders. However, the sequence is not appropriate for all target behaviors. For example, target behaviors for fluent speech or improved vocal quality will not lend themselves to intermixed and pure probes; conversational probes are used, and the untaught stimuli more appropriately consist of new audiences, new settings, and new situations.

Similarly, objectives for pragmatic language behaviors are checked for generalization in different ways. Behaviors such as eye contact, turn taking, initiating and maintaining conversation, and so forth may be established in the clinic room but, again, probed through observation of the client's interactions with other conversational partners in the natural environment. For example, a clinician might first teach a person with a pragmatic language

disorder conversational turn taking during one-on-one therapy. To probe to see if that behavior is generalizing, the clinician might invite other familiar individuals into the therapy room, such as parents, classmates, or friends, and observe whether the turn-taking behavior has generalized during conversations with others. A next step in probing for generalization would be to observe whether or not appropriate turn taking is occurring in conversations with others in the client's natural environment. Clinicians need to be able to "think outside the box" when planning procedures for probing for generalization of these types of target behaviors.

Chapter Summary

1. Discrete trial teaching (DTT) is an intensive behavioral approach to teaching specific skills and is possibly the behavioral-based procedure most relevant to the field of speech-language pathology.

2. A discrete trial is a brief (5–20 seconds) instructional unit designed to teach a specific skill and is well suited for teaching behaviors that are short-lived, with a clearly identified beginning and end, such as the production of a phoneme, grammatical structure, or fluent utterance.

3. Before conducting DTT, the clinician should conduct a full assessment, write and baserate appropriate target behaviors, prepare physical and verbal stimuli, prepare baseline and treatment data recording sheets, and conduct baseline trials for those target behaviors to be treated first.

4. The components of a discrete trial consist of the following five parts: (1) the

cue referred to hereafter as the *antecedent*, (2) the *prompt*, (3) the *response*, (4) the *consequence*, and (5) the *intertrial interval*.

5. The antecedent component of a discrete trial consists of a **discriminative stimulus**, annotated S^D; "a stimulus in the presence of which a particular response will be reinforced" (Malott, 2007, p. 202). In DTT for speech and language therapy, the antecedent is the physical and verbal stimuli prepared by the clinician to evoke a response from the client, which, if correct, can be reinforced.

6. Antecedent stimuli may also include irrelevant, or distractor, stimuli in the presence of which a response will *not* be reinforced, annotated S^Δ.

7. Prompts are the hints that a clinician gives a client to increase the probability of a correct response.

8. As soon as possible, prompts should be faded or gradually reduced so that the response is maintained in the presence of more natural stimuli.

9. The type of response given by the client in response to the antecedent will determine the next step in DTT—the consequence.

10. As a consequence for a correct response, reinforcement is given.

11. As a consequence for an incorrect response, the clinician can:
    a. Give corrective feedback or some other type of punishment
    b. Give a prompt to evoke a correct or more correct response; if the response is correct, reinforce and record the correct response and, if incorrect, record the incorrect response and move on to the next trial
    c. Ignore the incorrect response and move on to the next discrete trial

12. If the clinician chooses to deliver punishment as a consequence for an incorrect response, corrective feedback (positive punishment) and response cost (negative punishment) are commonly used techniques.

13. The intertrial interval is a brief pause, between 1 and 5 seconds, after one discrete trial has been presented and before another begins.

14. Criterion levels are set by the clinician to determine next steps in treatment; for example, it is recommended that after five correctly imitated modeled discrete trials, the clinician should switch to evoked trials, and after two consecutive incorrect responses to evoked trials, the clinician should switch back to modeled trials.

15. Criterion levels also determine when a clinician should probe for generalization, usually after the client has met the criterion level for dismissal set by the written target behavior over at least three consecutive sessions. There are three types of probe procedures that are particularly useful during DTT: an intermixed probe, a pure probe, and a conversational probe.

16. The intermixed probe, also called the initial probe, consists of discrete trials presented by the clinician alternating between taught and untaught stimuli; percentage correct is calculated only from the data collected for responses to untaught stimuli.

17. A pure probe, in which only untaught stimuli are presented, is conducted if the client reaches the criterion level required by the target behavior during the intermixed probe.

18. Final conversational probes are taken in natural settings after the client reaches the criterion level during a pure probe; speech and language samples

are taken and analyzed in much the same way as they are during initial assessment procedures to determine generalization of the target behavior in a natural setting.

19. When a client reaches criterion level during final conversational probes, it is an indication that (a) the client is ready to move on to a new level of the same target behavior, (b) the client is ready to move on to a different target behavior, or (c) the client is ready to be dismissed from treatment.

20. Although the sequence of probe procedures described is appropriate for many articulation and language target behaviors, it is not appropriate for all target behaviors, such as fluency, voice, and pragmatic language disorders.

Application Exercises

1. Prepare physical and verbal antecedent stimuli for the following expressive language target behaviors:
   a. Prepositional phrases at the sentence level
   b. Past tense *–ed* at the word level
   c. Possessive pronouns *his* and *hers* at the word level
   d. Irregular past tense verbs at the sentence level

2. Prepare physical and verbal antecedent stimuli for the following receptive language target behaviors:
   a. Identification of common objects
   b. Categorization of common objects (e.g., furniture, food, animals, clothes, etc.)
   c. Following two-step directions

3. What corrective feedback could you give to a client who has produced the following incorrect responses to picture cards and verbal stimuli?
   a. Responds /wop/ instead of /rop/
   b. Responds with the word *eated* instead of *ate*
   c. Responds with /kæ/ instead of /kæt/
   d. Responds with "She running" instead of "She is running"

4. Describe appropriate procedures for probing for generalization for the following target behaviors:
   a. Production of /l/ in initial word position
   b. Production of pronouns *my* and *your*
   c. Production of irregular past tense verbs
   d. Maintaining a topic of conversation
   e. Responding to bids for joint attention
   f. Production of fluent speech
   g. Production of appropriate vocal intensity

References

Behavior Analyst Certification Board. (2012). *Fourth edition task list.* Retrieved February 16, 2015, from http://www.bacb.com/Download files/TaskList/BACB_Fourth_Edition_Task_List.pdf

Cooper, J. O., Heron, T. E., & Heward, W. L. (2007). *Applied behavior analysis* (2nd ed.). Upper Saddle River, NJ: Pearson Education.

Hegde, M. N. (1998). *Treatment procedures in communicative disorders* (3rd ed.). Austin, TX: Pro-Ed.

Lovaas, O. I. (1987). Behavioral treatment and normal educational and intellectual functioning in young autistic children. *Journal of Consulting and Clinical Psychology, 55,* 3–9.

Malott, R. (2007). *Principles of behaviour.* Englewood Cliffs, NJ: Pearson Prentice-Hall.

Maul, C. A., & Ambler, K. L. (2014). Embedding language therapy in dialogic reading to teach morphologic structures to children with language disorders. *Communication Disorders Quarterly, 35,* 237–247.

McEachin, J. J., Smith, T., & Lovaas, O. I. (1993). Long-term outcome for children with autism who received early intensive behavioral intervention. *American Journal on Mental Retardation, 97,* 359–372.

National Professional Development Center on Autism Spectrum Disorders. (2010). *Discrete trial training: Data collection sheets.* Retrieved March 13, 2015, from http://autismpdc.fpg .unc.edu/sites/autismpdc.fpg.unc.edu/ files/imce/documents/Discrete-Trial-com plete10-2010.pdf

Pomaville, F., & Kladopoulos, C. (2013). The effects of behavioral speech therapy on speech sound production with adults who have cochlear implants. *Journal of Speech, Language, and Hearing Research, 56,* 531–541.

Skelton, S. L., & Hagopian, A. L. (2014). Using randomized variable practice in the treatment of childhood apraxia of speech. *American Journal of Speech-Language Pathology, 23,* 599–611.

Smith, T. (2001). Discrete trial training in the treatment of autism. *Focus on Autism and Other Developmental Disabilities, 16,* 86–92.

CHAPTER 6

Teaching New Behaviors

- ■ Negative Reinforcement
  - ■ Aversive Situations
  - ■ Escape and Avoidance
  - ■ Applications to Clinical Practice

After defining, measuring, and thoroughly assessing a client's communicative behaviors, a speech-language pathologist (SLP) develops a treatment plan to address the identified areas of need. As discussed in Chapter 1, one of the primary goals of speech-language treatment is to develop, rehabilitate, and/or strengthen desirable communicative behaviors. Across disorders, SLPs seek to establish new speech-language skills and increase those that occur at low rates. For example, clinicians teach children with lateral lisps to produce the /s/ and /z/ sounds appropriately. When working with adults who exhibit dysarthria, SLPs teach clients to exaggerate their production of consonant sounds in order to increase overall intelligibility of speech. For people who stutter, increased fluency is targeted. Additionally, clinicians work with clients' significant others in order to support the acquisition of new communicative behaviors.

SLPs seek to establish _____ speech-language skills and increase those that occur at _____.

When utilizing a behavioral approach to treatment, each of these tasks is accomplished through the manipulation of antecedent and consequence events. By rearranging antecedent and consequence events, SLPs are able to establish contingencies that will help develop new and strengthen existing desirable communicative behaviors.

Antecedent Manipulations

As is the case with all forms of behavior, communication occurs within the context of various antecedent stimuli. In many cases, SLPs are sought out because the naturally occurring antecedent stimuli do not serve to evoke desirable forms of verbal behavior. By rearranging antecedent stimuli, clinicians help enrich clients' environments to make the occurrence of certain communicative behaviors more likely. **Antecedent manipulations** involve altering the stimuli that occur prior to a behavior being exhibited. These techniques are particularly useful when a client does not yet display the target behavior. By utilizing antecedent manipulations, clinicians increase the likelihood that clients will exhibit a behavior that can be reinforced.

_____ _____ involve altering the stimuli that occur prior to a behavior being exhibited.

Modeling With Required Imitation

Modeling with required **imitation** is a frequently employed antecedent manipulation used in the field of speech-language pathology. It is a helpful tool to utilize when the client does not exhibit a desired communicative behavior or only does so at a minimal rate. According to Hegde

(1998), modeling is "the clinician's production or display of a target response the client is expected to learn" (p. 156). For example, a clinician models production of present progressive *–ing* (e.g., "He is walk*ing*," "She is smil*ing*," etc.) by describing what characters are doing while reading a storybook with a child. When working with an adult client who has dysphagia, the SLP may model use of a chin tuck posture prior to presenting a given food texture. Modeling can be used as a treatment technique when working with clients who exhibit a variety of speech-language needs.

> When SLPs display use of a target behavior for clients, they are using _____.

Modeling should be used in conjunction with imitation. As it applies to the field of communicative disorders, imitation involves the client repeating the model provided by the SLP. It is important to require imitation when using modeling because it provides the clinician with a behavior to reinforce. For example, an SLP may model use of waving hello when teaching a child to greet familiar adults; however, if imitation is not required, the clinician is unable to reinforce, and accordingly strengthen, the client's greeting skills. Similarly, modeling may be used to teach an individual with a voice disorder to adopt a more appropriate pitch, but the clinician is more likely to observe actual behavior change if imitation is required and subsequent reinforcement is provided upon correct production of the target behavior.

When using these techniques, imitated responses should take the same form as the clinician's model. The client's behavior should mirror that of the clinician's. For example, if the clinician models the phrase "two cats" when teaching plural *–s*, the client should respond by saying "two cats" as well. In this example, the clinician's model and the client's response are produced with point-to-point correspondence and formal similarity (see Chapter 2 for further information).

An additional characteristic of imitated responses is that they immediately follow the modeled stimulus. When using modeling to teach new forms of verbal behavior, the clinician seeks to evoke the imitative response within a couple seconds of the antecedent stimuli. If the temporal delay between the clinician's model and the client's response is too great, the behavior cannot be considered imitative in nature, and it is more likely that other controlling variables are at play.

As previously discussed, it is beneficial to use modeling and imitation when the client never or rarely produces the target behavior. Therefore, these techniques should be used during the initial stages of treatment to help the client establish new target behaviors. Also, in order to bolster clients' correct response rates, clinicians employ modeling if clients repeatedly misuse the target behavior. Finally, modeling is used when transitioning to a higher level of treatment (e.g., from the word to phrase level) to support the client's production of the more complex version of the target behavior.

When making the determination regarding whether to use modeling during the therapeutic process, SLPs should consider that some clients may not have the prerequisite imitation skills in order to benefit from this treatment method. Although many children learn to imitate at a young age, some clients have difficulty with imitation in general, which could limit the effectiveness of using this technique in treatment. In these cases, clinicians teach the skill of imitation (i.e., echoic behavior; see Chapter 2 for additional information) prior to utilizing modeling with required imitation during treatment sessions.

Prompts

Whereas models display use of the target behavior for the client to imitate, **prompts** supplement antecedent stimuli to make a correct response more likely to occur. In a general sense, prompts are like hints used to help evoke desirable behavior. Prompts take many forms; for example, there are verbal, visual, and tactile-kinesthetic prompts.

Verbal

Verbal prompts involve spoken words, or parts of words, used to help an individual produce a target behavior. Partial modeling is a type of verbal prompt frequently used by SLPs, particularly when attempting to fade the use of modeling in treatment. For example, during the initial stages of therapy, a clinician may use modeling to teach a child with a language disorder to answer *where* questions during play-based activities. As treatment progresses, the clinician may continue presenting the antecedent stimuli (i.e., the *where* questions) and then model part of the target behavior (e.g., "It is in _____."). By providing this partial model, the clinician increases the likelihood that the client will complete the sentence with the target behavior. Over time, partial modeling can continue to be faded so that the client is able to produce more complex forms of the target behavior independently. Fading is discussed in greater detail later in this chapter.

Verbal prompts involve _____ _____, or _____ ___ _____, used to help an individual produce a target behavior.

Phonemic cues, also known as partial verbal prompts, are another type of verbal prompt that can be used with clients who exhibit communicative disorders. When utilizing this type of prompt, clinicians provide their clients with the first phoneme of the target response to help evoke the desired behavior. For example, an adult with aphasia may have difficulty naming common objects in the environment. In order to help evoke this skill, the clinician could provide the antecedent stimulus (e.g., a toothbrush) along with a phonemic cue (e.g., saying /t/) in order to prompt use of the target behavior (e.g., the client saying "toothbrush").

Something as simple as vocal emphasis can also serve as a verbal prompt. Clinicians often supplement modeling with vocal emphasis to draw the client's attention to a critical component of the target behavior. In the previously presented example for teaching plural –s, the clinician may emphasize the bound morpheme (i.e., cats) in order to increase the likelihood that the client imitates the target behavior accurately.

Frequently used verbal prompts include _____ _____, _____ _____, and _____ _____.

Although the previously discussed examples all contain part of the target behavior, verbal prompts do not always include a component of the client's response. When working with a child who has autism, the clinician may use the verbal prompt, "What do you want?" in order to evoke a request for a desired item (e.g., "bubbles"). In this example, the clinician's prompt and the client's response would not necessarily be produced in a similar manner. Although frequently effective in evoking target behaviors, prompts of this type can change the nature of the verbal operant and make it multiply controlled (see Chapter 2 for further information regarding multiple control). Furthermore, clients can become dependent on these prompts to facilitate their responses. Consequently, prompts of this nature should also be used sparingly and faded as soon as possible.

Visual

Visual prompts include anything that clients can see that increases the probability that they will produce a target response. Frequently used visual prompts in the field of communicative disorders include textual prompts, gestural prompts, positional prompts, and facial expressions.

> Textual prompts, gestural prompts, positional prompts, and facial expressions are examples of _____ _____.

Textual prompts include written and printed stimuli, such as sentence strips, written instructions, scripts, checklists, and other similar methods, that serve as cues for desired verbal behavior. For individuals with dementia, SLPs can use a textual prompt in the form of a memory book to help clients recall their personal identification information. When teaching children to describe common objects, clinicians often use printed sentence strips

(e.g., "The _____ is _____." "The _____ can _____.") to help clients form their responses in complete sentences. Textual prompts are a useful tool to help evoke various forms of verbal behavior across a variety of clients.

Whereas textual prompts make use of printed stimuli, gestural prompts involve the use of body movements to help evoke a target behavior. These prompts include gestural actions, such as pointing, signing, or motioning, carried out by the clinician that serve to increase the likelihood a client will engage in a given behavior. For example, a clinician may use a "hushing" gesture by bringing her pointer finger up to her lips to help prompt production of the /ʃ/ sound. Similarly, gestural prompting in the form of pointing to a conversational partner could be used to help a client who is learning how to take conversational turns. It should be noted that gestural prompts do not involve the clinician making any form of physical contact with the client.

Positional prompts are another type of visual prompt that has applicability to the field of communicative disorders. These prompts involve physically moving the antecedent stimuli that clients are expected to engage with closer to them. These prompts are particularly useful when working on receptive vocabulary tasks. For example, a clinician may use positional prompts in order to help a child be able to identify basic objects in a field of two. In this case, when presenting the two objects, the SLP would place the target item closer to the child. Therefore, after being presented with the antecedent stimulus (e.g., "Show me the _____."), the client would be more likely to identify the named object correctly.

A final type of visual prompt is facial expressions. Various movements of the facial muscles can be used to help evoke target behaviors. Looking at a child expectantly serves as a prompt to engage in an appropriate mand form. Raising or lowering the eyebrows can also help a client answer yes/no questions accurately. By providing an articulatory posture (e.g., biting the lower lip to prompt production of /f/ or /v/), a clinician prompts correct production of certain speech sounds. Facial expressions can also be used in conjunction with the previously discussed prompting methods to increase the salience of the antecedent stimuli.

Tactile-Kinesthetic

Tactile-kinesthetic prompts include the use of physical contact to help the client engage in a target behavior. These prompts differ from gestural prompts because touch is used to help evoke a response. Tactile-kinesthetic prompts are used to teach a variety of different skills. For example, when working with an articulation client who demonstrates difficulty with production of /k/, the clinician may tap the juncture of the neck and chin to help signal correct placement of the posterior tongue against the soft palate. Tactile-kinesthetic prompts in the form of hand tapping can be used to help clients with fluency or motor speech disorders utilize a more appropriate rate of speech. Light taps on the hand could also be used to prompt a child with a pragmatic language disorder to make comments during conversation with a peer.

> Tactile-kinesthetic prompts include the use of _____ _____ to help the client engage in a target behavior.

The clinician should be careful to differentiate between tactile-kinesthetic prompts and **manual guidance**. Although both methods make use of physical contact, manual guidance involves the clinician guiding the client's motor movements through production of a target response. This technique is most frequently used in the initial stages of treatment to help a client who has difficulty imitating the clinician's model. For example, in order to help a nonverbal child use the sign "more" to make a request, the clinician may take the client's hands and physically guide them to form this sign. Similarly, when teaching production of the /m/ sound, the clinician may gently hold the client's lips together to attain correct placement. Manual guidance should be used with caution, as it is a very intrusive form of prompting.

Using Hierarchies of Prompts

As previously discussed, prompts are used to supplement antecedent stimuli to help evoke target behaviors. Depending upon the nature of the behavior being taught, certain prompting methods will be more or less effective in evoking a correct response from the client. Prior to selecting a method to utilize during therapy, the clinician should thoughtfully consider which prompting techniques will be most efficient for a given target behavior and client. By considering this information, the clinician can then develop a **hierarchy of prompts** to use during the treatment process. Although these hierarchies should be individualized for each client and target behavior, Figure 6–1 shows a general hierarchy that presents prompts from the most to least invasive.

After a prompting hierarchy has been developed, the clinician should then

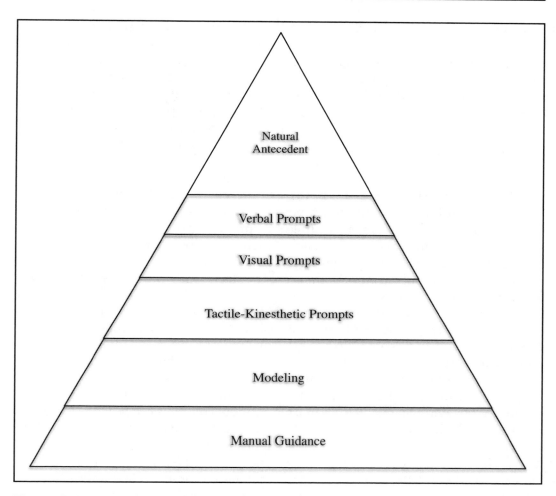

Figure 6–1. Prompt hierarchy.

decide whether a **least-to-most** or **most-to-least** prompting methodology will be used. When utilizing a least-to-most system, the clinician initially provides the least intrusive prompting method and then only offers more assistance if the target behavior is not evoked. For example, the clinician may start off by presenting the naturally occurring antecedent stimuli. If the client does not respond, verbal, visual, and tactile-kinesthetic prompts may be provided in a sequential manner until a response is evoked. If no response is obtained, modeling and/or manual guidance could be used to support the client's performance.

Although utilizing a least-to-most prompting method provides increased opportunities for the client to engage in independent responses, using prompts in this manner also runs the risk of having the client practice incorrect forms of the target behavior. As a result, the clinician may elect to present prompts in order from most to least intrusive. In this case, more invasive prompting methods such as manual guidance and modeling would be provided in the initial stages of treatment. Based on the client's progress, the clinician would then present less invasive prompting methods such as visual or verbal prompts.

Fading Prompts

Although prompts are a useful method to help support a client's success in the initial stages of therapy, they should be faded over the course of treatment. **Fading** involves making prompts less invasive. It includes reducing the properties of a prompt so that stimulus control is transferred to the natural antecedent stimuli. Fading is important because prompts are not always available in the client's natural environment. If fading is not utilized, it is unlikely that the client will engage in the target behavior spontaneously. Because the goal of treatment is to evoke socially significant behavior change, fading must be considered when utilizing prompts.

Fading plays a key role in ensuring that a client does not become **prompt dependent**. Prompt dependency occurs when the client engages in a target behavior only when the prompt is provided. For example, a client who is working on requesting using the sentence frame, "I want _____" could become dependent upon the clinician's verbal prompt "What do you want?" in order to facilitate use of the target behavior. Clinicians should fade the use of prompts in order to help clients become more independent in their use of the behaviors targeted during treatment.

In order to prevent prompt _____, the clinician should use _____ to help promote the client's independence.

Fading can be used with all of the previously discussed prompting techniques. When utilizing verbal prompts in treatment, the acoustic properties of the prompts should be reduced over time. Modeling and partial modeling can be faded to phonemic cues in order to help transfer stimulus control. Similarly, vocal emphasis can be faded by gradually reducing the stress or loudness placed on the specific words the clinician wants the client to imitate. By reducing these acoustic properties, the clinician increases the client's independence in producing the target behavior.

The visual properties of prompts should also be faded over the course of treatment. Figure 6–2 provides an example of how the visual properties of a textual prompt can be faded. By making the text lighter and lighter, the clinician helps transfer stimulus control to the naturally occurring antecedent stimuli. Similarly, positional prompts can be faded by slowly moving the antecedent stimuli back to their normal position. Gestural prompts and facial expressions are also faded by making the prompts less noticeable. For example, instead of pointing enthusiastically, the clinician may gesture more inconspicuously in order to fade a gestural prompt. Likewise, the use of facial expressions can be faded by making expectant looks, raised eyebrows, and/or articulatory postures less obvious over time.

Finally, the physical properties of tactile-kinesthetic prompts and manual guidance should also be faded. Tactile-kinesthetic prompts can be faded by gradually using lighter forms of touch to evoke the target behavior. Manual guidance can be faded from total assistance, to partial assistance, to a tactile-kinesthetic prompt that can be faded as discussed previously. Regardless of the type of prompting used

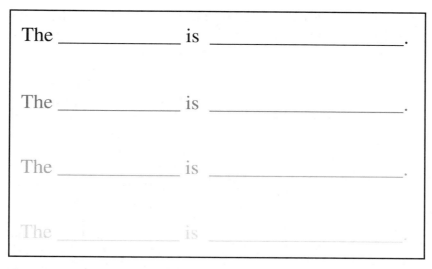

Figure 6–2. Prompt fading.

during treatment, fading is an important component of therapy that should not be overlooked.

Stimulus Manipulations

As previously discussed, modeling and prompting serve to supplement antecedent stimuli during speech and language therapy. Although these are beneficial techniques, in some cases it is necessary to alter naturally occurring antecedent stimuli altogether in order to facilitate behavioral change in the client's environment. These antecedent stimulus manipulations serve to rearrange environmental stimuli in a way that will more readily evoke a target behavior.

Particularly when working with the pediatric population, antecedent-based stimulus manipulations are helpful in supporting the child's performance in natural settings. For example, the clinician may teach a child's family to place preferred items out of reach or in locked cabinets

in order to evoke opportunities for mand behavior. A clinician may also teach the parents of a client with receptive language concerns to obtain the child's attention prior to providing directions, thus making it more likely that the child will comply with those directions. Within the classroom setting, an SLP may encourage the teacher to provide a student with preferential seating in the front of the classroom to support the student's understanding of instruction.

Antecedent-based stimulus manipulations have applicability to the adult population as well. By recommending a change in a dysphagia patient's diet, an SLP is implementing an antecedent stimulus manipulation (i.e., the change in food or liquid texture) to help the patient swallow more safely. Furthermore, by instructing a caregiver to provide directions in a slower, more concrete manner, the clinician is able to arrange the antecedent stimuli in a way that helps a client with aphasia understand instructions. By considering stimulus manipulations that can be put in place in a client's environment, the clinician helps support the acquisition of target behaviors.

Priming

An additional antecedent manipulation that can be used to help evoke desired communicative behaviors is priming. **Priming** involves previewing a task with clients to help prepare them for participation in the actual activity. Priming is conducted prior to a given situation in order to familiarize the client with the setting, materials, and/or information involved in a given activity. For example, a school-based SLP uses priming when preteaching vocabulary words that a student would be expected to learn during a classroom lesson. Similarly, priming could be used when a college student who stutters needs to give a speech in a communications class. The SLP could preview the auditorium and practice various aspects of the speech (e.g., finding the podium, setting up the presentation materials, etc.) with the client in order to help the client become more familiar with this potentially difficult activity. By familiarizing clients with activities before they encounter them, SLPs help increase their clients' opportunities for success in using taught skills in new environments.

Shaping New Behaviors

The previously discussed antecedent-based methods are useful techniques for establishing and strengthening the use of target behaviors. However, is some cases, the client may be unable to produce a socially acceptable form of the target

behavior when provided with antecedent-based support. For example, even with extensive modeling and prompting, a client who distorts production of the /r/ phoneme may still have difficulty producing this sound appropriately. In this case, the clinician could utilize shaping to help the client develop appropriate use of the target behavior.

Shaping involves successively reinforcing approximations of a target behavior over time. In a general sense, shaping simplifies the target behavior so that the clinician has something to reinforce and build upon. When using shaping, the clinician initially accepts less desirable responses and then gradually expects better performance from the client prior to providing reinforcement. If shaping was used in the previously discussed example, the clinician would initially reinforce production of /r/ if there was a slight reduction in the severity of the distortion of the client's production. Over time, the clinician would provide reinforcement only after responses that more closely approximated correct production of the target phoneme. This shaping procedure would be continued until production of the /r/ phoneme was acoustically correct.

> The process of successively reinforcing approximations of a target behavior over time is called
> _____.

Although shaping is a useful tool in therapy, it should not be utilized haphazardly or without thought. Accordingly, clinicians take several steps to adequately define the shaping procedure prior to implementing this technique. The guidelines discussed below outline steps commonly used when implementing a shaping procedure.

Defining the Terminal Form of the Target Behavior

When electing to use shaping during the treatment process, the clinician first develops a clear definition of the terminal form of the target behavior. This terminal behavior is the final response that the clinician wants the client to be able to use at the end of treatment. As discussed in Chapter 3, this definition should be both operational and measureable so that the clinician is able to obtain reliable data. Although the client may not be able to engage in the terminal response at the beginning of treatment, defining this behavior ahead of time helps set a goal for the client that the clinician can then shape down to address more effectively.

Defining Successive Approximations of the Target Behavior

After the terminal response has been defined, a clinician then outlines the intermediary responses that will receive reinforcement during the shaping procedure. These intermediary responses, or successive approximations, should be directly tied to the terminal goal. Ideally, the defined successive approximations would also already be in the client's repertoire. If the client is unable to exhibit the successive approximations of the target behavior, additional antecedent support may be used to help evoke the intermediary responses.

Using Additional Antecedent Support When Necessary

Any of the previously discussed antecedent manipulations can be used in conjunction with shaping to help evoke correct production of successive approximations of the target behavior. The clinician could choose to model an intermediary response to help support a client's production. Similarly, prompting and/or manual guidance may also be needed to evoke a response from the client. If excessive antecedent support is needed to facilitate the client's production of a successive approximation, the clinician should consider further shaping the intermediary responses down in order to evoke a form of the target behavior that can be reinforced.

Reinforcing Successive Approximations of the Target Behavior

Throughout the shaping procedure, reinforcement is provided for successive approximations of the target behavior. Once the client establishes production of one of the intermediary responses, the clinician then shifts to evoking and reinforcing the next successive approximation. Although reinforcement plays an important role in shaping, the clinician should be careful not to reinforce a given successive approximation for too long. The ultimate goal of shaping is to evoke, reinforce, and strengthen the terminal response. Accordingly, clinicians move fairly rapidly across intermediary responses in order to help the client produce the target behavior.

Collecting Data and Monitoring Progress

As discussed in Chapter 3, data are collected throughout therapy to guide the treatment process. This is true when implementing a shaping procedure as well. The clinician monitors the data collected while utilizing shaping to determine when to introduce a new successive approximation. Once the clinician documents a few consecutive correct responses at a given level, treatment progresses to the next successive approximation toward the terminal response. If a review of the data indicates slow improvement with shaping, the clinician may need to further simplify the intermediary responses to support progress.

Chaining: Forward and Backward

As previously discussed, shaping involves reinforcing successive approximations that lead up to a terminal response. Accordingly, the clinician builds toward production of the target behavior when using shaping. A similar technique that involves building toward production of the target behavior is chaining. **Chaining** involves reinforcing successive components of a target behavior. Chaining is most applicable to communicative behaviors that involve multiple steps.

_____ is the process of reinforcing successive components of a target behavior.

The two types of chaining procedures that can be used during treatment include **forward chaining** and **backward chaining**. When using forward chaining, the clinician initially teaches the first component of the target behavior and then gradually includes subsequent components of the terminal response. Accordingly, the clinician starts off by providing reinforcement after the client produces the first component of the target behavior. Once

this component is established, reinforcement is then provided for production of the first and second steps of the target behavior produced sequentially. This process then continues until all components of the target behavior are produced correctly in order.

Forward chaining is often used in the initial stages of articulation therapy. For example, forward chaining can be used to establish production of the /s/ sound in initial word position of consonant-vowel-consonant (CVC) words. First, reinforcement would be provided upon production of the initial sound in isolation (i.e., the first step in the target behavior). Once this step was established, treatment would then progress to production of initial /s/ in consonant-vowel (CV) syllables (i.e., the second step in the target behavior). Finally, reinforcement would only be provided upon correct production of initial /s/ in CVC words (i.e., the terminal response).

Backward chaining also has applicability to the field of communicative disorders. When using this procedure, the clinician initially teaches the last component of a target behavior. Once this task has been established, the client is then expected to perform the last and second to last steps in succession prior to receiving reinforcement. Again, this process continues until all components of the target behavior are produced correctly in order. For example, when teaching use of plural –s, an SLP may utilize backward chaining to help build production of this skill up to the sentence level. Initially, the clinician may use a verbal prompt in the form of a sentence frame (e.g., There are two _____.) to evoke production of plural –s at the word level (i.e., the last component of the target behavior). Once the client was successful in producing plural –s at this level, the backward chaining procedure could be continued so that the client is able to produce more of the target behavior independently (i.e., the sentence frame would fade from "There are two _____," to "There are ___ _____," to "There __ ___ ____," to "__ __ ___ ____" so that the client would ultimately produce the target behavior at the sentence level).

Task Analysis

When utilizing a chaining procedure, it is beneficial to outline all of the components involved in performing the target behavior. This process of defining each of the sequential steps included in a complex target behavior is known as developing a **task analysis**. Display Box 6–1 presents an example of how a task analysis can be outlined for teaching basic conversational skills. Task analyses can also be used when training direct care providers to use treatment techniques in the natural setting. Display Box 6–2 provides an additional example of how a task analysis can be used to teach preschool staff to implement language tasks during snack time. Once developed, such task analyses help clinicians more successfully implement chaining during the treatment process.

Positive Reinforcement: Delivering the Consequence for Desired Responses

Thus far, this chapter has presented information regarding antecedent manipulations, shaping, and chaining. Although these techniques play an important role in teaching new communicative skills, the primary method for increasing desirable behaviors is reinforcement. As discussed in Chapter 1, reinforcement is the process of strengthening a target behavior through manipulation of consequence stimuli. This section begins with a discussion of positive reinforcement.

Display Box 6–1. Task Analysis for Greeting

Step 1: Establish and maintain eye contact with the communicative partner.

Step 2: Smile toward the communicative partner.

Step 3: Establish an appropriate distance away from the communicative partner.

Step 4: Say "Hello" to the communicative partner.

Step 5: Respond to the communicative partner's greeting.

Step 6: Make comments and/or ask questions based on the communicative partner's response.

Step 7: When the conversation is over, say, "It was nice talking to you" and "Goodbye."

Display Box 6–2. Task Analysis for Snack Time Setup

Step 1: Obtain boxes with food and utensils to be used at snack time.

Step 2: Prompt students to transition to snack table.

Step 3: Teacher/instructional assistant distributes utensils while practicing receptive identification of objects in a field of two.

Step 3a: Focus the child's attention.

Step 3b: Present items in a field of two.

Step 3c: Provide the antecedent stimulus "Show me _____."

Step 3d: If the child responds correctly, provide verbal praise paired with the identified object.

Step 3e: If the child responds incorrectly, re-present the trial with a positional prompt. If he or she responds correctly with the positional prompt, provide verbal praise paired with the identified object.

Step 3f: If the child responds incorrectly with the positional prompt, re-present the trial with manual guidance. If he or she responds correctly with manual guidance, provide verbal praise paired with the identified object.

Step 4: When all children have utensils, briefly describe food/drink options (e.g., We have apples and grapes today. They are both fruit. They are yummy. Etc.).

Step 5: Restrict access to snack items and solicit requests from the children throughout the remainder of snack time.

Positive reinforcement is the process of providing consequence stimuli contingent upon a behavior that serve to increase the future occurrence of that behavior. Positive reinforcement involves adding or presenting a stimulus to support the client's acquisition of a target behavior. Therefore, positive reinforcement is the consequence that clinicians typically provide for desired responses.

Identifying Possible Reinforcers Through Preference Assessment

Although positive reinforcement is a powerful tool used to establish desirable behaviors, reinforcers vary from client to client. Therefore, **preference assessments** may be needed to help determine potential reinforcers to use with individual clients. These measures help identify a pool of stimuli that the client prefers.

> Preference assessments can be used to help determine _____ reinforcers to use with individual clients.

There are a variety of well-documented methods for conducting preference assessments (see Cooper, Heron, & Heward, 2007, for a review). In general, clinicians tend to determine possible reinforcers through three primary approaches: interview, direct observation, and/or assessment trials. Initially, the clinician simply asks the client and/or significant others regarding potential preferences. This is accomplished through asking open-ended questions or interviewing the client. In some cases, the clinician presents the client with a reinforcer menu to complete. Table 6–1 provides an example of a reinforcer menu that may be used to identify potential reinforcers. If an interview fails to identify potential reinforcers, the clinician may elect to conduct a direct observation of the client during a time when he or she has free access to a variety of preferred stimuli. By measuring the amount of time that the client engages with each stimulus, the clinician can identify the client's preferences. In select cases, an SLP may decide to present stimuli in a series of assessment trials and record the client's responses. Preferences would then be determined based on which stimuli the client selected most frequently.

Preference assessments only identify *possible* reinforcers. Although a client may

Table 6–1. Example of a Reinforcer Menu

Client's Name: _____   Date: _____

Target Behavior(s): _____

Instructions: Please read the items below to your child and ask them to identify activities/prizes they would like to earn. Place an "X" next to items your child selects.

_____ 1. Computer	_____ 7. Pencils
_____ 2. Coloring	_____ 8. Erasers
_____ 3. Reading book	_____ 9. Candy
_____ 4. Bubbles	_____ 10. Play Dough
_____ 5. Blocks	_____ 11. Tops
_____ 6. Bouncy balls	_____ 12. Stickers

show a preference for a certain stimulus, it is only considered a reinforcer if data indicate an increase in the target behavior once the consequence is introduced. Therefore, even though a client may show a strong inclination toward a certain stimulus during a preference assessment, it should only be used if its presentation results in an actual increase in the target behavior. If this does not occur, the preferred stimulus cannot be considered a positive reinforcer.

Types of Positive Reinforcers

The stimuli that serve as positive reinforcers fall into one of two categories: uncon-

ditioned or conditioned. Figure 6–3 provides a summary of the various types of unconditioned and conditioned reinforcers. Both categories are described in further detail below.

Unconditioned Reinforcers

Unconditioned reinforcers do not depend upon prior conditioning to support their effectiveness. Therefore, the effects of these reinforcers do not have to be taught. They inherently serve as reinforcers because they support the survival of a species. Examples of unconditioned reinforcers include food, water, shelter, and sensory stimulation.

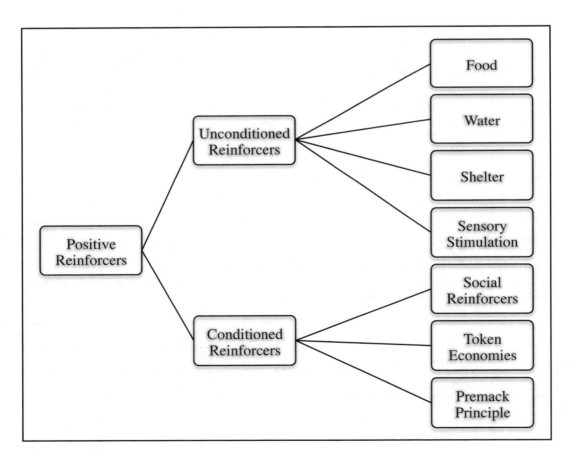

Figure 6–3. Types of positive reinforcers.

One of the benefits of unconditioned reinforcers is that they have strong reinforcing value. Hence, they serve to increase target behaviors fairly rapidly if used judiciously. Although unconditioned reinforcers are powerful in increasing a desired behavior, there are also several weaknesses involved with their use. Unconditioned reinforcers may only be effective when the client is in a state of deprivation; for example, a client must be at least a little hungry in order to work for food as a reinforcer. Furthermore, unconditioned reinforcers are often not a natural reinforcer to use while teaching many speech-language skills. For example, it is unlikely that the client would be offered a bite of food or drink of water upon correct production of a speech sound in a typical environment. Therefore, the use of unconditioned reinforcers in this manner could seem rather contrived and unnatural.

Conditioned Reinforcers

There is a second category of reinforcers as well. Over time, individuals learn the reinforcing value of certain stimuli based on their previous pairing with other reinforcers. These consequences are known as **conditioned reinforcers**. Conditioned reinforcers may take many forms, several of which are discussed in the following section.

Social Reinforcement. **Social reinforcement** is a type of conditioned reinforcement that is mediated by a listener. The client's communicative partner provides the consequence that serves as a social reinforcer. Within the field of speech-language pathology, verbal praise is a frequently used method of social reinforcement that can be applied when teaching a variety of behaviors. Upon correct use

of the target skill, simple statements such as "You're right" or "That was great" increase the likelihood that a client will exhibit that behavior again in the future. Although clinicians frequently rely on verbal praise when providing treatment, additional social reinforcers such as attention, eye contact, head nods, and smiling can also serve as social reinforcers for some clients.

Social reinforcement can be paired with **informative feedback**, a way to further reinforce a correct response by giving clients information regarding their performance of a target behavior (Hegde, 1998). Informative feedback lets the client know what was correctly done. For example, if a client has an interdental lisp and finally produces a correctly articulated /s/, the clinician might say something such as, "Good! You kept your tongue tip up and away from your teeth that time!"

Informative feedback can be effectively delivered by the clinician for many target behaviors. For other target behaviors, however, informative feedback is best delivered via mechanical means. For example, mechanical devices that measure vocal frequency or intensity can give visual feedback to clients who have target behaviors for production of appropriate pitch or loudness of voice. In these cases, a range of frequency or intensity is specified by an upper line and a lower line on a computerized display. The client then speaks into a microphone, attempting to keep the graphic display of running speech between the two lines. An added benefit to this type of mechanically generated informative feedback is the objective, accurate accumulation of data to monitor the client's progress. Because there is little evidence to indicate informative feedback is effective as the sole method of reinforcement, it should always be used in conjunction with social reinforcement or other reinforcement methods.

> Social reinforcement is mediated by a
> _____.

There are many benefits to using social reinforcers in the treatment of communicative disorders. First, social reinforcement plays a primary role in many of the verbal operants (see Chapter 2). Using social reinforcers is a more natural consequence to use during the treatment sequence. For example, when working on building a child's tact repertoire, a clinician uses social reinforcement to help establish and maintain the client's commenting skills, because this type of reinforcing consequence is directly associated with tacting. In cases where primary reinforcement is needed to help develop certain speech-language skills, social reinforcers can also be paired with bites of food or sips of drink (i.e., primary reinforcers) in the initial stages of treatment. Over time, the primary reinforcers are then faded while the more natural social reinforcers are maintained.

Although social reinforcers are often beneficial, there are some limitations associated with their use. The primary concern regarding social consequences is that they may not serve as reinforcers for clients with severe speech-language needs. In a general sense, social consequences are typically not as effective for clients with a limited history of vocal verbal behavior (Hegde, 1998). Although social reinforcement plays a key role in most verbal operants, it is not as directly applicable to mand behavior. For example, when a child asks for a drink of water, the parent is unlikely to provide verbal praise (e.g., saying, "Good job asking") without providing access to the reinforcer specified

by the child. In these cases, social consequences may need to be paired with primary reinforcers as discussed above.

Token Economies. Token economies are based on the principle of **generalized conditioned reinforcement**. Generalized conditioned reinforcers are conditioned reinforcers that can be effective in a myriad of situations. They are effective because they can provide an individual access to a wide variety of other reinforcers and are not dependent upon a state of deprivation. The most commonly encountered generalized conditioned reinforcer in the natural environment is money. Money serves as a generalized conditioned reinforcer because its value has to be learned, and it can provide access to a wide variety of other reinforcers (e.g., food, clothing, services, etc.).

> Money is an example of a
> _____ _____
> _____.

A **token economy** is a specific technique that makes use of generalized conditioned reinforcement. Token economies include three primary components: the target behavior, the generalized conditioned reinforcer, and the backup reinforcer. When clients engage in the defined target behavior, they are provided with generalized conditioned reinforcers. These reinforcers may take many forms, such as tokens, stickers, points, and/or happy faces. Once clients obtain a predetermined number of generalized conditioned reinforcers, they can then exchange them for a backup reinforcer. Backup reinforcers could include a variety of preferred items, such as small toys, edibles, or desirable activities. Figure 6–4 demonstrates an example of a token economy that may be

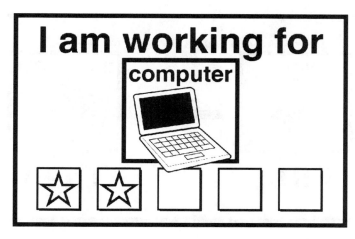

I am working for

computer

Figure 6–4. Token economies.

used during treatment. Upon correct production of the target behavior, the client is provided a star (i.e., a token) to put on his chart. Once five stars are obtained, the client is allowed access to a preselected backup reinforcer—in this case, time on the computer.

There are many benefits associated with using token economies during therapy. Because clients have the opportunity to select a backup reinforcer from a pool of preferred stimuli, token economies do not depend on a state of deprivation and are not susceptible to the satiation effect. Furthermore, tokens can be easily administered and typically do not interrupt the flow of treatment sessions. Although token economies have many strengths, using this technique can become costly if the clinician needs to purchase a variety of backup reinforcers to support the client's performance (Hegde, 1998).

Premack Principle. First defined in the late 1950s, the **Premack principle** is based on the concept that high-probability behaviors can serve as reinforcers for low-probability behaviors (Premack, 1959). In other words, preferred activities can be used to reinforce behaviors that are less frequently exhibited. Colloquially known as "first/then" or "if/then" contingencies, the Premack principle is particularly useful to support the acquisition of participation behaviors such as appropriate sitting, attention, and effort. Figure 6–5 provides an example of a visual support based on the Premack principle. Using a chart of this nature would help a clinician prompt and ultimately reinforce a client's participation during speech-language sessions.

Schedules of Reinforcement

Regardless of the type being provided, all reinforcers are administered at specific times contingent upon the client's behavior. When a reinforcer is provided should be outlined by the **schedule of reinforcement** selected by the clinician. Schedules of reinforcement specify the number of correct responses, amount of elapsed time, or number of different responses needed prior to earning a reinforcer. The primary types of reinforcement schedules used in the field of communicative disorders include continuous schedules, intermittent schedules, and lag schedules.

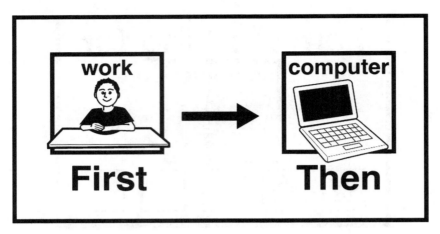

Figure 6–5. Premack principle.

_____, _____, and _____ schedules are the primary types of reinforcement schedules used by SLPs.

Continuous schedules of reinforcement involve the client receiving a reinforcer after every correct response. Clinicians typically utilize continuous schedules of reinforcement in the initial stages of treatment because they can be used to quickly establish production of new behaviors. Accordingly, continuous schedules result in high response rates. Although continuous schedules do have a place in treatment, they must be faded in order to promote generalization of the behavior to natural environments. In order to promote generalization, clinicians move to more intermittent schedules of reinforcement over time.

Whereas continuous schedules provide reinforcement after every instance of a behavior, **intermittent schedules of reinforcement** make reinforcers available for only some occurrences of a target skill. The target behavior will go unreinforced at predetermined times. The primary types of intermittent schedules of reinforcement are ratio schedules and interval schedules.

Ratio schedules of reinforcement are based upon the number of correct responses exhibited by the client. Ratio schedules can be either fixed or variable in nature. When utilizing a **fixed ratio** schedule of reinforcement, the clinician provides a reinforcer after a predetermined number of correct responses. Fixed ratio schedules are often abbreviated "FR" and followed by the number of times a client must exhibit a behavior prior to receiving reinforcement. For example, when using a FR4 schedule of reinforcement, the clinician provides a reinforcer after every fourth correct response from the client.

A **variable ratio** (VR) schedule of reinforcement involves providing reinforcement after an average number of correct responses. For instance, when using a VR4 schedule of reinforcement, the clinician may initially provide a reinforcer after the client's fourth correct response. The next reinforcer may then be provided after six correct productions. On the subsequent set of trials, reinforcement may be delivered for the second instance of the target behavior. In this example, the clinician would be providing a reinforcer after an average of four responses (12 total instances of the target behavior divided by three reinforcers).

Whereas ratio schedules rely on the number of responses produced by the client, **interval schedules of reinforcement** are based on time. Both fixed and variable interval schedules of reinforcement may be utilized during treatment. A **fixed interval** (FI) schedule of reinforcement provides an opportunity to earn a reinforcer for the first correct response after a set amount of time. Therefore, when using an FI 45-second schedule, clients have the opportunity to obtain reinforcement after 45 seconds have elapsed from their previous response.

When using **variable interval** (VI) schedules of reinforcement, an opportunity to earn a reinforcer is provided after an average amount of time. For example, when using a VI 3-minute schedule, the client has a chance to earn a reinforcer after an average duration of 3 minutes. The time between reinforcers may vary; however, the session is arranged in a way so that the client has an opportunity to receive a reinforcer for the first instance of a target behavior that occurs after an average of 3 minutes.

The **lag schedule of reinforcement** is a more recently developed technique that has applicability to speech-language pathology (Esch, Esch, & Love, 2009; Koehler-Platten, Grow, Schulze, & Bertone, 2013; Lee, McComas, & Jawor, 2002; Susa & Schilinger, 2012). Although the previously discussed reinforcement schedules serve to increase the frequency and consistency of a response, lag schedules of reinforcement are used to increase the variability of a target behavior. When using this technique, reinforcement is provided only if the client's response varies in some way from previous responses. For example, lag schedules may be used to teach request-based mands to children with autism. Initially, the clinician reinforces a specific mand sentence (e.g., I want _____) with the reinforcer specified by the client. In subsequent trials, reinforcement would be provided only for different mand sentences (e.g., "I need _____"; "Please give me _____"). Although lag schedules of reinforcement may not be appropriate for teaching all speech-language skills, they play an important role in treatment when the clinician is concerned with increasing the client's ability to exhibit various forms of a target behavior.

This section on positive reinforcement and reinforcement schedules was designed to give SLPs some basic information regarding these important concepts. Knowing what kind of reinforcer to deliver and when to deliver it are critical clinical skills. Display Box 6–3 presents various scenarios to illustrate clinical applications of methods of reinforcement and reinforcement schedules.

Display Box 6–3. Clinical Scenarios

Consider the following scenarios and answer the following questions:

   a. What type of reinforcement is being used? In some cases, there will be more than one.
   b. What reinforcement schedule is being used?

Scenario 1

A clinician is working with her client on production of /f/ in initial position at the word level. For every correct response, she says, "Hey! You got it! Your teeth really made contact with your lower lip—perfect!" or something of that nature. She then reinforces the client's production by dropping a token into a cup. If the client has 50 tokens at the end of the session, she allows him to pick a toy or a piece of candy from her "treasure chest."

Scenario 2

A client is allowed to jump on a small trampoline for 2 minutes after producing present progressive *–ing* correctly 20 times at the sentence level.

Scenario 3

To begin fading reinforcement, the clinician charted correct responses for production of plural *–s* at the phrase level and, after 6, 8, 4, 5, and 7 correct responses, said, "You're doing a great job—keep it up!" to the client.

Scenario 4

Daniel had been having trouble sitting in his chair during speech therapy sessions. The clinician determined how long he seemed to be able to sit in his chair easily. She found he could sit nicely for 2 minutes before he got fidgety or exhibited out-of-seat behavior. The clinician decided to say, "Way to go! I like how nicely you are sitting," or something of that nature for every 2 minutes of good in-seat behavior. If Daniel was not sitting nicely at the 2-minute mark, the clinician would wait until the first sign of good sitting behavior and say something like, "Oh! There you go, sitting so nice and tall" before beginning the next 2-minute block of time.

Scenario 5

As treatment progressed, Daniel started sitting nicely for 2 minutes with no difficulty. The clinician then decided she would encourage good sitting behavior by making a comment such as, "Keep it up! You're still sitting nice and straight and tall" at 5 minutes, then at 4 minutes, then at 6 minutes, then at 3 minutes, and then at 7 minutes.

See Item 7 in Application Exercises for correct answers.

Negative Reinforcement

Although speech-language pathologists are primarily concerned with increasing target behaviors through the use of positive reinforcement, negative reinforcement is also used to teach some communication skills. **Negative reinforcement** is the process of removing a stimulus contingent upon a behavior to increase its future occurrence. Consequently, negative reinforcers allow a client to escape or avoid an aversive situation.

Aversive Situations

Aversive situations may take a variety of forms. Some aversive states, such as pain, noise, and extreme cold or heat, serve as unconditioned antecedent stimuli. As a result, behaviors that serve to cease such stimuli will be negatively reinforced without the need for previous learning. Behaviors such as turning on the heater when it is cold or turning down a blaring television set are negatively reinforced because they result in the cessation of aversive stimuli.

Over time, individuals also learn that certain situations can be aversive. For example, some children find the classroom setting aversive based on the difficulty of the curriculum. By engaging in off-task behavior, the child may be sent to the principal's office, thus terminating participation in the classroom activities. Hence, the client's undesirable behavior is negatively reinforced because it resulted in a removal of an aversive situation.

Negative reinforcers allow an individual to _____ or _____ an aversive situation.

Escape and Avoidance

Behaviors are maintained by negative reinforcement because they either allow the individual to escape or avoid an aversive stimulus. When people come in contact with aversive situations, they often engage in specific behaviors in order to terminate those stimuli. The previously discussed example of being off task to terminate participation in classroom activities is an illustration of how escape can maintain undesirable behavior through negative reinforcement. In cases of **escape**, the client initially comes in contact with the aversive situation and then engages in a behavior that serves to terminate the nonpreferred stimulus. **Avoidance** occurs when a client engages in specific behaviors to avoid coming in contact with the aversive stimulus altogether. Some clients who stutter avoid speaking with certain conversational partners because they have stuttered more when around those individuals in the past. As a result, their avoidance behavior is maintained through negative reinforcement because it prevents participation in the aversive situation.

Applications to Clinical Practice

A variety of inappropriate speech-language and interfering behaviors may be maintained through negative reinforcement. By understanding the role negative reinforcement plays in maintaining these behaviors, clinicians are able to make better use of response reduction techniques to invoke behavior change (this topic is discussed in greater detail in Chapter 8).

In terms of its application to teaching new behaviors, negative reinforcement is most frequently used when working on protest-based mands. Many clients must be taught to use appropriate protesting behavior (e.g., asking for a break). By utilizing nonpreferred tasks during treatment sessions, the clinician uses negative reinforcement to teach the client more appropriate forms of verbal behavior that provide escape and/or avoidance of aversive situations.

Also, clinicians need to be aware of the fact that many clients find speech and language therapy to be at least mildly aversive. Clinicians might observe that children ask an increasing amount of questions, which, if attended to, may provide them with escape from therapy. Similarly, adult clients may strive to spend more and more time during a therapy session engaging the clinician in irrelevant conversation, again because such idle chit-chat relieves them of the demands of therapy. When this happens, clinicians need to apply a behavior reduction technique, such as extinction or differential reinforcement of low rates of responding (see Chapter 8), to keep therapy on track.

Chapter Summary

1. After completing the assessment process, SLPs seek to establish new speech-language skills and increase those that occur at low rates.
2. Speech-language therapy involves the manipulation of antecedent and consequence stimuli.
3. Antecedent manipulations involve altering the stimuli that occur prior to a behavior being exhibited.
4. Modeling with required imitation is an antecedent-based treatment technique that can be used to teach a variety of communicative behaviors.

5. Prompts supplement antecedent stimuli to make a response more likely to occur.
6. Examples of verbal prompts include:
   a. Partial modeling
   b. Phonemic cues
   c. Vocal emphasis
7. Examples of visual prompts include:
   a. Textual prompts
   b. Gestural prompts
   c. Positional prompts
   d. Facial expressions
8. Tactile-kinesthetic prompts include the use of physical contact to help the client engage in a target behavior. This differs from manual guidance, which involves the clinician guiding the client's motor movements through production of the target response.
9. Shaping is the reinforcement of successive approximations of a target behavior. Chaining is the reinforcement of successive components of a target behavior. Task analyses can be used with chaining to further define the components of a target behavior.
10. Positive reinforcement involves adding or presenting a stimulus to increase the frequency of a target behavior. Preference assessments can be conducted to identify potential reinforcers.
11. Reinforcers may be unconditioned (e.g., food, water, shelter, sensory stimulation) or conditioned (e.g., social reinforcers, token economies, the Premack principle) in nature.
12. Reinforcement can be provided on continuous, intermittent, or lag schedules.
13. Examples of intermittent schedules of reinforcement include fixed ratio, variable ratio, fixed interval, and variable interval schedules.
14. Negative reinforcement involves removing a stimulus to increase the

frequency of a target behavior. Behaviors may be negatively reinforced through escape or avoidance of aversive situations.

Application Exercises

1. A speech-language pathologist (SLP) is working with a 3-year-old preschool student with a significant intellectual disability who has minimal imitation skills. How might the SLP work on the child's use of echoic behavior so that modeling and imitation can be used during treatment?
2. Write an operational definition of a target behavior per the guidelines included in Chapter 3. After you have defined the target behavior, discuss at least three prompting techniques that could be used to address the goal.
3. Discuss the similarities and differences between shaping and chaining.
4. Differentiate between unconditioned and conditioned reinforcers.
5. An SLP finds that social consequences in isolation are not serving as positive reinforcers for a specific client. What are some courses of action the SLP could take in order to positively reinforce the target behavior?
6. How might an SLP use negative reinforcement during treatment? Can you think of any applications to treatment not discussed in this chapter?
7. Answers to clinical scenarios in Display Box 6–3:

   Scenario 1: Social reinforcement, informative feedback, token economy

   Continuous schedule of reinforcement, FR1

   Scenario 2: Premack principle (high probability behavior)

   Fixed ratio schedule of reinforcement, FR20

   Scenario 3: Social reinforcement

   Variable ratio schedule of reinforcement, VR6

   Scenario 4: Social reinforcement, informative feedback

   Fixed-interval schedule of reinforcement, FI2min

   Scenario 5: Social reinforcement, informative feedback

   Variable-interval schedule of reinforcement, VI5min

References

Cooper, J. O., Heron, T. E., & Heward, W. L. (2007). *Applied behavior analysis* (2nd ed.). Upper Saddle River, NJ: Pearson Education.

Esch, J. W., Esch, B. E., & Love, J. R. (2009). Increasing vocal variability in children with autism using a lag schedule of reinforcement. *The Analysis of Verbal Behavior, 25*(1), 73–78.

Hegde, M. N. (1998). *Treatment procedures in communicative disorders* (3rd ed.). Austin, TX: Pro-Ed.

Koehler-Platten, K., Grow, L. L., Schulze, K. A., & Bertone, T. (2013). Using a lag schedule of reinforcement to increase phonemic variability in children with autism spectrum disorders. *The Analysis of Verbal Behavior, 29*(1), 71–83.

Lee, R., McComas J. J., & Jawor J. (2002). The effects of differential and lag reinforcement schedules on varied verbal responding by individuals with autism. *Journal of Applied Behavior Analysis, 35*(4), 391–402.

Premack, D. (1959). Toward empirical behavior laws I: Positive reinforcement. *Psychological Review, 66*(4), 219–233.

Susa, C., & Schilinger, H. D. (2012). Using a lag schedule to increase variability of verbal responding in an individual with autism. *The Analysis of Verbal Behavior, 28*(1), 125–130.

CHAPTER 7

Generalizing and Maintaining Behaviors

The procedures discussed in Chapter 6 are used to develop and strengthen a variety of communicative behaviors. After using these techniques to establish target behaviors in the structured treatment setting, beginning clinicians may be tempted to think that their job is complete. However, recall that the purpose of providing behaviorally based speech-language services is to have a socially significant effect on the client's life. If the effects of treatment do not generalize to appropriate settings, communicative partners, and other antecedent stimuli, socially significant change has not occurred. As a result, behavior change must generalize and be maintained prior to considering cessation of treatment services. It is not enough to be able to exhibit a response with the speech-language pathologist in the clinic room; the client must be able to use the target behavior in a variety of antecedent conditions across time.

Stimulus Discrimination Versus Generalization

Verbal behavior often must occur within the context of a very specific set of antecedent stimuli. For example, upon seeing his mother walking into the classroom to pick him up from school (i.e., the antecedent stimuli), a preschool-aged child may wave and provide the response, "Hi, Mom." Such a response would not be socially acceptable for the child to engage in when presented with other antecedent stimuli, such as seeing his father or another student's parent coming through the door. This process of responding to different antecedent stimuli in different ways is known as **discrimination**.

> Discrimination is the process of responding to _____ antecedent stimuli in _____ ways.

Discrimination occurs when individuals learn to respond appropriately to discriminative stimuli (S^D) and stimulus deltas (S^Δ; see Chapter 5 for additional information). Children engage in discrimination when they use an "outside voice" at recess but not in the classroom. In this example, the playground serves as the S^D, and the classroom serves as the S^Δ for using an "outside voice." Similarly, drivers demonstrate stimulus discrimination when they stop at a red light (the S^D) and continue driving when the light is green (the S^Δ for stopping behavior). Discrimination often plays a key role during speech-language therapy as well. Clients must learn to discriminate between stimuli in order to correctly label vocabulary pictures, follow directions, produce speech sounds correctly, and so forth.

Although teaching stimulus discrimination is often an important component in the treatment process, clinicians must also guard against their clients becoming overly discriminative across stimuli. A common obstacle that clinicians encounter is clients successfully engaging in a target behavior in the treatment room and then failing to exhibit that response in other settings. In such cases, the therapeutic environment serves as an S^D for the response while other settings become S^Δs. This is often due to the lack of available reinforcement for engaging in the target behavior in nontreatment settings.

In order to avoid inappropriate discrimination between antecedent stimuli, clinicians attempt to promote **generaliza-**

tion of taught skills. According to Chance (2006), "Generalization is the tendency for the effects of training to transfer or spread" (p. 303). Generalization occurs when, without specific teaching, target behaviors are exhibited in new settings, with new people, in response to new antecedent stimuli, or in new ways. A child who has been taught to label pictures of vehicles during treatment sessions may generalize this skill to expressive identification of the actual items (e.g., cars, planes, trains, etc.). When an adult client who stutters uses fluency strategies that have been taught in the clinical setting at home, generalization is at play. While clinicians must monitor their clients' progress to prevent **overgeneralization** (e.g., a child labeling all females as "mom," an aphasia client calling all vehicles "cars," etc.) of taught skills, they must carefully plan treatment sessions to ensure that generalization of the target behavior to all relevant situations occurs. In other words, clinicians must actively program generalization rather than passively expect it to occur as the result of the success of their treatment methods in the clinic setting (Stokes & Baer, 1977).

Types of Generalization

Speech-language pathologists (SLPs) are concerned with three types of generalization: stimulus generalization, setting generalization, and response generalization. **Stimulus generalization** occurs when the client produces a target behavior in response to untaught, although typically similar, antecedent stimuli. This phenomenon can be observed throughout our daily lives. An individual who test drives a new car is able to start the vehicle, accelerate, and stop because of stimulus generalization. Although a new antecedent stimulus (i.e., the new car) is being encountered, the person is able to generalize to this new condition what had previously been learned by driving other vehicles.

Within the field of speech-language pathology, stimulus generalization occurs when articulation clients produce sounds correctly in response to untaught stimuli. Similarly, a child who has been taught to locate objects in a field of three may generalize this skill to picture identification as well. In this type of generalization, the client's response stays the same; however, there is a change in the evoking antecedent stimuli. Clinicians should address stimulus generalization throughout the treatment process because there is rarely enough time to teach all relevant exemplars that the client may encounter.

When a target behavior is exhibited in the presence of untaught antecedent stimuli, _____ generalization has occurred.

Setting generalization is a concept closely related to stimulus generalization. Setting generalization occurs when clients exhibit taught skills under very specific antecedent conditions, new settings. Setting generalization happens when a target behavior is produced outside of the location where teaching has taken place. A collegiate student is able to use studying skills he or she learned in high school because of setting generalization. This event is also observed when college graduates apply the knowledge obtained during their coursework upon entering the workforce.

SLPs are concerned with generalizing target behaviors taught in the clinical setting to more natural environments. Again, this is pivotal to ensuring the social significance of the treatment provided. For example, production of fluent speech within the clinical setting is not adequate for clients who stutter; this skill should also be generalized to natural settings (e.g., home, classroom, cafeteria, library, etc.). Likewise, inpatient dysphagia clients must be able to generalize safe swallowing techniques across settings in order to promote their well-being. SLPs should strive to arrange treatment sessions in ways to promote setting generalization as well.

> When a target behavior is exhibited in untaught settings, _____ generalization has occurred.

Although stimulus and setting generalization are both characterized by the effects of treatment spreading to new antecedent conditions (i.e., stimuli and settings), **response generalization** refers to the effects of treatment transferring to untaught, although typically similar, forms of the target response. Response generalization accounts for clients exhibiting new forms of target behaviors. As a result of response generalization, a student who has been taught to sound out words when reading may be able to use this skill to write novel words as well. Children who have been taught production of specific speech sounds (e.g., /f/) may demonstrate response generalization to be able to produce the phoneme's cognate pair (e.g., /v/). Addressing response generalization during treatment can make the therapeutic process more efficient.

> When a client exhibits new forms of a target behavior, _____ generalization has occurred.

Techniques for Promoting Generalization During Treatment

As previously discussed, generalization plays a paramount role during treatment. Without addressing generalization, SLPs are unable to effect socially significant behavior change. Far too often, clinicians assume that generalization is a passive, automatic process. Because the client is able to exhibit a specific target behavior during speech-language sessions, SLPs may think that further support is unnecessary. Beginning clinicians should not make this assumption. SLPs should not expect generalization to occur unless treatment has been specifically designed to address it from the beginning. The following sections describe various methods for enhancing generalization throughout treatment.

Choosing Functional Target Behaviors

The first step for addressing generalization should occur before treatment sessions have even been initiated. After completing a thorough assessment, clinicians use the available data, including client input, to select functional target behaviors to teach during treatment. SLPs strive to select goals that will be useful to clients in their everyday lives. For example, when working with the school-aged population, school-based SLPs select goals tied to classroom standards because these skills will be more functional for their clients. Similarly, when working with adults with traumatic brain injury, target behaviors should be relevant to helping them attain communicative skills that will bring them as close as possible to premorbid status in their vocational and social activities.

In most cases, clinicians should ensure that clients have adequate use of the various verbal operants, such as mands or tacts, prior to addressing response topography (e.g., syntactic or morphological structure; see Chapter 2 for a full description of verbal operants). For example, a minimally verbal child should be taught to mand for highly preferred items prior to teaching formal properties such as plural *–s*, present progressive *–ing*, or syntactic structures. Having adequate functional communication skills helps individuals contact reinforcement in natural environments, thus enhancing the likelihood that generalization will occur.

Varying the Stimuli

Varying the type of antecedent stimuli presented during treatment sessions can enhance generalization as well. When an assortment of antecedent stimuli is used during treatment, clients are more likely to exhibit the target behavior in untaught conditions. Using a variety of exemplars helps ensure that clients are not responding to an irrelevant component (e.g., color, shape, size) of the antecedent stimulus, and clinicians can be more confident that clients are obtaining a good grasp of the concept being taught during treatment. For example, a clinician might be working with a client on naming common objects, such as *ball*. The clinician might start out by showing a picture of a striped beach ball to evoke the client's response. As soon as the response has been established, according to the clinician's predetermined criterion, stimuli should be varied to include pictures of baseballs, basketballs, soccer balls, tennis balls, golf balls, and so forth. By varying the stimuli in this manner, the clinician promotes appropriate generalization of the word *ball*.

In addition to varying the immediate antecedent stimuli, clinicians may also change the settings in which treatment is provided, thus promoting setting generalization. There are many ways in which a clinician can teach a target behavior across settings. After teaching a student to answer *wh–* questions in the speech room, an SLP may provide treatment in the child's classroom to promote generalization to that environment as well. Clinicians may work across settings with clients who have experienced left visual field neglect following right hemisphere brain damage in order to ensure that they are attending to items on the left side in all environments. SLPs can accompany fluency clients on outings to fast-food restaurants or social events, giving them some prearranged signal to remind them to use their fluency strategies when they become dysfluent. Adults and children who have been taught to use a system of augmentative and alternative communication (AAC) must be given extensive support in all of their natural environments; the clinician in this case gives direct treatment in each relevant setting (e.g., home, school, community) and also consults with all the significant persons in the client's life. By providing therapy in a variety of settings, clinicians increase the probability that their clients will respond correctly when they come in contact with other antecedent conditions.

Another way in which stimuli can be varied is for SLPs to engage other individuals in the treatment process. Clinicians want their clients to use taught skills appropriately with everyone they come in contact with, such as parents, guardians, care providers, teachers, peers, or even other clients. By including others in the treatment sessions, clinicians put their clients in contact with different antecedent conditions where they will be expected to use the target behaviors taught during therapy. Having others present and participating during treatment sessions further supports the client's ability to generalize taught skills. This is strengthened even further when clinicians teach others in the client's natural environment techniques used in the clinic to support production of the target behavior—an approach that is closely related to another technique for promoting generalization, programming common stimuli.

Programming Common Stimuli

There is often little about the clinical setting that resembles conditions clients encounter in their everyday lives, which may be a serious obstacle to generalization of target behaviors. Generalization will be more likely if stimuli presented during treatment are also present in the client's natural environment. Therefore, utilizing common stimuli that are present in both clinical and extra-clinical settings is one way clinicians can promote generalization of target behaviors. Clinicians can provide common social stimuli, as well as common physical stimuli (Falcomata & Wacker, 2013).

Common Social Stimuli

Clinicians who bring others into the clinic room to provide varying stimuli can also teach them to continue to evoke target behaviors in extra-clinical environments. In this way, others become discriminative stimuli to the client in training and generalization settings. Peers are especially well suited to serve as social stimuli common to clinic and natural settings. For example, a clinician targeting social skills in a child with autism might teach turn taking between herself and the child first, then bring peers into the clinic room to practice turn taking, teaching the peers to use the same methods to evoke the turn-taking behavior. When the child with autism encounters the peers in the natural environment, and they evoke turn-taking behavior from the child, generalization of turn-taking behavior might be more likely to occur.

Common Physical Stimuli

Common physical stimuli may include assistive devices, materials from the classroom setting, items brought from the client's household, and so forth. People who require AAC systems may be taught by an SLP in a clinical setting to access a speech-generating device (SGD). If they do not have the SGD available in other settings, generalization is not at all likely to occur. Target behaviors such as the initiation of communicative interaction, requesting, commenting, and so forth will generalize to other settings only if the SGD is present. This seems like an obvious necessity, but many school districts do not support transporting an expensive SGD between school and home, thereby ensuring a lack of generalization in settings other than the classroom.

SLPs working in the public schools can teach target behaviors using antecedent stimuli that are commonly encountered in the classroom setting, such as textbooks, worksheets, and writing materials. For example, to teach appropriate responses to *wh*– questions, clinicians might read a passage from a textbook, or have the child read it silently, and then ask questions about the passage. To teach increased expressive vocabulary, the clinician can consult with the classroom teacher to determine words that the child must understand to function better academically; for example, if the teacher is planning a unit on weather, words such as *cumulus*, *temperature*, *humidity*, and *meteorologist* could be targeted. School-based SLPs might also arrange their clinical space to resemble more closely the classroom setting with similar furniture, seating arrangements, and bulletin board displays (Rincover & Koegel, 1975).

Providing common physical stimuli includes the typical stimulus cards or objects that clinicians use during therapy to evoke the target behavior. Pictures shown should be realistic color photographs of objects or actions the client can recognize in other settings; line drawings or anthropomorphic cartoon drawings of animals performing human functions should be avoided. Objects that the client or the client's significant other brings from home to the clinic setting may also be incorporated into therapy. A child's favorite toys from home, for example, can be used to evoke targeted behaviors, which may then generalize when the child plays with those toys in the home setting. Using stimulus materials from a client's natural setting is especially important when the client is from a culturally or linguistically diverse (CLD) background. Commercially available stimulus items may be strange and confusing to those who are CLD and do little to promote generalization of target behaviors to natural settings.

Teaching Loosely

When teaching target behaviors in the clinic setting, if clinicians present just a few stimuli, with no variation whatsoever, the client's response may become stimulus bound, produced only when confronted with the exact same stimuli presented in the exact same way by the same person, in the clinic setting. In this case, generalization of the target behavior to other settings is not likely to take place. Therefore, researchers have suggested that teaching more loosely will diminish the strong discriminative control exerted by specific stimuli presented in the clinic setting upon the target behavior. Loose teaching is a characteristic of various naturalistic approaches to teaching language, such as milieu teaching (Charlop-Christy & Carpenter, 2000; Hart & Risley, 1975) and pivotal response training (Koegel, Carter, & Koegel, 2003).

It is almost always necessary to establish a target behavior using the type of very tightly controlled teaching methods exemplified in discrete trial teaching (DTT), described in Chapter 5. However, clinicians should seek to vary the physical and verbal stimuli they provide as the client nears the criterion level for correct responses. For example, a clinician who is teaching a child to mand may begin by presenting a very specific verbal stimulus, such as, "What do you want?" However, as the child's intraverbal mand behavior increases, the clinician might vary the verbal stimuli given, saying, "What do you need?" "Do you see something you like?" or "Can I help you?"

Baer (1999) further suggested that teaching loosely entails varying nonessential clinical stimuli, which, if left constant, may become discriminative stimuli for production of the target behavior. He recommended, among many other suggestions, that clinicians dress very differently on different days, vary the tone of their voice, vary the angle at which they hold the stimulus items, set the lighting in the clinic room at various degrees of brightness, and vary the location of the furniture. Not all of these recommendations should be carried out at once, of course, but building an adequate amount of "looseness" into the clinic setting may help to promote generalization to the natural environment.

Providing an Adequate Number of Exemplars

Clinicians should provide enough stimulus exemplars to teach a response to a client. There is no one number of adequate exemplars that will result in a client learning and generalizing a targeted response. Factors influencing the number of exemplars necessary include the level and complexity of the target behavior, the type of target behavior (e.g., articulation, pragmatic language, etc.), the aptitude of the client, and so forth.

Stimulus exemplars can refer to the specific stimulus items (e.g., photocards, objects), settings in which the target behavior must generalize, and the people who are responsible for teaching the client (Cooper, Heward, & Heron, 2007). The number of exemplars required is dependent to a great extent on the nature of the target behavior. For articulation target behaviors, the stimulus is often a picture

card accompanied by verbal stimuli to evoke production of specific sounds. The clinician might decide to limit stimulus items to 4 or 5 exemplars at the beginning of therapy to get the behavior established, or to present as many as 10 to 20 exemplars. There is no research to indicate which is better—fewer stimulus items with each item presented repeatedly or a greater number of stimulus items presented one at a time. No matter what decision is made, data collected will indicate whether the number of stimulus items presented is sufficient in teaching the target behavior to the client.

For other target behaviors, as few as one or two examples might be sufficient. Pragmatic language skills might be taught in the clinic room with just the clinician and then show generalization to other people in the client's natural environment. For example, Stokes, Baer, and Jackson (1974) taught four institutionalized children to wave "hello." The children were taught the response during one-on-one therapy in a small room. Probes for generalization were conducted by having others wave to the children during the course of a day. Three of the children showed no generalization of the waving behavior until they were taught by a second therapist. One child, however, showed generalized hand waving after being taught by just the first therapist, thereby indicating that just one exemplar in her case was sufficient.

Similarly, if the target behavior has to do with production of a communicative response in the client's natural environment, it may be necessary to teach the behavior within multiple exemplar settings. For example, a person with a newly acquired SGD might first receive instruction on its use in the clinic room. However, that one environment almost certainly will not provide enough of an exemplar stimulus to ensure generalization of the use of the SGD in other settings. The clinician might then teach the client to use the SGD in the classroom setting and then probe to see if use of the SGD has generalized to other settings. If it has not, then the clinician might decide to teach a third exemplar setting, such as a fast-food restaurant. After receiving instruction in three settings, the client might then begin to spontaneously use the SGD in other settings, such as at home or at social events.

Teaching an adequate number of response exemplars is also important to help promote generalization. For example, when working with a child who exhibits a phonological disorder, generalization is typically more likely to occur if production of several maximally different phonemes (i.e., an adequate number of response exemplars) is taught to address the process rather than just one or two phonemes. In another example, a child with a target behavior for greeting skills can be taught to say, "Hello!" However, the child should also practice waving, making eye contact, nodding, and saying "good morning" to promote generalization to other greeting behaviors. Failure to teach an adequate number of response exemplars may result in robotic, stimulus-bound responses, such as the client who only produces the taught carrier phrase, "I want _____" without producing other manding phrases or sentences, even though the student is capable of doing so.

Fading Reinforcement

A major desired outcome of treatment is for the client to produce the target behavior without all the special stimuli that are provided by the clinician in the clinic setting. These special stimuli include the clinician's reinforcement of correct responses, which must be **faded**, or gradually withdrawn, as soon as possible. Clinicians employ a variety of reinforcement techniques delivered according to a predetermined reinforcement schedule to effectuate an increase in clients' correct response rate (see Chapter 6 for a description of reinforcement techniques and schedules). The correct response should show an increase; if it does not, whatever technique the clinician is using is not serving as a reinforcer, and the clinician must find another technique that will result in an increase in the correct response rate.

> Part of the definition of a reinforcer is that it results in an _____ of the correct response rate; if it does not, then it is not a reinforcer.

At the beginning of treatment, a continuous schedule of reinforcement in which every correct response is reinforced (fixed ratio 1; FR1) is commonly used. It is assumed that correct responses will not be produced at a very high rate in the beginning of treatment, so whenever a correct response is produced, it should be reinforced. However, as the correct response rate becomes established, according to a predetermined criterion level set by the clinician, the amount of reinforcement the client receives should be gradually thinned. The clinician should move to an intermittent schedule of reinforcement, in which some correct responses are not reinforced. For example, if the client has received reinforcement on a continuous fixed ratio (FR1) schedule, the clinician could consider thinning that schedule to an FR2 schedule in which every other response is reinforced. If the client has received reinforcement according to an interval schedule of reinforcement, in which reinforcement is given to the first correct response produced after a certain period of time, the interval can be gradually increased. For example, if a client has been reinforced on a fixed interval of 2 minutes (FI2min), the time interval might be increased to 3 minutes (FI3min).

Clinicians might also switch from fixed ratio or interval schedules to a variable schedule, which is easier to fade (Hegde, 1998). With a variable schedule of reinforcement, the client usually cannot detect a pattern as to when a correct answer may receive reinforcement, which may result in a more consistent response rate in the absence of reinforcement. There are numerous examples of behaviors that are maintained on intermittent schedules of reinforcement in the natural environment. Consider the compulsive slot machine player. Slot machines pay out according to an intermittent, variable ratio schedule of reinforcement. Because the players never know when they are going to receive a payoff, the slot-playing behavior is exhibited for long periods of time in the complete absence of reinforcement—in this case, a jackpot. Consider also the employer who checks on his employees on a variable-interval schedule of reinforcement to give them a "thumbs up" if they are found to be diligently working. If employees do not know when they are going to receive such a visit, their working behavior is more likely to be consistently maintained. Similarly, in the clinic room, clients working on target behaviors such as correct articulation of sounds, correct production of language structures, fluency of speech, and so forth continue to work hard when the clinician switches

from a fixed ratio or interval schedule to a variable one.

_____ schedules of reinforcement are easier to fade than _____ schedules of reinforcement.

When clinicians begin to thin a schedule of reinforcement, they need to be aware of the possibility of **ratio strain**, which occurs when the correct response rate decreases as a result of too abruptly thinning a reinforcement schedule. Data collection is always important during treatment; it is especially important to document the maintenance of a correct response rate when less and less reinforcement is given. If the correct response rate begins to drop, the clinician should reinstate a denser schedule of reinforcement to reestablish the behavior.

_____ _____ occurs when the reinforcement schedule is thinned too abruptly, and the correct response rate decreases.

Also, there are some target behaviors for which the reinforcement schedule should not be thinned at all. For many pragmatic language behaviors, for example, thinning of reinforcement should not take place. Appropriate eye contact is reinforced by conversational partners returning eye contact and giving their attention to the speaker. Topic initiation is reinforced by a conversational partner following the initiator's lead and engaging in conversation regarding that topic. Rituals of social politeness are reinforced by the responses that are given by others (e.g., introductions, leave takings, etc.). These are behaviors that are continuously reinforced in the natural environment and should also be continuously reinforced in the clinic setting.

Probing for Generalization in the Clinic Setting

Clinicians from time to time need to probe for generalization of the target behavior in the clinic setting, after the client has reached a predetermined criterion level. Probes are conducted to determine generalization of the target behavior in response to novel stimuli not previously presented during treatment. A probe can be intermixed, in which taught stimuli are presented with untaught stimuli, in an alternating fashion. For intermixed probes, a correct response rate is calculated based only on responses to untaught stimuli. If the client reaches criterion level based on analysis of data collected during an intermixed probe, a pure probe should be conducted. During a pure probe, *only* untaught exemplars are presented, and the correct response rate is calculated based on all responses given. If the criterion is met, then a final conversational probe will determine whether or not the target behavior has generalized and is spontaneously produced in conversation. Probe procedures are an integral part of DTT and are therefore discussed in more detail in Chapter 5.

Techniques to Promote Maintenance in Natural Settings

According to Hegde (1998), the final goal of treatment is not generalization but maintenance of the behavior in the natural setting. In other words, the job of the clinician should not be considered done when the client reaches criterion level for production of the target behavior in the clinic setting. The target behavior is mastered only when it is produced by the client in natural settings and reinforced by the natural contingencies the client encounters in the environment. Probes for generalization in natural settings should be conducted before dismissal. If the client reaches criterion level during probes in natural settings, then it can be assumed that the target behavior has generalized; however, that does not necessarily indicate the target behaviors will be maintained over time in the absence of clinical treatment. It is therefore necessary to plan not just for generalization of the target behavior but also for maintenance. Some of the strategies previously discussed (e.g., using common physical and social stimuli) are designed to promote generalization in the clinic room and also generalization and maintenance in the natural environment. However, there are further maintenance strategies that, in effect, first result in the client receiving ongoing treatment in the natural environment and then lead to maintenance in the absence of treatment. These strategies can be implemented by the clients themselves and by clients' significant others.

Self-Monitoring

Self-monitoring involves clients learning to systematically observe and record their own behavior (Finn, 2003). This has been shown to be an effective technique in effectuating behavior change, possibly due to the influence of **reactivity**, a behavioral term referring to the extent to which an observation or assessment procedure results in a modification in the usual behavior of the person being observed or assessed. Reactivity is much more likely if the observation or assessment measure is **obtrusive**—meaning that the person is aware of the fact that an observation or measurement is being conducted. Professionals try to be as unobtrusive as possible when observing and assessing a client, to keep reactivity to a minimum. However, in the case of self-monitoring, obtrusiveness may work to the benefit of the client. Because the assessor and the assessed are one and the same, self-monitoring provides a maximum degree of obtrusiveness, which may result in quicker behavior change due to the client's heightened awareness of correct and incorrect responses (Cooper et al., 2007).

> _____-_____ involves clients learning to systematically observe and record their own behavior.

> _____ occurs when an observation or assessment procedure results in a modification in the usual behavior of the person being observed or assessed.

> Reactivity is more likely to occur when the observation or assessment procedure is _____, meaning the person is aware he or she is being observed or assessed.

Clinicians who teach clients to self-monitor help them to become their own therapists, providing ongoing treatment in their natural settings. There are a vari-

ety of ways that clinicians can help clients achieve self-monitoring skills. The clinician can make an audio recording of a few of the client's responses and then play the audiotape back, encouraging the client to judge whether the responses heard are correct or incorrect. This technique is most commonly employed for clients working on articulation or fluency target behaviors. For example, a clinician can simultaneously take data and make an audio recording of responses evoked during DTT for production of /r/ in initial position. After a block of 10 responses, the clinician can then play the recording back to the client and encourage the client to judge whether the response is correct or incorrect. After the client has demonstrated good skill in judging whether responses are correct or incorrect, the clinician can then provide the client with a copy of the same data chart being kept by the clinician and explain to the client the method of data collection (usually a "plus" for correct and a "minus" for incorrect; for younger children, data can be kept using happy face/sad face stamps). Then, when the audiotape is played back, the client can identify correct and incorrect responses and chart them. A comparison of the client's chart can then be made with the clinician's chart.

Clients should be encouraged to continue to listen to their productions outside of the clinic setting during their daily routines. Clinicians can require clients to gather data on their own productions outside of the clinic setting as homework. Clicker counters, iPhone apps, and communication diaries are methods of data collection that lend themselves nicely to the natural environment. Clinicians can then build into the clinical therapy session a review of the data the client has collected in extra-clinical situations.

Contingency Priming

Clients who have been taught to self-monitor can also learn **contingency priming**, a technique that involves asking for reinforcement when significant others in their natural environment fail to give it. Examples of contingency priming in everyday life include the spouse who asks, "Don't I look nice?" when an ignoring partner fails to make such a comment spontaneously, or the employee who feels a job has been done well and asks, "What did you think about how I completed that project?" expecting to receive reinforcement that had not otherwise been forthcoming.

> Asking for reinforcement for correct productions of target behaviors when others in the natural environment do not give it is called _____
> _____.

In the same way, clients can prime significant others to give reinforcement to correct productions of target behaviors in natural settings. The child who has learned to produce a good /r/ sound might say something like, "Hey! Did you hear that /r/?" to prime parents to give reinforcement. An adult stutterer who has properly applied a breathing or speech rate reduction technique to work through a dysfluency might say, "Well, I guess I got through that one, didn't I?" Although some may consider such statements to be "fishing for compliments," it is critically important that everything possible be done to ensure that clients' productions of newly learned target behaviors are reinforced in natural environments, especially when those productions are just starting

to show up in natural settings. If they are not, generalization and maintenance of the target response are not likely to occur.

Working With Significant Others

Of course, significant others who have been involved in a client's therapy and have learned to give reinforcement will not always have to be primed in order to deliver it. To extend treatment to the natural setting, eventually leading to generalization and maintenance, people who spend a lot of time with the client (e.g., parents, spouses, caregivers, teachers, etc.) should be shown how to evoke, prompt, and reinforce target behaviors. The involvement of the client's significant others in implementing a treatment plan is critical; without it, there is much less chance of a successful outcome (Cooper et al., 2007). The clinician should, from the onset of the therapeutic relationship, approach significant others with respect, caring, and a sincere willingness to take input from them and incorporate that input when devising target behaviors and devising a treatment plan. Establishing a good rapport with significant others will increase the likelihood that they will be receptive to the clinician's suggestions as to how they can support the client's production of targeted behaviors in the natural environment. In effect, clinicians should enter into a partnership with significant others to support and maintain target behaviors in the natural setting. When this occurs, the problem of generalization to natural settings is greatly alleviated, and target behaviors are more likely to be maintained over time.

Some may advocate that parents, spouses, and others should learn to deliver DTT in much the same manner as the SLP does (Hegde, 1998). It is the experience of the author that this can be effective when significant others are highly motivated to learn DTT and make the time at home to do it. There have been cases, especially before home-based applied behavior analysis (ABA) therapy was widely available to families, when parents took it upon themselves to learn the DTT procedure, spending up to 40 hours a week delivering DTT to their children with autism. However, if clinicians attempt to direct significant others who are not as motivated to conduct formal therapy sessions at home, compliance with that type of intervention plan may not take place and, in any event, will be difficult to monitor. Also, instructing significant others in this way requires the clinician to adapt an "expert model" in which professionals engage in a "one-way direction of information sharing" (Bruce, DiVenere, & Bergeron, 1998, p. 85).

Other models of service delivery in the helping professions suggest that family members and others may be more likely to carry out a plan of intervention at home when clinicians approach them from a family-centered perspective (Crais, Roy, & Free, 2006; Dunst, 2002; Dunst, Boyd, Trivette, & Hamby, 2002; Moes & Frea, 2000; Polmanteer & Turbiville, 2000; Woods, Wilcox, Friedman, & Murch, 2011). As Allen and Petr (1996) stated, "Family-centered service delivery, across disciplines and settings, recognizes the centrality of the family in the lives of individuals. It is guided by fully informed choices made by the family and focuses upon the strengths and capabilities of these families" (p. 64). Professionals working within family-centered service delivery models serve the whole family and specifically support improvement in children's developmental outcomes by designing assessment and intervention programs that take

into consideration individual families' strengths, values, cultural traditions, and routines of everyday life. The model can also be extended to working with adults who need to have newly established or re-established communicative skills supported in natural settings.

It is difficult to operationally define family-centered service delivery, and, therefore, experimental research documenting its effectiveness in furthering developmental outcomes for children and sustained improvement for adults is lacking. There is, however, some evidence that intervention plans are more likely to be carried out by family members and others if:

- They are congruent with the cultural beliefs and values of the client's household.
- They capitalize on already existing strengths in interactions between the client and significant others in the client's environment.
- They reflect the input of clients' significant others.
- They are embedded in daily routines.

Although the first bullet has but a scant experimental research base (e.g., Wang, McCart, & Turnbull, 2007), there are logically assumed benefits to be had by incorporating clients' cultural beliefs and values into a plan for generalization and maintenance. The next three bullets, capitalizing on already existing strengths, taking input, and embedding maintenance strategies into daily routines, have some experimental evidence supporting their efficacy in enhancing treatment outcomes (e.g., Kashinath, Woods, & Goldstein, 2006; Lucyshyn et al., 2007; Lucyshyn, Albin, & Nixon, 1997; Moes & Frea, 2000,

2002; Vaughn, Clarke, & Dunlap, 1997; Vaughan, Wilson, & Dunlap, 2002).

Cultural Beliefs and Values

van Kleeck (1994) has written an extensive tutorial regarding the manner in which advice commonly given by SLPs for supporting children's speech and language development in home settings might conflict greatly with the cultural beliefs and values of culturally and linguistically diverse (CLD) family members. According to van Kleeck, early intervention SLPs often encourage parents to

> . . . follow the child's lead when interacting . . . to respond quickly and enthusiastically to any attempts the child makes to communicate . . . and to achieve a balance in turn taking so that the child is learning to initiate and be as equal a participant in the interaction as possible. (p. 67)

van Kleeck (1994) pointed out that these suggested methods for supporting children's speech and language development are based on assumptions made from an American White, middle-class perspective. It is assumed that adults are welcome to the idea of having the child take the lead and be an equal conversational partner, that adults believe it is possible to infer what another intends to communicate, and that adults value children's talk. These are not assumptions that are universally shared across cultures. To name just a few differences, it has been documented that people in many cultures value quietness in a child, do not permit children to direct topics of conversation, and believe that any accommodations should be made by the child to conform to the needs of the family and not vice

versa (e.g., Johnston & Wong, 2002; Maul, 2015; Roseberry-McKibbin, 2014; Wang et al., 2007).

There is little experimental research regarding the ethnocultural generality of treatment methods, behavioral or otherwise. It is logical, however, to assume that clients' significant others would have difficulty following a maintenance plan that might be in direct conflict with their cultural beliefs and values Therefore, SLPs should be aware of cultural differences they might encounter in their clients and plan for intervention accordingly.

Capitalizing on Strengths

Researchers in family-centered practices have emphasized the need to acknowledge strength in families—to support that which is good about how the families have adapted to their children with disabilities and build upon those strengths when designing assessment procedures and programs of intervention (Cosden, Koegel, Koegel, Greenwell, & Klein, 2006; Maul & Singer, 2009). A strength-based model can also be extended to working with clients' significant others in putting together and implementing a maintenance program for newly taught communicative skills. It begins, as planning for generalization and maintenance always should, before treatment, with a **strength-based assessment** (SBA; Cosden et al., 2006).

To make a strength-based assessment, SLPs look at not only what a client cannot do but what the client can do. Utilizing a family-centered model, SLPs also look for family strengths. What is it that the family is already doing that might be capitalized upon in devising maintenance strategies? For a nonverbal child, for example, the SLP may observe that a parent waits at least a little while to require some kind of manding behavior from the child (e.g., a vocalization or a gesture) before giving a desired item to him. If so, that is a behavior that can be reinforced (e.g., "I really like the way you waited for Johnny to ask for his iPad before you gave it to him") and included in a maintenance strategy. For an adult with aphasia, the SLP may observe that a spouse is good about attending to the client attempting to speak. Again, that behavior can be reinforced (e.g., "I notice you really pay attention when Mary tries to speak") and included as a systematic maintenance strategy for the spouse to continue to use.

Although there is little experimental evidence showing the efficacy of a strength-based approach, there are benefits that may accrue by taking such a perspective. Often, family members are distraught over the communicative difficulties of their loved ones. They may have been through a number of deficit-based assessments delivered by other professionals who have not been encouraging and may feel a sense of helplessness regarding their ability to be of help. An SLP who notices and comments upon what the client can do and what the family members are already doing that is supportive of the client can give a real boost to the morale of the family. A strength-based approach might change significant others' depressed, pessimistic attitudes and motivate them by increasing a general sense of hope and facilitating satisfying relationships among the SLP, the client, and the clients' significant others.

Taking and Acting Upon Input

At the very outset of the therapeutic relationship, SLPs should strive to listen to the input of the client and the clients' significant others and act upon it. This means that the client and all involved with the client should have some say as to what behaviors should be taught and how they will be involved with helping the client in extra-clinical settings. If the SLP devises a plan that reflects input, it is more likely that there will be "buy-in" on the part of significant others. People who have had a part in making a plan are more likely to carry out that plan. There is at least a small amount of research indicating the efficacy of this approach.

Moes and Frea (2000) conducted a case study in which they contrasted the results obtained when using a "prescriptive" approach versus a "contextualized" and "family-directed intervention" to address problem behaviors in a 3-year-old boy with autism, Matthew (p. 40). The parents expressed a desire to increase Matthew's on-task behavior to complete everyday routines (e.g., getting dressed, brushing teeth, sitting at the dinner table, etc.). The researchers began with a prescriptive approach and decided to focus on reducing Matthew's disruptive behavior by teaching functional communication; in this case, teaching Matthew the sign for "I need a break," when family members demanded compliance. The family diligently followed the plan, and Matthew's functional communication (e.g., producing the sign for "I need a break") increased and disruptive behavior decreased. However, on-task behavior, the goal desired by the family, showed no improvement.

The researchers then switched to a contextualized, family-directed approach. They sat down with the parents and asked them what modifications they would suggest for the treatment plan. The parents stated that they preferred Matthew be taught to ask for help instead of for a break. The father also stated that he wished to incorporate a technique that he had been using with at least a small amount of success—giving a direction and then counting to three to prompt Matthew to comply (a common parental ploy professionals would not be likely to recommend). The parents also requested that Matthew's older brother be included in the intervention package, so he could learn how to support his brother. The treatment package was modified in accordance with the input of the parents, and Matthew's on-task behavior then showed significant improvement.

Although this was a single case study, it perfectly illustrated the clinical usefulness of including family input when devising plans for intervention and maintenance of a target behavior. The revised treatment plan focused on a target behavior of the family's choosing. The father let it be known that a preexisting strength that had been ignored—his three-count technique—should be reinstated. The inclusion of Matthew's older brother ensured that all in the family would be involved in supporting the newly acquired targeted skill. Also, because this was an initial intervention that was carried out in the natural setting, generalization and maintenance were addressed congruently throughout the treatment procedure.

Daily Routines

Increasingly, the daily routines of a household have been regarded as a unit of analysis in the assessment and treatment of children with communicative disorders that are secondary to severe disabilities, such as autism spectrum disorder and intellectual disability. Intervention programs that are embedded in daily routines may be more likely to be sustained by busy families who might find it diffi-

cult to set aside specific times during the day to work directly with their children on speech and language goals. In addition, embedding intervention in the daily routines of a household is in accordance with legal mandates to carry out early intervention in the child's natural setting. Again, because the intervention and generalization setting are one and the same, generalization and maintenance of targeted speech and language skills are likely to occur.

There is some evidence supporting the use of daily routines as a context for intervention. In their review of evidence-based intervention practices for infants and toddlers at risk for autism spectrum disorders, Woods and Wetherby (2003) concluded that intervention should be embedded within the context of typical daily routines and community activities to facilitate generalization and to reduce the "stress of specialized training activities that are irrelevant to the child's problem behaviors for families" (p. 187). They reviewed specific empirically supported techniques for embedding intervention in daily routines. These techniques included (a) arranging the environment, (b) using natural reinforcers, (c) using time delay, and (d) imitating the child contingently.

Adults can arrange the environment in ways that encourage communicative interactions with children, such as placing desired objects out of reach, serving food at the dinner table bit-by-bit, interrupting or obstructing familiar routines, or doing something unexpected. Natural reinforcers are logical consequences of a child's communicative interactions. For example, the natural reinforcer for a request is to give the child that which has been asked for. The natural reinforcer for eye contact is to give the child attention and enter into an interaction with the child—saying "Good looking!" is not a natural reinforcer for eye contact. Adults use time delay when they wait for a reasonable amount of time for a child to respond to their attempts to interact, instead of immediately giving a prompt to evoke the response. Finally, adults imitate the child contingently when they imitate a child's utterance or action, immediately after the child has spoken or acted. Such contingent imitation encourages interactive play and turn taking and also serves as a model of imitative behavior for children who need help developing imitation skills (DeThorne, Johnson, Walder, & Mahurin-Smith, 2009). Teaching parents to implement such techniques may result in increased generalization and maintenance of speech and language skills.

Kashinath et al. (2006) examined the effects of teaching parents to embed within their daily household routines the generalized use of various strategies, such as modeling and the use of natural reinforcement, to increase the communicative behavior of their children with autism. Five mother-child dyads participated in this study; the children ranged in age from 33 to 65 months. The mothers participated in identifying daily routines that occurred most frequently and offered opportunities for interaction and communication as contexts for the experimental implementation of their newly learned strategies. Routines identified included getting dressed, snack time, dinner time, handwashing, putting on shoes, and various play routines. For each dyad, two routines were targeted for direct intervention, and two different routines were identified to check for generalization of the mother's strategy use. The primary dependent variable was the frequency with which the mothers implemented the strategies during the selected daily routines, and the secondary dependent variable was the frequency of single words produced by the children.

Results indicated an increase in parental use of the strategies taught and an increase in the frequency with which children produced single-word utterances. It was found that the mothers maintained their frequency of using the first strategy after the second strategy was taught. Also, during the two routines selected for generalization probes, mothers applied the strategies without returning to baseline levels, and the children's production of single words showed an increase in frequency, as in the two routines selected for direct intervention.

In general, working with significant others to support speech and language goals in natural environments may be the most critical component of a plan to facilitate generalization and ensure maintenance. SLPs will enhance the possibility of successful outcomes for clients if they take input from the clients' significant others, act upon that input, consider cultural values and beliefs, capitalize on existing strengths, and devise a maintenance plan that is embedded in the daily routines of clients' natural environments.

Chapter Summary

1. To effectuate socially significant change for the client, taught communicative behaviors must generalize and be maintained in the client's natural environment.

2. Discrimination is the process of responding to different antecedent stimuli in different ways; clinicians must guard against their clients becoming overly discriminative to the extent a

response is only produced in the presence of stimuli presented in the clinic setting.

3. Generalization occurs when, without specific teaching, target behaviors are exhibited in new settings, with new people, in response to new antecedent stimuli, or in new ways.

4. Stimulus generalization occurs when the client produces a target behavior in response to untaught, though typically similar, antecedent stimuli.

5. Setting generalization happens when a target behavior is produced outside of the location where teaching has taken place.

6. Response generalization refers to the effects of treatment transferring to untaught, though typically similar, forms of the target response.

7. Clinicians must actively plan for the generalization and maintenance of target behaviors taught in the clinic setting.

8. Techniques for promoting generalization and eventual maintenance of target behaviors during treatment in the clinic setting include:
   a. Choose target behaviors that are functional for the client
   b. Vary stimuli presented, so that clients are more likely to exhibit the target behavior in untaught conditions
   c. Utilize common social and physical stimuli that are present in both clinical and extra-clinical settings
   d. After establishing a behavior with tightly controlled teaching, teach more loosely, varying verbal and physical stimuli
   e. Provide enough stimulus and response exemplars to teach a response to a client

   f. Gradually fade reinforcement so that eventually the response is maintained in the absence of reinforcement provided by the clinician

9. Periodically probe for generalization of the target behavior, using intermixed, pure, and conversational probes.

10. Techniques for promoting generalization and maintenance of the target behavior in clients' natural environments include:
    a. Teaching the client to self-monitor
    b. Teaching contingency priming
    c. Working with significant others
       i. Consider the cultural beliefs and values of clients' households
       ii. Capitalize on existing strengths in clients' interactions with significant others
       iii. Take input from significant others and act upon it
       iv. Embed extension of treatment and maintenance plans in daily routines

Application Exercises

1. Give everyday examples of:
   a. Discrimination
   b. Generalization
   c. Overgeneralization
2. How could a clinician vary stimuli when teaching a client with aphasia to name common objects?
3. A child in first grade is being treated for stuttering. Describe generalization and maintenance strategies for including common social and physical stimuli while teaching fluent speech.
4. Write a target behavior for each of the following clients. Devise a plan for

promoting generalization and maintenance of the target behavior in natural settings.

Name: Joe Smith

Age: 18

Injury: Fell from his skateboard at high speed; scalp lacerations, temporal bone fracture, subdural hemorrhage, and hematoma. Cognitive rehabilitation recommended

Deficits: Poor memory and attention skills; deficits in organization, planning, and impulse control (e.g., tends to blurt out inappropriate comments, including swearing)

Name: Zachary Martin

Age: 12

Diagnosis: High-functioning autism; verbal, with severe pragmatic language deficits, including lack of turn-taking skills, inability to read social cues, no conversational repair, lack of awareness regarding proxemics, and perseveration on one high-interest topic of conversation, namely, Star Trek.

Name: Marisa Lopez

Age: 2.5 years

Diagnosis and Background Information: Marisa has Down syndrome. She resides with her mother, father, and three older siblings. The primary language of the household is Spanish. The family has strong ties to Mexico, has many relatives living there, and makes frequent visits to that country. Marisa knows only six words in

Spanish: *mama, papa, no, leche, agua,* and *gato.* Mr. and Mrs. Lopez work seasonally at a cantaloupe packing plant in the California Central Valley, and resources are limited in the household. However, Mr. and Mrs. Lopez place a very high value on their children's education and work hard to give them opportunities that they themselves never had. They are eager to learn how to support their daughter's speech and language development.

References

Allen, R. I., & Petr, C. G. (1996). Toward developing standards and measurements for family-centered practice in family support programs. In G. H. S. Singer, L. E. Powers, & A. O. Olson (Eds.), *Redefining family support: Innovations in public-private partnerships* (pp. 57–85). Baltimore, MD: Paul H. Brookes.

Baer, D. M. (1999). *How to plan for generalization* (2nd ed.). Austin, TX: Pro-Ed.

Bruce, M. C., DiVenere, N., & Bergeron, C. (1998). Preparing students to understand and honor families as partners. *American Journal of Speech-Language Pathology, 7,* 85–94.

Chance, P. (2006). *First course in applied behavior analysis.* Long Grove, IL: Waveland Press.

Charlop-Christy, M. H., & Carpenter, M. H. (2000). Modified incidental teaching sessions: A procedure for parents to increase spontaneous speech in their children with autism. *Journal of Positive Behavioral Interventions, 2,* 98–112.

Cooper, J. O., Heron, T. E., & Heward, W. L. (2007). *Applied behavior analysis* (2nd ed.). Upper Saddle River, NJ: Pearson Education.

Cosden, M., Koegel, L. K., Koegel, R. L., Greenwell, A., & Klein, E. (2006). Strength-based assessment for children with autism spectrum disorders. *Research and Practice for Persons With Severe Disabilities, 31*(2), 134–143.

Crais, E. R., Roy, V. P., & Free, K. (2006). Parents' and professionals' perceptions of the implementation of family-centered practices in child assessments. *American Journal of Speech-Language Pathology, 15,* 365–377.

DeThorne, L. S., Johnson, C. J., Walder, L., & Mahurin-Smith, J. (2009). When "Simon Says" doesn't work: Alternatives to imitation for facilitating early speech development. *American Journal of Speech-Language Pathology, 18,* 133–145.

Dunst, C. J. (2002). Family-centered practices: Birth through high school. *Journal of Special Education, 36,* 139–147.

Dunst, C. J., Boyd, K., Trivette, C. M., & Hamby, D. W. (2002). Family-oriented program models and professional helpgiving practices. *Family Relations, 51,* 221–229.

Falcomata, T. S., & Wacker, D. P. (2013). On the use of strategies for programming generalization during functional communication training: A review of the literature. *Journal of Developmental and Physical Disabilities, 25,* 5–15.

Finn, P. (2003). Self-regulation and the management of stuttering. *Seminars in Speech and Language, 24,* 27–32.

Hart, B., & Risley, T. R. (1975). Incidental teaching of language in the preschool. *Journal of Applied Behavior Analysis, 8,* 411–420.

Hegde, M. N. (1998). *Treatment procedures in communicative disorders* (3rd ed.). Austin, TX: Pro-Ed.

Johnston, J. R., & Wong, M. Y. A. (2002). Cultural differences in beliefs and practices concerning talk to children. *Journal of Speech, Language, and Hearing Research, 45,* 916–926.

Kashinath, S., Woods, J., & Goldstein, H. (2006). Enhancing generalized teaching strategy use in daily routines by parents of children with autism. *Journal of Speech, Language, and Hearing Research, 49,* 466–485.

Koegel, L. K., Carter, C. M., & Koegel, R. L. (2003). Teaching children with autism self- initiations as a pivotal response. *Topics in Language Disorders, 23*(2), 134–145.

Lucyshyn, J. M., Albin, R. W., Horner, R. H., Mann, J. C., Mann, J. A., & Wadsworth, G. (2007). Family implementation of positive behavior support for a child with autism: Longitudinal, single-case, experimental, and descriptive replication and extension. *Journal of Positive Behavior Interventions, 9,* 131–150.

Lucyshyn, J. M., Albin, R. W., & Nixon, C. D. (1997). Embedding comprehensive behavioral

support in family ecology: An experimental, single-case analysis. *Journal of Consulting and Clinical Psychology, 65,* 241–251.

Maul, C. A. (2015). Working with culturally and linguistically diverse students and their families: Perceptions and practices of school speech-language therapists in the United States. *International Journal of Language and Communication Disorders.* doi:10.1111/1460-6984.12176

Maul, C., & Singer, G. H. S. (2009). "Just good different things": Specific accommodations families make to positively adapt to their children with disabilities. *Topics in Early Childhood Special Education, 29,* 155–170.

Moes, D. R., & Frea, W. D. (2000). Using family context to inform intervention planning for the treatment of a child with autism. *Journal of Positive Behavior Interventions, 2,* 40–46.

Moes, D. R., & Frea, W. D. (2002). Contextualized behavior support in early intervention for children with autism and their families. *Journal of Autism and Developmental Disorders, 23,* 521–534.

Polmanteer, K., & Turbiville, V. (2000). Family-responsive individualized family service plans for speech-language pathologists. *Language, Speech, and Hearing Services in Schools, 31,* 4–14.

Rincover, A., & Koegel, R. (1975). Setting generality and stimulus control in autistic children. *Journal of Applied Behavior Analysis, 8,* 235–246.

Roseberry-McKibbin, C. (2014). *Multicultural students with special language needs: Practical strategies for assessment and intervention* (4th ed.). Oceanside, CA: Academic Communication Associates.

Stokes, T. F., & Baer, D. M. (1977). An implicit technology of generalization. *Journal of Applied Behavior Analysis, 10,* 349–367.

Stokes, T. F., Baer, D. M., & Jackson, R. L. (1974). Programming the generalization of a greeting response in four retarded children. *Journal of Applied Behavior Analysis, 7,* 599–610.

van Kleeck, A. (1994). Potential cultural bias in training parents as conversational partners with their children who have delays in language development. *American Journal of Speech-Language Pathology, 3,* 67–78.

Vaughn, B. J., Clarke, S., & Dunlap, G. (1997). Assessment-based intervention for severe behavior problems in a natural family context. *Journal of Applied Behavior Analysis, 30,* 713–716.

Vaughn, B. J., Wilson, D., & Dunlap, G. (2002). Family-centered intervention to resolve problem behaviors in a fast-food restaurant. *Journal of Positive Behavior Interventions, 4,* 38–45.

Wang, M., McCart, A., & Turnbull, A. (2007). Implementing positive behavior support with Chinese American families: Enhancing cultural competence. *Journal of Positive Behavior Interventions, 9,* 38–51.

Woods, J. J., & Wetherby, A. M. (2003). Early identification of and intervention for infants and toddlers who are at risk for autism spectrum disorder. *Language, Speech, and Hearing Services in Schools, 34,* 180–193.

Woods, J. J., Wilcox, M. J., Friedman, M., & Murch, T. (2011). Collaborative consultation in natural environments: Strategies to enhance family-centered supports and services. *Language, Speech, and Hearing Services in Schools, 42,* 379–392.

CHAPTER 8

Decreasing Undesirable Behaviors

Chapter 6 presented extensive information regarding methods for increasing desirable communicative behaviors. Through the use of antecedent manipulations, shaping, chaining, and reinforcement, speech-language pathologists (SLPs) help their clients develop new and rehabilitate lost speech-language skills. Although the process of strengthening desirable behaviors is a core component of the therapeutic process, it is rarely the only task that clinicians are expected to complete. SLPs are also called upon to help decrease undesirable behaviors exhibited by their clients. This is accomplished through the use of treatment methods that involve making changes to antecedent and consequence events. Several procedures for reducing undesirable behaviors are discussed in this chapter.

> In addition to strengthening desirable communicative skills, SLPs also seek to _____ undesirable forms of verbal behavior.

Types of Undesirable Behavior for Reduction

Undesirable communicative behaviors are the primary responses SLPs attempt to reduce during treatment. Examples of undesirable communicative behaviors include erred production of speech sounds, dysfluencies, aberrant vocal characteristics, answering questions incorrectly, omission of grammatical morphemes, inappropriate syntactic structure, and so forth. Clients may also demonstrate undesirable forms of the various verbal operants (see Chapter 2 for additional information), such as mand behavior in the form of hitting, crying, or screaming, that may need to be addressed. In addition to teaching desired

forms of verbal behavior, clinicians also strive to simultaneously decrease these undesirable communicative responses.

An additional category of responses that clinicians may need to address during treatment is **interfering behaviors** (Hegde, 1998). Interfering behaviors disrupt the provision of speech-language services. Behaviors such as noncompliance, inattention, crying, and off-task responses can affect the client's ability to participate during treatment sessions. Some clients may also engage in **elopement**, defined as attempts to physically leave the therapeutic environment. Examples of elopement include crawling under the table or running out of the clinic room. If present, interfering behaviors often must be addressed prior to teaching use of the desirable target behavior. Adequate compliance and participation are prerequisite skills that facilitate a client's participation in treatment. Therefore, clinicians strive to decrease interfering behaviors in order to support their clients' progress.

Having a solid understanding of the functions of these responses plays a significant role in the clinician's ability to reduce interfering behaviors. Clients frequently engage in interfering behaviors in order to escape or avoid what they perceive as an aversive treatment task. However, a client may also engage in undesirable responses in order to receive the clinician's attention or obtain automatic reinforcement. As the functions of interfering behaviors vary across clients, a formal assessment of the functions of undesirable behaviors is often necessary.

Assessment of Undesirable Behaviors

Recall that behaviors are exhibited due to a history of receiving reinforcement in specific antecedent conditions. Therefore, the behaviors that clients engage in serve specific functions for them. This holds true for most undesirable forms of behavior as well. For example, a client may ask the clinician repetitive, off-topic questions in an attempt to avoid treatment activities. In this case, the client's behavior may be being maintained through negative reinforcement. A child's crying behavior may be positively reinforced if an adult offers that child a variety of preferred items (e.g., toys, snacks, etc.) to calm him or her down. Some clients may engage in self-injurious behavior such as head hitting, hand biting, or eye gouging in order to obtain automatic reinforcement. Clinicians are able to most effectively address undesirable behaviors when they understand the functions of these responses.

Functional behavior assessments (FBAs) can be used to identify the stimuli that maintain undesirable behaviors (see Chapter 4 for additional information on this topic). Should an FBA be conducted, SLPs should work closely with board certified behavior analysts (BCBAs) to identify the maintaining functions of behaviors. Once these functional relationships have been identified, the SLP and BCBA can collaborate to modify the maintaining contingencies and, consequently, reduce the undesirable behavior itself.

Antecedent Interventions

The results of an FBA may indicate that an undesirable behavior is exhibited in specific contexts or situations. In such cases, **antecedent interventions** may be needed in order to help reduce the frequency of the behavior. Antecedent interventions used to reduce undesirable behaviors involve altering the environmental events that occur prior to the response in order to decrease the occurrence of the behavior. Table 8–1 provides examples of specific antecedent interventions for commonly encountered undesirable behaviors. Antecedent interventions frequently used in the field of speech-language pathology include environmental manipulations, noncontingent reinforcement, and high-probability request sequences.

> _____ _____ for undesirable behaviors involve altering the environmental events that occur prior to the response in order to decrease the occurrence of the behavior.

Environmental Manipulations

Environmental manipulations involve antecedent changes made to treatment and/or naturalistic settings that serve to decrease the undesirable behavior. Examples may include removing specific antecedent stimuli that serve as "triggers" for the response. A variety of undesirable speech-language behaviors may be addressed through environmental manipulations. For instance, an individual who exhibits a hoarse, strained-strangled vocal quality (the undesirable behavior) due in part to poor hydration may be instructed to drink more water (the environmental manipulation). Similarly, an SLP may prescribe nectar-thick liquids (the environmental manipulation) for a patient with dysphagia who aspirates (the undesirable behavior) on thin liquids.

Environmental manipulations have applicability to interfering behaviors as well. Antecedent supports such as reduced background noise or room dividers can be used when working with clients who

Table 8–1. Examples of Antecedent Manipulations for Undesirable and Interfering Behaviors

Undesirable or Interfering Behavior	Antecedent Intervention
A client has difficulty interacting with peers during recess.	Social narratives are developed and reviewed with the client to help facilitate socialization.
A child has difficulty complying with the clinician's directions during treatment sessions.	The child is provided choices to select from during treatment sessions (e.g., "Do you want to do the cards or the book?").
An individual who experienced a traumatic brain injury has difficulty completing tasks in an organized manner at work.	A visual task analysis is developed for the individual to use while at work.
The client reaches for the clinician's treatment materials and attempts to play with them without consent.	Treatment materials are placed in a box with a locking lid that the clinician can easily control.
A child has difficulty sitting in his assigned area during whole-group floor time activities.	Colored tape is used to section off the area on the carpet where the child is expected to sit.
A student has difficulty attending to instruction in the classroom.	The student is provided with preferential seating near the teacher.

have difficulty attending to instruction. Similarly, clients who protest during transitions between clinical tasks may benefit from a visual schedule depicting each of the activities they will be expected to complete during the session. Children who are hypersensitive to visual or auditory stimuli may benefit from dimmed lights or quieter treatment settings. Another technique frequently employed by school-based SLPs is strategic grouping. Clinicians may find that the presence of certain other students may evoke undesirable behavior from a child. In such cases, school-based SLPs plan treatment groups to help reduce behaviors that interfere with treatment sessions.

Noncontingent Reinforcement

Noncontingent reinforcement is an antecedent intervention procedure that involves providing time-based reinforcement that is unrelated to the client's responses (Cooper, Heron, & Heward, 2007). Clinicians who utilize this procedure administer reinforcing stimuli on an interval schedule regardless of the behavior exhibited by the client. Noncontingent reinforcement serves to enhance the reinforcing value of the clinical environment, thus making it less likely that the client will engage in an undesirable behavior that serves the same function. This procedure can be used with behaviors that are positively, negatively, or automatically reinforced. For example, a clinician may observe that a client tries to grab her pen and scribble on the table during treatment sessions. After determining that this behavior was being positively reinforced by access to the pen, the clinician may allow the client noncontingent writing time in order to help decrease the client's use of the undesirable behavior. When working with a client who attempts elopement from the clinic setting every 10 to 12 minutes, a clinician may elect to provide a noncontingent break every 8 minutes in an attempt to reduce the need for this potentially negatively reinforced behavior. Similarly, a clinician may observe that a client presses firmly on his eyes every 8 to 10 minutes, presumably in an attempt to obtain automatic visual reinforcement. In such cases, the clinician may allow the client to play with visually stimulating toys, such as pom-poms, tops, or spinning lights, on a noncontingent interval schedule in an attempt to fulfill the same automatic function.

> Noncontingent reinforcement can be used with behaviors that are
> _____, _____, or _____ reinforced.

Noncontingent reinforcement is particularly useful in helping maintain a client's effort during assessment and baseline sessions. As discussed in Chapter 3, statements such as, "You're working so hard," "Thank you for paying attention," or "You are doing just what I need to have you do" can be provided noncontingently to support a client's participation. Such statements make it more likely that the clinician will obtain data that represent the client's true speech-language capabilities

rather than performance that was affected by noncompliance or inattention.

High-Probability Request Sequences

Another antecedent intervention is **high-probability (high-p) request sequences.** High-p request sequences can be used to increase a client's ability to respond to antecedent stimuli appropriately. Also known as behavioral momentum (Mace et al., 1988; Nevin, Mandell, & Atak, 1983), this technique involves presenting several requests that the client is likely to comply with (the high-p requests) prior to introducing the target antecedent stimulus (the low-p request). The high-p requests should be presented in rapid succession, and the responses should be present in the client's behavioral repertoire.

This method is particularly helpful when clients are capable of responding correctly to the clinician's requests; however, they have difficulty with compliance (Davis, Brady, Williams, & Hamilton, 1992). This can be observed when working with clients who are learning to follow functional one-step compliance directions. For example, instead of complying with directions to "come here," "clean up," or "stop playing," a client may respond to the clinician's requests by saying "no." In such instances, the clinician may rapidly present several high-p requests (e.g., "clap hands," "get the car," "put it in," etc.) prior to introducing the low-p request (e.g., "clean up"). Introducing such high-p requests may help facilitate the client's compliance with the target low-p request.

High-p request sequences can also be used when working with adult clients. For example, clinicians can use this technique to help facilitate the word-finding skills of individuals with aphasia. Clinicians can present several high-p requests (e.g., "look at me," "say _____," etc.) prior to presenting a more challenging confrontation naming task (i.e., the low-p request). Presenting antecedent stimuli in this sequence can sometimes help facilitate more fluent responses from the client.

A Clinical Definition of Punishment

The previous sections discussed various antecedent based interventions that can be used to reduce undesirable behaviors. The prevalence of such responses can also be decreased through the manipulation of consequence stimuli. **Punishment** is the process of manipulating consequences contingent upon a behavior that serves to decrease its future occurrence. This definition varies somewhat from the traditional view of punishment, which suggests the infliction of physical pain, restraint, harsh reprimands, and so forth. This dichotomy between the clinical and popular definitions of punishment has led to confusion and concern surrounding the use of this treatment method. This lack of clarity has been further multiplied due to confusion regarding the differences in the definitions of negative reinforcement and punishment. Although these terms sound similar, clinicians must remember that negative reinforcement serves to increase the frequency of a behavior while punishment decreases response rates. Although SLPs prefer to rely on the use of reinforcement techniques during treatment, clinical applications of punishment can play a key role in reducing undesirable communicative and interfering behaviors. Figure 8–1 presents a summary of various clinically applicable types of punishment.

_____ is the process of manipulating consequences contingent upon a behavior that serve to decrease its future occurrence.

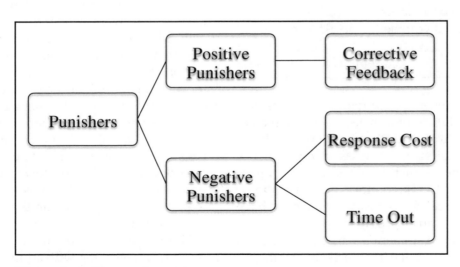

Figure 8–1. Types of punishers.

Positive Punishment

Positive punishment involves the presentation of consequence stimuli contingent upon a behavior that serves to decrease its future occurrence. Therefore, when using positive punishment, clinicians are adding a stimulus as a consequence in order to decrease the frequency of a given behavior. Early research studies within the field of speech-language pathology used more aversive forms of positive punishment, such as loud noises (Brookshire, 1969) or electric shock (Marshall, 1970), to reduce undesirable communicative behaviors. As the field has progressed, clear ethical concerns have caused clinicians to abandon such practices for less aversive punishment procedures. Today, corrective feedback is the primary form of positive punishment that clinicians use.

Corrective Feedback

Corrective feedback involves providing clients with information that describes why a response was in error. Corrective feedback is consistent with positive punishment because it involves adding something to the environment (i.e., the clinician's corrective feedback) in order to facilitate a reduction in the client's response. Clinicians use statements such as "no" or "incorrect" to signal to clients when they fail to use a target behavior correctly. For example, Quist and Martin (1967) found that providing a response-contingent "wrong" resulted in decreased frequency of stuttering across the three participants included in their study. When made contingent upon incorrect responses, corrective feedback can serve as a positive punisher that results in a decrease in the frequency of an undesirable behavior.

> involves providing clients with information that suggests an incorrect response was in error.

According to Hegde (1998), corrective feedback can be verbal, nonverbal, or mechanical in nature. Verbal corrective feedback includes the examples discussed in the previous paragraph. Additional examples of verbal corrective feedback include "that's not right," "you need to try again," and so forth. When providing verbal corrective feedback, it is beneficial to be as specific as possible regarding the nature of the client's incorrect response. For instance, when a child produces the word *tat* in response to a picture of a cat, the clinician may state, "Oh no, you didn't get your tongue to the back to say 'cat.' Try again." Such feedback helps clients understand the specific component of their behavior that needs to change in order to obtain reinforcement. By making corrective feedback unambiguous, clinicians increase the likelihood that their corrective feedback will serve not only as a positive punisher but also as a prompt for improved performance in subsequent trials.

Corrective feedback can also be provided via nonverbal means. A common example of nonverbal corrective feedback is when parents give their children "the look" when they misbehave in public. Similar nonverbal gestures such as shaking the head, lowering the eyebrows, or holding up a hand can be used as positive punishment during treatment sessions as well. Nonverbal corrective feedback may not be effective for clients who struggle with eye contact or have difficulty attending to their conversational partners. In such cases, nonverbal gestures are paired with verbal corrective feedback in order to help decrease undesirable behaviors.

Finally, mechanical methods can be used to provide corrective feedback for incorrect responses. Advances in technology have made the use of biofeedback more feasible for clinicians. Electropalatography can be used to provide clients with objective feedback regarding articulatory placement. Nasometry can be used with clients who have a history of cleft palate to reduce hypernasality. Similarly, sound level meters can help individuals with voice disorders decrease their intensity levels. Various apps have also been developed that clinicians can use to provide mechanical feedback to their clients. Although mechanical measurement devices can be expensive and difficult to maintain, biofeedback provides objective measures of behavior that can be used as positive punishment for some clients.

Negative Punishment

Undesirable behaviors can also be reduced through stimulus removal. **Negative punishment** is the process of removing a desirable stimulus in order to decrease the frequency of a behavior. Forms of negative punishment used in society include loss of privileges, fines, and incarceration. Within the field of speech-language pathology, the primary forms of negative punishment that clinicians use are response cost and time-out procedures.

Response Cost

Response cost is a negative punishment procedure that involves the removal of reinforcers contingent upon a behavior. This stimulus removal then serves to decrease the future frequency of the

undesirable behavior. Each instance of the undesirable behavior "costs the client a reinforcer" (Hegde, 1998, p. 226). For example, an individual who is trying to stop swearing may be expected to put a dollar in a glass jar each time a swear word is uttered. A child who has difficulty participating in class may lose 1 minute of recess every time she is out of her seat during instruction.

In order to use response cost effectively, the client must already have access to a bank of reinforcers. This is typically best facilitated through the use of generalized conditioned reinforcers, such as tokens, points, money, and so forth (see Chapter 6 for additional information regarding generalized conditioned reinforcement). In the previous example, instances of swearing could not be reduced if the individual did not have money available to put in the jar. Similarly, the child's out-of-seat behavior would be unlikely to decrease if there were no minutes of recess left to take away. Therefore, when using this technique during treatment, clinicians ensure that their clients are able to accumulate a number of reinforcers prior to implementing a response cost procedure.

In terms of its direct application to undesirable communicative behaviors, the majority of research on response cost as a treatment technique has been conducted in the field of fluency disorders (Bloodstein & Bernstein Ratner, 2008; Halvorson, 1971). For example, a clinician may provide a child who stutters with a token following every smooth utterance (i.e., positive reinforcement). Then, each time the client engages in a dysfluency (e.g., a part word repetition, sound prolongation, phrase interjection, broken word, etc.), a token would be removed (i.e., the response cost). If the client's dysfluency rate decreased over the course of treatment, the use of response cost acted as a negative punisher that resulted in a reduction of the frequency of the undesirable communicative behavior.

Time-Out

Whereas response cost procedures result in the removal of a previously earned reinforcer contingent upon a response, **time-out** involves terminating an individual's ability to earn positive reinforcement for a set time period following an undesirable behavior. For example, a child who hits his sibling while watching television may be sent to his room for 5 minutes. Although there is temporal separation between the behavior and resulting consequence, the concept of time-out applies to individuals convicted of crimes who have to serve prison sentences as well.

> _____ is a negative punishment technique that involves terminating an individual's ability to earn positive reinforcement for a set time period.

As is the case with response cost, the majority of the research conducted on applications of time-out to communicative disorders has centered on dysfluency (Bloodstein & Bernstein Ratner, 2008; Costello, 1975; Onslow, Packman, Stocker, van Doorn, & Siegel, 1997). Use of time-out for stuttering involves clinicians removing their attention from the client contingent upon instances of dysfluency. Following dysfluencies, a clinician may instruct the client to stop, turn away and break eye contact with the client, and ensure that reinforcement is not provided for a short period (typically no

longer than 5 seconds). After the time-out period has been completed, eye contact is reestablished, and the client and clinician continue with their conversation. This example constitutes negative punishment because the clinician removes her attention from the client to decrease the overall rate of dysfluency.

Several details must be thoughtfully considered when using time-out. In order to use this method effectively, the "time in" environment must be reinforcing. Therefore, using time-out is not effective for behaviors that are maintained by escape or avoidance. If time-out is used for behaviors that have this function, the client will be positively reinforced, and the undesirable behavior will be maintained. Furthermore, there should be no opportunities to access reinforcement in the time-out setting. Parents who send their children to their room for a time-out may be surprised to observe increased instances of the undesirable behavior. This may occur because the child has free access to a variety of positive reinforcers, such as toys, books, games, television sets, computers, and so forth, in their room. Finally, the duration of time-out should be brief. It is important to remember that time-out is not used for retribution or vengeance. Rather, it is a clinical technique that should be used conscientiously.

Possible Side Effects of Punishment

In addition to the moral objections previously discussed, punishment can result in several undesirable side effects. Some clients may be sensitive to punishing stimuli. In such cases, the use of punishment may evoke emotional responses such as fear or anger from the client. If punishment is being used exclusively, the clinician and/or treatment setting may become a conditioned punisher. If this occurs, the client may engage in further undesirable behaviors in an attempt to avoid or escape treatment sessions. In order to prevent these undesirable side effects, clinicians must consider the characteristics of their individual clients and ensure that adequate opportunities for reinforcement are available during therapy.

Guidelines for Using Punishment

Although many individuals, including behaviorists, find punishment objectionable, it can be used appropriately when several guidelines are followed. First, clinicians must determine whether or not the behavior can be addressed using less aversive techniques such as extinction or differential reinforcement (both topics are discussed in greater detail later in this chapter). Similarly, if punishment procedures are deemed necessary, clinicians should use the mildest effective punisher possible. For example, in most cases, corrective feedback can adequately reduce undesirable communicative behaviors without the need for harsh reprimands or extended time-outs. As with all consequence-based treatment methods, clinicians should ensure that punishers are administered immediately after an undesirable response. If the punisher is not provided contingently, it is unlikely to have any measurable effect on the target behavior. Finally, clinicians must remember that a stimulus can only be considered a punisher if it results in a decrease in the client's use of a specific behavior. As is the case with reinforcers, the punishing value of a stimulus is not determined by subjective feelings. Clinicians must consult the collected data to determine if an undesirable response decreases with the introduction of positive or negative punishment. If a decrease in the data is not indicated, the stimulus is not serving as a punisher.

Extinction

Punishment is not the only method by which response rates can be reduced. Because all behaviors serve specific functions for clients, withholding the consequences that reinforce undesirable behaviors can help reduce their frequency. This procedure is known as **extinction**. If the clinician arranges the environment so that the behavior no longer pays off, the client is less likely to engage in the undesirable response. Table 8–2 provides examples of how positively, negatively, and automatically reinforced behaviors can be subjected to extinction.

> Withholding the consequences that reinforce undesirable behaviors to reduce their frequency is called _____.

In order to use extinction effectively, clinicians must understand the function the undesirable behavior serves for the client. This is accomplished through collaboration with BCBAs who conduct FBAs to help determine the functions or behavior (see Chapter 4 for additional information on this topic). A common misconception is that extinction is simply planned ignoring. Although many undesirable behaviors are exhibited in order to obtain attention, it is possible that the

Table 8–2. Extinction of Positively, Negatively, and Automatically Reinforced Behaviors

Positively reinforced behavior	A preschool-aged client cries during treatment sessions and repeatedly asks for her mother. Whenever this happens, the mother comes into the clinic room to console the child. The client's crying appears to be maintained by her mother's attention. In order to put this behavior on extinction, the clinician meets with the client's mother to discuss that she should not positively reinforce the crying behavior by coming into the clinic room.
Negatively reinforced behavior	An adult client asks repeated off-topic questions during therapy sessions in order to avoid treatment activities. In order to put this behavior on extinction, the clinician continues presenting treatment activities when the client asks off-topic questions, thus preventing the behavior from being negatively reinforced by avoidance.
Automatically reinforced behavior	A client forcefully bangs his head on the table during treatment sessions in order to obtain sensory feedback. The clinician places a foam cover over the table in order to put this automatically reinforced behavior on extinction.

client's behavior could have a different function. Consider the following example:

A student yells at her teacher each time she is presented with a math worksheet. The teacher assumes the function of the behavior is attention and decides to use planned ignoring to address the yelling. Each time the student yells, the teacher ignores the behavior but does not require the student to complete the math worksheet. Over time, the teacher realizes that an increase in yelling behavior is being observed. The teacher calls in a BCBA who works at the school who conducts an FBA that suggests the yelling behavior is being maintained through negative reinforcement by escape from nonpreferred tasks (i.e., completing the math worksheet). A new extinction procedure is then applied in which the student is required to complete the math worksheet, regardless if yelling is exhibited or not. Over time, the student's yelling behavior decreases.

This example illustrates the importance of knowing a behavior's function prior to implementing an extinction procedure. If the function is not known, extinction may not serve to decrease the frequency of the undesirable behavior.

Even when the function of the behavior is known, several problems may arise while using extinction. During the initial stages of using extinction, clinicians may observe a sudden increase in the client's use of an undesirable response. This is known as **extinction burst**, which is a commonly occurring phenomenon. A person who has been greatly reinforced in the past through access to attention or escape from a task for an undesirable behavior will not easily give that behavior up; therefore, it is highly likely that the behavior will escalate until it finally decreases as a result of the successful application of the extinction procedure. The extinction burst is especially likely when an undesirable behavior has been reinforced lavishly over a long period of time on an intermittent schedule of reinforcement. For example, if a 5-year-old child's tantrum behavior has been reinforced since the child was 2 years old by the parent picking the child up, walking around, generally fussing over the child, and giving the child whatever he wants, then the child is likely to display a fierce extinction burst when the parent begins to ignore the tantrum behavior. If the behavior has received such reinforcement intermittently (e.g., sometimes the parent pays much attention to it, and sometimes the parent does not), the extinction burst is likely to be more extreme, because the child does not know when tantrums will be reinforced and will keep escalating that behavior, hoping for the intermittent payoff. Although it seems paradoxical, an undesirable behavior that has been continuously reinforced will be easier to extinguish because the person performing that behavior will notice right away when it no longer results in reinforcement. In any event, once an extinction procedure has been put into effect, it must be applied consistently, even when the extinction burst occurs. Otherwise, the person simply learns the level at which the targeted undesirable behavior must be exhibited in order to receive reinforcement.

Clinically, SLPs must also ensure that uncontrolled reinforcement is not being provided for the behavior in other settings (e.g., the classroom, home, etc.) as this can affect the success of using extinction during treatment. Although complications may occur, they are not significant threats as long as the extinction procedure is followed with accuracy. SLPs should plan for these complications and inform all relevant parties from the onset of treatment that they may occur. A final caution is that extinction should not be used for behaviors that may cause the client or others physical harm. For example, behaviors such as head banging, chair throwing, or eye gouging pose significant risk to the client if they are not addressed directly. Therefore, extinction is not recommended in such cases.

Differential Reinforcement

Although punishment and extinction can be used to decrease undesirable behaviors, they have minimal impact in helping the client develop more appropriate responses. Therefore, there is a need for further procedures that will provide positive behavior support (Zurawski, 2015) to increase appropriate responses while simultaneously reducing their undesirable counterparts. **Differential reinforcement** is a treatment method that helps address this area of need.

Differential reinforcement is a treatment method that involves placing one behavior on extinction while concurrently providing reinforcement for another. Therefore, differential reinforcement serves to decrease one behavior while, at the same time, increasing another. SLPs use differential reinforcement to strengthen desirable communicative behaviors while decreasing undesirable responses.

> When using differential reinforcement, one behavior is placed on _____ while the other is _____.

The four primary methods of differential reinforcement (Table 8–3) used by SLPs include:

1. Differential reinforcement of other behaviors
2. Differential reinforcement of low rates of responding
3. Differential reinforcement of incompatible behaviors
4. Differential reinforcement of alternative behaviors

Differential Reinforcement of Other Behaviors (DRO)

Differential reinforcement of other behaviors (DRO) involves placing an undesirable response on extinction while reinforcing all other behaviors. Therefore, reinforcement is essentially provided for not engaging in the undesirable behavior (Cooper et al., 2007). When using DRO, the clinician defines the undesirable behavior in objective terms and then withholds reinforcement from that specific response. All other behaviors exhibited by the client are then reinforced. These behaviors are typically unspecified and represent a wide variety of responses. For example, when working with a client who crawls under the table for attention, the clinician may choose to ignore this behavior while providing attention for a variety of other desirable responses whenever that behavior is not occurring (e.g., making eye contact, sitting down, answering questions, looking at treatment materials, etc.). DRO can be particularly helpful when addressing behaviors that interfere with the client's ability to successfully participate

Table 8–3. Differential Reinforcement Techniques

Differential Reinforcement of Other Behaviors	Differential Reinforcement of Low Rates of Responding
• Involves placing an undesirable response on extinction while reinforcing all other behaviors • The undesirable behavior is defined in objective terms • The reinforced behaviors are typically unspecified and represent a wide variety of responses	• Involves providing reinforcement contingent on the client exhibiting the undesirable response at a lower rate • Can be used to shape down the frequency or intensity of a response
Differential Reinforcement of Incompatible Behaviors	**Differential Reinforcement of Alternative Behaviors**
• Involves placing an undesirable response on extinction while reinforcing an incompatible behavior • The selected incompatible response cannot be produced at the same time as the undesirable behavior	• Involves putting the undesirable behavior on extinction and reinforcing a defined alternative behavior that serves the same function

during treatment services. Examples of such behaviors include inattention, yelling, off-topic questions, and so forth.

When using DRO during treatment, clinicians should not inadvertently reinforce other undesirable behaviors the client may exhibit. This has the potential to occur because, although the undesirable response is identified, the behaviors that receive reinforcement are not clearly defined. For instance, a clinician who uses DRO to address out-of-seat behavior may provide reinforcement once the client has stayed seated for 5 minutes. However, although the child was sitting, he may have engaged in other undesirable behaviors, such as throwing treatment materials or aggression toward the clinician (Hegde, 1998). If this problem arises, clinicians must ensure that each of the undesirable behaviors observed is clearly defined and put on extinction.

Differential Reinforcement of Low Rates of Responding (DRL)

Occasionally, it may not be feasible to place an undesirable behavior on extinction. This is particularly true when a client exhibits an undesirable response with great frequency. In such cases, the clinician can reduce the overall rate of the behavior in a stepwise fashion. **Differential reinforcement of low rates of responding (DRL)** involves providing reinforcement contingent on the client exhibiting the undesirable response at a lower rate. Therefore, DRL can be used to shape down the frequency or intensity of a response. For example, DRL may be used to help individuals with voice disorders decrease their vocal intensity. In the initial stages of treatment, clients may be rein-

forced for a vocal intensity that is slightly lower than their habitual loudness level (e.g., 80 dB). As treatment progresses, reinforcement would only be provided for progressively more appropriate intensity levels (e.g., 75 dB to 70 dB to 65 dB and so forth. In addition to addressing undesirable communicative behaviors, DRL can also be used to address interfering behaviors, such as repetitive requests (Austin & Bevan, 2011) or responses (Handen, Apolito, & Seltzer, 1984) that affect the provision of treatment.

Differential Reinforcement of Incompatible Behaviors (DRI)

Like DRO, **differential reinforcement of incompatible behaviors (DRI)** also involves placing undesirable behaviors on extinction; however, the responses that receive reinforcement during DRI cannot be produced at the same time as the undesirable behavior. Therefore, the reinforced responses are said to be incompatible with the undesirable behavior. Examples of incompatible behaviors include sitting and standing, silence and verbalizing, making eye contact and looking around the room, and so forth. In order to use DRI effectively, clinicians must objectively define both the undesirable behavior and the incompatible response.

Although the previously discussed examples focused on responses that were incompatible with interfering behaviors, DRI also has broad applicability in addressing undesirable communicative behaviors. Because clients cannot simultaneously produce correct and incorrect forms of speech-language skills, DRI can be used to increase desirable verbal responses while also reducing undesirable communicative behaviors. DRI is a core component of fluency shaping techniques used to address stuttering. By teaching responses that are incompatible with the act of stuttering, such as easy onset of phonation, reduced rate of speech, or light articulatory contacts, SLPs can help clients reduce their overall rate of dysfluency (Bloodstein & Bernstein Ratner, 2008; Wagaman, Miltenberger, & Arndorfer, 1993).

Differential Reinforcement of Alternative Behaviors (DRA)

Clients may exhibit undesirable behaviors because they have not been taught to use socially acceptable responses that serve the same function (Hegde, 1998). In such cases, **differential reinforcement of alternative behaviors (DRA)** can be used. DRA involves putting the undesirable behavior on extinction and reinforcing a defined alternative behavior that serves the same function. This contrasts with DRI in that the alternative behavior is not necessarily incompatible with the undesirable response. For example, a child who engages in elopement to escape tabletop activities may be taught to ask for a break instead. Although elopement and asking for a break are not incompatible behaviors, they could serve the same function for the child. The difference between DRA and DRO is that in DRA, the alternative response must be clearly defined, whereas in DRO, other reinforced behaviors remain unspecified.

Clinicians follow several rules when using DRA. These guidelines apply to the selection of incompatible responses in DRI as well. In choosing an alternative response to reinforce, the clinician must first ensure that the behavior is present in the client's repertoire. For example, clinicians would not expect nonverbal or minimally verbal clients to say, "I need a break" when addressing elopement via DRA. Instead, behaviors consistent with the client's current level of functioning, such as pointing to a time away area or exchanging a break card, would be used. Accordingly, the alternative response should also be easier for the client to perform than the undesirable behavior. Finally, the alternative behavior should allow the client to contact reinforcement more quickly and consistently than the undesirable response. When these guidelines are followed, the clinician increases the likelihood that the client will adopt the alternative response rather than continue using the undesirable behavior.

Clinicians should select alternative and incompatible responses that:

1. Are present in the client's
   _____

2. Are _____ for the client to perform than the undesirable behavior

3. Allow the client to contact reinforcement more _____ and _____ than the undesired response

---

Differential Reinforcement and Positive Behavior Support

Techniques involving differential reinforcement are the cornerstone of an approach to reducing undesirable behaviors called **positive behavior support**, which has been defined as "a set of research-based strategies used to increase quality of life and decrease problem behavior by teaching new skills and making changes in a person's environment" (Association for Positive Behavior Support, n.d.). The approach rejects the use of punishment and has wide applicability to all types of undesirable behavior exhibited by any person in any setting, including in the SLP's clinic room.

Functional Communication Training

Functional communication training (FCT) is a specific type of DRA that involves teaching the use of communicative responses that serve the same function as the undesirable behavior. FCT has a broad research base (Brown et al., 2000; Carr & Durand, 1985; Frea & Hughes, 1997; Tiger, Hanley, & Bruzek, 2008; Worsdell, Iwata, Hanley, Thompson, & Kahng, 2000) and has been used to address a variety of undesirable responses. Figure 8–2 presents a summary of the primary steps involved in FCT.

> Functional communication training (FCT) is a specific type of _____ that involves teaching the use of communicative responses that serve the same function as the undesirable behavior.

FCT starts with developing an objective definition of the undesirable behavior. After this definition is developed, an FBA is performed to identify the function of the undesirable behavior. As previously discussed, this step is completed by BCBAs who have training and experience in conducting FBAs. Although carrying out formal FBAs is outside of an SLP's scope of practice, clinicians may consult with BCBAs to identify specific antecedent situations in which the behavior occurs. BCBAs may also call upon SLPs to collect data on behaviors that occur during speech-language sessions.

Once the BCBA analyzes the FBA data and determines the stimuli that are maintaining the behavior, SLPs and BCBAs can collaborate to develop an alternative

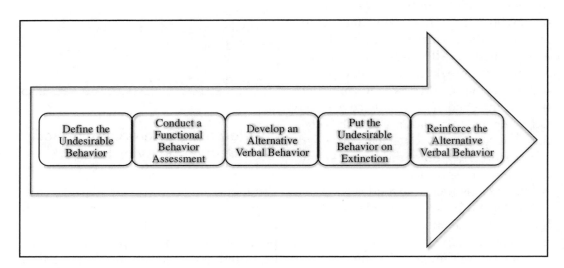

Define the Undesirable Behavior → Conduct a Functional Behavior Assessment → Develop an Alternative Verbal Behavior → Put the Undesirable Behavior on Extinction → Reinforce the Alternative Verbal Behavior

Figure 8–2. Functional communication training.

response that serves the same function as the undesirable behavior. SLPs play a key role in selecting and defining the alternative behavior to be used during FCT. Although BCBAs are experts in the field of behavior, they typically do not have extensive background in speech-language development. As a result, SLPs can be particularly effective in helping define the selected alternative verbal behavior based on their knowledge of communication development and the client's current functional level. Table 8–4 provides examples of various alternative communicative responses that can be used during FCT.

The verbal responses selected during FCT must also follow the guidelines outlined for defining alternative or incompatible behaviors. Clinicians must make sure that engaging in the alternative communicative behavior is within the client's behavioral repertoire. This helps ensure that the verbal response will not require more effort to perform than the current undesirable behavior. Furthermore, clini-

cians should make certain that the selected verbal response will result in consistent reinforcement that is provided in a time-efficient manner. For example, if a child is being taught to use sign language to request food items instead of exhibiting tantrum behavior when hungry, the clinician should instruct all relevant people in the client's life in the meaning of these signs so that they can be reinforced across settings. This consistency will help support the generalization of the verbal response.

The next step in FCT is to put the undesirable behavior on extinction. Clinicians use the results of the FBA in order to make sure that the undesirable behavior is not being reinforced. For example, if the FBA demonstrated that the client engaged in aggression to obtain attention, the clinician would not provide attention contingent upon instances of aggression. Similarly, if the client throws treatment materials in an attempt to escape clinical activities, the clinician would continue presenting antecedent stimuli and not

Table 8–4. Examples of Alternative Responses During Functional Communication Training

Undesirable Behavior	Function	Alternative Verbal Response
The client hits peers in order to get their attention.	Attention from peers	The client is taught to request the attention of peers by verbalizing their names.
The client elopes from her desk during extended academic tasks.	Escape nonpreferred tasks	The client is taught to say "all done" in order to escape nonpreferred tasks.
The client climbs up on a chair to access toys placed on a high shelf.	Access to preferred toys	The client is taught to point to preferred toys in order to gain access to them.
During snack time, the client yells when he wants more food.	Access to food items	The client is taught to sign "more" in order to access additional food.

allow the client to get out of participating in treatment activities contingent upon the undesirable behavior.

The final step of FCT involves transferring reinforcement from the undesirable response to the alternative verbal behavior. The provided reinforcer should be consistent with the function of the behavior documented during the FBA. For the client who engaged in aggression for attention, reinforcement may be transferred to verbal responses such as "Look" or "Watch" that serve to gain the clinician's attention. In the example of the client who threw treatment materials in order to escape clinical activities, the client may be taught a more socially acceptable way to ask for a break, such as just saying, "I need a break," or, in the case of a nonverbal individual, exchanging a card with an icon indicating a break is needed. These are more socially acceptable responses that should receive continuous negative reinforcement when being established, by allowing the client to escape from therapeutic trials for a short amount of time. However, there is a possibility the client may overuse these new communicative skills to request more and more time away from therapeutic tasks. In that case, the clinician should require the client to perform a specified amount of work before being allowed to take a break. A "wait" card or some other signal can indicate to the client that he needs to work a bit more before his request for a break is reinforced.

Chapter Summary

1. SLPs attempt to decrease undesirable communicative and interfering behaviors during treatment.

2. Assessment of undesirable behaviors is important because it can identify possible functions of the responses.

3. Antecedent interventions involve altering the environmental events that occur prior to the response in order to decrease the occurrence of the behavior. Frequently used antecedent interventions for undesirable behaviors include environmental manipulations, noncontingent reinforcement, and high-probability request sequences.

4. Punishment involves presenting or removing a stimulus contingent upon a behavior that serves to decrease its future occurrence.

5. There is often confusion between the clinical and popular definitions of punishment. Punishment and negative reinforcement are frequently confused as well.

6. Positive punishment involves the presentation of consequence stimuli contingent upon a behavior that serves to decrease its future occurrence. Corrective feedback is the primary form of positive punishment used by SLPs.

7. Negative punishment is the process of removing a desirable stimulus in order to decrease the frequency of a behavior. Examples of negative punishment procedures include response cost and time-out.

8. Punishment may be associated with several undesirable side effects that clinicians must guard against during treatment.

9. When using punishment, the least aversive effective technique should be used immediately following the client's behavior.

10. A stimulus is only a punisher if it results in a decrease in the frequency of the undesirable behavior.

11. Extinction involves withholding the consequence stimuli that maintain a response.
12. Differential reinforcement is a treatment method that involves placing one behavior on extinction while concurrently providing reinforcement for another.
13. The primary methods of differential reinforcement include:
    a. Differential reinforcement of other behaviors
    b. Differential reinforcement of low rates of responding
    c. Differential reinforcement of incompatible behaviors
    d. Differential reinforcement of alternative behaviors
14. Functional communication training is a specific type of differential reinforcement of alternative behaviors that involves defining the undesirable behavior, determining the function of the undesirable behavior through a functional behavior assessment, defining an alternative verbal response, putting the undesirable behavior on extinction, and providing reinforcement for the alternative verbal behavior.

Application Exercises

1. Jackson is a 4-year-old preschool student who has difficulty participating in and transitioning between academic centers. During instruction, his teacher reports that he is easily distracted by what is happening in other areas of the classroom. When it is time to transition, Jackson runs around the room and protests going to his next center activity. Discuss antecedent interventions that could be used to decrease these interfering behaviors.
2. Give examples of how corrective feedback could be provided for the following responses:
    a. During storybook reading, a child says, "He is walk" when asked, "What is the boy doing?"
    b. A student says "wed" when shown the written word *red*.
    c. When asked, "Where do you go to school?" the client says, "To learn."
    d. A patient who exhibits left visual field neglect reads "wing" when shown the word *drawing*.
3. Discuss the reason why using extinction to address undesirable behaviors with unknown functions is not recommended.
4. How could you use differential reinforcement to address the interfering behaviors listed below:
    a. Asking off-topic questions
    b. Crawling under the table
    c. Jumping up and down on a chair
    d. Throwing the clinician's treatment materials
5. Given the undesirable behaviors and corresponding functions listed below, develop alternative verbal responses that could be used during FCT:
    a. Hitting peers in order to gain their attention
    b. Yelling in order to request specific food items while grocery shopping
    c. Crying in order to protest separation from parents when dropped off at preschool
    d. Turning over desks, tables, and chairs in order to escape nonpreferred academic tasks

References

Association for Positive Behavior Support. (n.d.). *What is positive behavior support?* Retrieved May 6, 2015, from http://www.apbs.org/new_apbs/genIntro.aspx#definition

Austin, J. L., & Bevan, D. (2011). Using differential reinforcement of low rates to reduce children's requests for teacher attention. *Journal of Applied Behavior Analysis, 44*(3), 451–461.

Bloodstein, O., & Bernstein Ratner, N. (2008). *A handbook in stuttering* (6th ed.). Clifton Park, NY: Delmar Cengage Learning.

Brookshire, R. H. (1969). Effects of random and response contingent noise upon disfluencies of normal speakers. *Journal of Speech, Language, and Hearing Research, 12,* 126–134.

Brown, K. A., Wacker, D. P., Derby, K. M., Peck, S. M., Richman, D. M., Sasso, G. M., . . . Harding, J. W. (2000). Evaluating the effects of functional communication training in the presence and absence of establishing operations. *Journal of Applied Behavior Analysis, 33*(1), 53–71.

Carr, E. G., & Durand, V. M. (1985). Reducing behavior problems through functional communication training. *Journal of Applied Behavior Analysis, 18*(2), 111–126.

Costello, J. M. (1975). The establishment of fluency with time-out procedures: Three case studies. *Journal of Speech and Hearing Disorders, 40,* 216–231.

Cooper, J. O., Heron, T. E., & Heward, W. L. (2007). *Applied behavior analysis* (2nd ed.). Upper Saddle River, NJ: Pearson Education.

Davis, C. A., Brady, M. P., Williams, R. E., & Hamilton, R. E. (1992). Effects of high-probability requests on the acquisition and generalization of responses to requests in young-children with behavior disorders. *Journal of Applied Behavior Analysis, 25*(4), 905–916.

Frea, W. D., & Hughes, C. (1997). Functional analysis and treatment of social-communicative behavior of adolescents with developmental disabilities. *Journal of Applied Behavior Analysis, 30*(4), 701–704.

Halvorson, J. A. (1971). The effects on stuttering frequency of pairing punishment (response cost) with reinforcement. *Journal of Speech and Hearing Research, 14*(2), 356–364.

Handen, B. L., Apolito, P. M., & Seltzer, G. B. (1984). Use of differential reinforcement of low rates of behavior to decrease repetitive speech in an autistic adolescent. *Journal of Behavior Therapy and Experimental Psychiatry, 15*(4), 359–364.

Hegde, M. N. (1998). *Treatment procedures in communicative disorders* (3rd ed.). Austin, TX: Pro-Ed.

Mace, F. C., Hock, M. L., Lalli, J. S., West, B. J., Belfiore, P., Pinter, E., & Brown, D. K. (1988). Behavioral momentum in the treatment of noncompliance. *Journal of Applied Behavior Analysis, 21*(2), 123–141.

Marshall, R. C. (1970). The effects of response contingent punishment upon a defective articulation response. *Journal of Speech and Hearing Disorders, 35*(3), 236–240.

Nevin, J. A., Mandell, C., & Atak, J. R. (1983). The analysis of behavioral momentum. *Journal of the Experimental Analysis of Behavior, 39,* 49–59.

Onslow, M., Packman, A., Stocker, S., van Doorn, J., & Siegel, G. M. (1997). Control of children's stuttering with response-contingent time-out: Behavioral, perceptual, and acoustic data. *Journal of Speech, Language, and Hearing Research, 40*(1), 121–133.

Quist, R. W., & Martin, R. R. (1967). The effect of response contingent verbal punishment on stuttering. *Journal of Speech and Hearing Research, 10*(4), 795–800.

Tiger, J. H., Hanley, G. P., & Bruzek, J. (2008). Functional communication training: A review and practical guide. *Behavior Analysis in Practice, 1*(1), 16–23.

Wagaman, J. R., Miltenberger, R. G., & Arndorfer, R. E. (1993). Analysis of a simplified treatment for stuttering in children. *Journal of Applied Behavior Analysis, 26*(1), 53–61.

Worsdell, A. S., Iwata, B. A., Hanley, G. P., Thompson, R. H., & Kahng, S. W. (2000). Effects of continuous and intermittent reinforcement for problem behavior during functional communication training. *Journal of Applied Behavior Analysis, 33*(2), 167–179.

Zurawski, L. (2015). Utilizing positive behavioral interventions and supports to reinforce therapeutic practices in the schools. *Perspectives on School-Based Issues, 16,* 4–10.

CHAPTER 9

Establishing the Evidence Base: Single-Case Experimental Designs

Chapter Outline

- What Is Science?
  - A Philosophy
  - A Disposition
  - A Set of Methods
- Formulating a Research Question
- Scientific Experimentation Versus Routine Clinical Work
- Characteristics of Single-Case Research Designs
  - Participant Selection
  - Data Collection and Analysis
  - Establishment of Experimental Control
- Types of Single-Case Research Designs
  - ABA Withdrawal or Reversal
  - ABAB Withdrawal or Reversal
  - Multiple Baseline Research Designs
    - Multiple Baseline Across Participants
    - Multiple Baseline Across Behaviors
    - Multiple Baseline Across Settings
  - Alternating Treatments Research Design
- External Validity in Single-Case Research

Throughout this textbook, behavioral principles have been described as evidence based, without much explanation regarding the process by which that evidence base was established. In this chapter, basic scientific concepts are discussed, followed by a description of specific research designs that have been employed to investigate the efficacy of treatment methods based on behavioral principles.

What Is Science?

The origin of the word **science** is the Latin word *scientia*, meaning knowledge; science is therefore the process through which a body of knowledge is created. Science can be explained in terms of the behavior of scientists who act according to a certain philosophy, display characteristics of a certain disposition, and follow a set of procedures that are referred to as the **scientific method**.

A Philosophy

In Chapter 1, the concepts of **determinism** and **empiricism** were described as foundational to the science of behaviorism; those philosophical concepts are in fact foundational to science, in general. Scientists in all fields believe nothing happens without a cause, consistent with determinism, and they also believe those causes can best be discovered by the examination of phenomena through sensory experience, consistent with empiricism. Those phenomena that can be directly observed and measured are suitable for scientific exploration.

A Disposition

An individual's disposition consists of personal qualities that are cultivated through his or her learning history. Accordingly, scientists develop certain character traits and beliefs based on their experiences in the field of experimentation. As a result of these experiences, scientists display personal characteristics that are consistent with the scientific disposition, which include the qualities of neutrality, objectivity, and skepticism. A position of **neutrality** requires scientists to have no preconception as to the results of their inquiries. Scientific experimentation should be entered into with an open mind, and a definite result should not be anticipated. **Objectivity** is obtained when scientists explain an experiment in enough detail so that other scientists in other settings with other participants can replicate the experiment, indicating objectivity. **Skepticism** is a mental attitude that results in questioning everything (especially those notions that are commonly taken for granted) and preferring no explanation to a poor one. Skepticism is especially important when considering treatment methods that may be pseudoscientific, lacking empirical evidence, and promoted by those who falsely claim them to be effective.

When scientists have no preconceived notion as to the results of their studies, they have taken a position of _____.

When scientists have explained their experiment in enough detail that it can be replicated by other scientists in other settings, with other participants, they have established _____.

> A mental attitude that leads a person to question everything others may take for granted is called
>
> _____.

Distinguishing between science and **pseudoscience** is sometimes difficult. Finn, Bothe, and Bramlett (2005) described pseudoscientific treatment methods as having certain characteristics, some of which are highlighted in Display Box 9–1. Clinicians should understand the difference between a scientifically supported treatment method and a pseudoscientific one, and they should take a skeptical position until they have done the necessary research to verify efficacy. The field of communicative disorders is, unfortunately, rife with pseudoscientific treatment methods, especially for children with autism spectrum disorder (ASD). It is highly likely that clinicians will be approached by parents desperate for any treatment that may lead to normalization of their child with ASD. Treatment methods such as facilitated communication, sensory integration training, auditory integration therapy, and so forth have fervent advocates but are little supported by peer-reviewed scientific evidence (American Speech-Language-Hearing Association, 1995; Maglione, Gans, Das, Timbie, & Kasari, 2012).

A Set of Methods

The scientific method describes procedures scientists employ to discover explanations for natural phenomena. There are various types of research, such as statistical, qualitative, correlational, and descriptive studies, that involve different sets of methods. However, the research base for behavioral principles has been established through experimental studies, specifically through a subcategory of experimental study called single-case research. Therefore, while recognizing the value of other types of research, the emphasis of this discussion is on single-case research design.

Generally, the steps set forth in the scientific method are as follows:

1. Formulation of a research question
2. Researching background information
3. Constructing a hypothesis
4. Testing the hypothesis through experimentation
5. Analyzing results of the experiment and drawing conclusions
6. Disseminating results through peer-reviewed journals

These are the steps that scientists take when conducting single-case experimental research, with one exception: Formal hypotheses are seldom stated in single-case research design. Instead, scientists conducting single-case research usually begin with a research question and then conduct an experiment designed to provide an answer to that research question.

Formulating a Research Question

Scientists formulate a question that they seek to answer by conducting their experiment. In single-case research, the research question usually substitutes for the hypothesis. Researchers in the field of communicative disorders are likely to ask questions regarding:

- The effectiveness of a treatment method

Display Box 9–1. Characteristics of Pseudoscientific Treatment Methods

■ Proponents of the treatment method state that it is "untestable," and there is no way, therefore, that the treatment's benefits can be disproved (p. 173).

■ The treatment method remains unchanged, even when experimental evidence indicates a lack of efficacy. The method continues based on the charisma of the proponents and on the belief and convictions of the method's followers.

■ There is a strong "confirmation bias"; when available evidence is conflicting, followers of the method will embrace the positive evidence and ignore the negative (p. 174).

■ The treatment method is supported mostly by anecdotal reports on personal experiences of clients who have received the treatment.

■ Extraordinary treatment effects are claimed without sufficient evidence to support those claims. Pseudoscientists are likely to claim efficacy based only on their expert opinion.

■ There is a lack of peer-reviewed evidence. Scientists report results of experiments to peer-reviewed journals to be critically examined before publication. Pseudoscientists often disseminate information directly to the public regarding treatment methods through other means, such as the Internet or news media.

■ There is a disconnection between the claims about treatment effectiveness and well-established scientific principles. Claims are "rarely connected to a scientific or empirical tradition" (p. 176).

■ Treatment methods are described in terms that may appear to be scientific but are not. Often, the terms that are applied result in concepts that are unobservable and unmeasurable; in other words, they do not lend themselves to an operational definition.

■ Extravagant or poorly specified claims are made regarding the treatment's effectiveness. Benefits may be described in terms of, for example, a "miracle cure" (p. 177).

■ Proponents of pseudoscientific treatment methods often state they are taking a holistic approach that addresses the whole person, not just the specific complaint.

Source: Finn, Bothe, and Bramlett (2005).

- The relative effectiveness of a treatment method when compared to another
- Possible interactive effects of combined treatment methods
- The manner in which participant or clinician characteristics interact with a treatment method to produce varied effects
- The effectiveness of a treatment method across individuals

Sometimes, when reporting the results of a study, researchers will write a paragraph or two stating the purpose, or aim, of their research rather than using a research question format. In either case, a well-constructed research question or statement of purpose should clearly set forth the purpose of the inquiry, often including a brief description of participants, and identify an **independent variable** and a **dependent variable.**

Independent and dependent variables can be explained in terms of cause and effect; the ultimate goal of an experimental research study is to determine if a cause-effect relationship exists between the two variables. The independent variable is the cause the scientist investigates to see what kind of effect it has on a dependent variable, if any. A researcher conducting a single-case design efficacy study in the field of communicative disorders seeks to determine the effect a treatment method, the independent variable, has on a targeted communicative behavior, the dependent variable. Possible independent variables would be treatment methods such as time-out, response cost, verbal praise, token reinforcement, corrective feedback, and so forth. Possible dependent variables would be fluency of speech, expressive language, pragmatic behaviors, vocal quality, and so forth. Display Box 9–2 gives examples of research questions or statements of purpose.

In scientific research investigating the efficacy of a treatment method, the behavior to be treated is the _____ variable, and the treatment method being investigated is the _____ variable.

Scientific Experimentation Versus Routine Clinical Work

There are many similarities between what researchers do when applying the scientific method to perform an experiment and what speech-language pathologists (SLPs) do when performing routine clinical work in treating their clients. The scientist starts out with a research question. The SLP also begins with a question— what is the best way to treat a client's communicative difficulties?

Once the question is formulated, the scientist then performs background research, reading and searching the literature for any information or published studies relevant to their question. The clinician starts off with a thorough assessment of the client and might also spend some time reading professional journals or other published documents if the client has some kind of condition the clinician has little experience in treating. Also, if the client or the client's significant others have asked for an unfamiliar approach to therapy, the wise clinician will scour the professional literature to determine if there is an evidence base supporting that type of therapy.

After gathering background information, the scientist formulates a hypothesis

---

Display Box 9–2. Examples of Research Questions or Statements of Purpose

"Will repeated practice treatment result in increased accuracy of sound production in trained and untrained utterances for speakers with AOS [apraxia of speech] and aphasia?" (Wambaugh, Nessler, Cameron, & Mauszycki, 2012, p. S7)

"What is the effect of the parents' use of least-to-most prompting strategy on the turn-taking skills of their children who use AAC [augmentative and alternative communication]?" (Kent-Walsh, Binger, & Hasham, 2010, p. 98)

"The purpose of this research was to explore the effectiveness of utilising MIT [melodic intonation therapy] to improve expressive language in a person with global aphasia following right hemisphere stroke" (Morrow-Odom & Swann, 2013, p. 1322).

"Will children with severe SSD [speech sound disorders] increase the quantity, or amount, of their naturally produced speech and AAC [augmentative and alternative communication] speech following the IMI [integrated multimodal intervention]?" (King, Hengst, & DeThorne, 2013, p. 197)

"The aim of this study was therefore to develop, implement, and describe an aided language stimulation program and determine its effect on the acquisition of target vocabulary items of 4 children with LNFS [limited or no functional speech]" (Dada & Alant, 2009, p. 53).

"One purpose of the current study is to examine the effect of SpeechEasy on stuttering during spontaneous conversational speech in SDL [situations of daily living] over time and as a function of situation and/or speaking context" (O'Donnell, Armston, & Kiefte, 2008, p. 100).

---

or, in single-case research, formulates a research question or a statement of purpose. Similarly, the clinician writes an assessment report, formulates target behaviors, and writes a treatment plan that, it is hoped, will result in improved performance of the target behaviors. Therapy is much like

conducting experimentation. The clinician applies a treatment method, the independent variable in routine clinical work, hoping to have an effect on the dependent variable, the client's target behaviors.

Scientists and clinicians carefully take data (see Chapter 3), which they then analyze to make conclusions regarding the effects of the independent variable (the treatment method) on the dependent variable (the communicative behavior). Scientists seek to disseminate the results of their studies by writing articles to submit for publication in peer-reviewed journals. Clinicians write treatment summary reports and discuss results of treatment with the client and the client's significant others, somewhat analogous but, of course, much more limited in scope compared to the widespread dissemination of a scientist's published findings. Similarities between scientists and clinicians, then, include starting with a question, performing background research, conducting experimentation/treatment, collecting and analyzing data, and disseminating results.

There are, however, very significant differences between scientific research and routine clinical work. The scientist must strive to isolate an independent variable to determine its effect on a specific, isolated dependent variable. The experiment must be constructed in a way that ensures the effect observed is caused by the independent variable and nothing else. Therefore, scientists seek to control for **extraneous variables**, those variables that may contribute to the effect seen in a dependent variable and thereby confound the results of the study. Scientists seeking to determine a cause-effect relationship between a treatment method and a communicative behavior make sure the participants have received no past therapy, or at least are not receiving concurrent therapy, for the communicative behavior, the dependent variable. Furthermore, scientists do not welcome the efforts of parents, teachers, spouses, or others in trying to help the participants learn the communicative behavior under scientific investigation. When the experiment is being con-

ducted, there can be no, or at least very little, adjustment in the treatment procedures, or methodology, of the study. All of these factors—past or concurrent therapy, the efforts of others, and variations in the treatment methodology—are extraneous variables that may invalidate a study and prevent scientists from making definite conclusions regarding the existence of a cause-effect relationship between the independent and dependent variables they have attempted to isolate.

> When conducting an experiment, scientists take great care to rule out _____ _____.

Compare the amount of care scientists take to rule out extraneous variables to what happens in routine clinical work. There are many extraneous variables that clinicians typically welcome when treating their clients. They may consider past or concurrent therapy to be helpful in facilitating improvement in their clients—the more therapy the client has received or is receiving, the better. To establish the target behavior in settings other than the clinic room, clinicians encourage significant others in the client's life to participate in therapy. Parents are taught techniques to support speech and language development in their children. Teachers are given instruction in how to support children's speech and language target behaviors in the classroom. Spouses are shown how to evoke responses from individuals with aphasia or dementia. Also, clinicians are not bound to follow strictly the original treatment plan they set up for a client. If data indicate the client is not making expected progress, clinicians make necessary adjustments. For example, a clinician working with a child may switch from a play-based approach to an at-the-table discrete trial regimen, or vice versa. A clinician working with a client with aphasia might find it necessary to switch from pictured stimuli to object stimuli in teaching naming skills. There are a myriad of possibilities open to clinicians during routine clinical work in adjusting treatment methods to meet the needs of the clients they serve.

These differences are attributable to the different goals scientists and clinicians seek to achieve. Scientists work to determine a cause-effect relationship that may exist between a treatment method and improved communicative behavior, and they adopt a neutral position regarding the possible results of their experiments. Clinicians work to effectuate improvement in clients through whatever means that may be available, and they are absolutely not neutral in their approach to treatment—they want and expect their clients to improve. In other words, scientists carefully control against the influence of extraneous variables, whereas clinicians often invite in some extraneous variables they feel will be helpful to their clients.

When an experiment is carefully controlled and produces positive results, the researchers have established the effectiveness of the treatment method under scientific investigation. However, when clients undergoing routine clinical treatment show improvement, clinicians cannot similarly claim that the treatment methods used were effective, because no effort was made to rule out extraneous variables. It may be that a particularly diligent parent, talented teacher, or devoted spouse had more to do with client improvement. If the clinician made several major adjustments to the treatment plan or used a variety of approaches or a combination of different prompts, there is no way to tell which of those components of therapy caused improvement in the client. The most

that the clinician can claim is accountability, because the goal of helping the client improve was accomplished (Hegde, 1998).

Characteristics of Single-Case Research Designs

In seeking to establish cause-effect relationships, researchers employ specific research designs. A research design is a planned methodology, or strategy, scientists use to conduct an experimental study. Single-case research design is the main strategy employed by behavioral scientists and may also be employed by researchers in the field of communicative disorders seeking to establish the efficacy of treatment methods. Regardless of the name, there can be, and often is, more than one participant involved in single-case research, but there are seldom more than three or four. Therefore, these designs are also often designated **small *n* research designs** —the *n* standing for the word *number*. The designs are distinguished in many ways from **group research design**, another category of commonly employed experimental designs, which involve much greater numbers of participants. The following paragraphs will explain some of the important differences between single-case, or small *n*, research designs and group research design.

Another term for single-case research design is _____ _____ research design.

Participant Selection

Researchers conducting group research design and single-case design experiments both begin by specifying required characteristics of potential participants. A list of **inclusion** criteria sets forth required characteristics of participants, and a list of **exclusion** criteria sets forth those characteristics that would preclude participation in the study. For example, researchers interested in the effects of self-monitoring on increasing fluency of speech in adult stutterers in their work settings might draw up a list of inclusion criteria, as follows:

Participants must be:

- Between 18 and 30 years of age
- At least 7% dysfluent; a fluency level of 93% or less
- Employed in a setting requiring customer contact

Exclusion criteria might specify that there be no concurrent condition, such as an expressive language disorder, intellectual disability, or hearing loss, that may confound results of the study.

> Participants for single-case and group research designs are selected based on _____ and _____ criteria.

After potential participant characteristics have been specified, however, there are major distinctions in participant selection between single-case research design, involving small numbers of participants, and group research designs, involving large numbers of participants. In group research design, the concept of **randomization** is critically important. Randomization occurs when participants are randomly selected (e.g., through a lottery process or other means of random selection) from a large population of accessible participants and then again randomly assigned to either a control group, which does not receive the treatment method (the independent variable), or an experimental group, which does receive the treatment method.

In the basic pretest/posttest control group design, participants in both groups are then given a pretest to measure the targeted communicative behavior (the dependent variable). A mean (average) measure is calculated for the control group and for the experimental group. After pretest measures have been taken, the treatment method is then applied to the participants in the experimental group. At the conclusion of the experiment, a posttest identical to the pretest is given to measure progress made in both groups. A gain score (e.g., the score of the posttest measure minus the score of the pretest measure) is calculated for each individual in each group. The average of the gain scores for individuals in the experimental group and, separately, for individuals in the control group is then calculated. Data are commonly analyzed through administration of a *t*-test, which determines if there is a statistically significant difference between the average gain scores of the control and experimental groups. If there is, and the average gain score of the experimental group is greater than the average gain score of the control group, it is established that there is a cause-effect relationship between the treatment method and improvement in the targeted communicative behavior. Thus, the only important data points in this type of group research design are the average score gains in the control and experimental groups. The results are considered valid and applicable to the larger population only if the process of randomization has been faithfully carried out in selecting and assigning participants.

> The concept of _____ in selecting participants is critically important in group research design but not at all important in single-case research design.

In single-case research design, randomization is not at all important. There is no large pool of accessible participants to randomly select and no control or experimental group requiring random assignment of participants. After inclusion and exclusion criteria have been specified, the researcher then just looks for individuals who fit the criteria—any individual who fits the criteria is considered a suitable participant for the study. Often, individuals may volunteer to participate in single-subject research experiments. This is referred to as **self-selection** and is strictly frowned upon in group research design but poses no problem in single-case research design, because statistical testing relying on randomized selection of a large number of participants is not conducted to analyze the results (Hegde, 2003). Participants in single-case research projects are often self-selected.

> When people volunteer to participate in a research study, they are considered to have been _____-_____.

Data Collection and Analysis

Unlike data collection in group research design, data collection in single-case research design is ongoing. Multiple measures are taken to establish a steady and reliable baseline, and then measures are taken for every session conducted or observation made in a natural setting when the treatment method is introduced. Therefore, every data point is important—before, during, and, if there is a follow-up phase, after the treatment method is employed.

Data collected during single-case research are analyzed quite differently, compared to the manner in which data are analyzed for group research. Results in single-case research design are not analyzed through statistical testing. Instead, results are analyzed through visual inspection of the data, which are presented graphically. At the conclusion of the experiment, data points for measures taken during baseline and treatment phases are displayed on a graph. If an upward trend is documented after the introduction of a treatment method, then that method has been demonstrated to be effective. If the treatment method is meant to decrease an undesirable behavior, and the behavior shows a downward trend after introduction of a treatment method, then, again, that method has been demonstrated to be effective.

> Results of single-case research are analyzed through _____ _____ of the data.

Establishment of Experimental Control

In group research design, if participants in the control and experimental groups have been randomly selected and assigned, **equivalency** of the two groups is assumed. Control is established because the presence of the control group, whose participants do not receive treatment, is believed to rule out extraneous variables that may confound the results of the study.

In single-case research design, control is demonstrated when there is no change in a dependent variable until the independent variable is introduced. The scientist conducting single-case research manipulates the independent variable in a manner that demonstrates control over the dependent variable, thus establishing a cause-effect relationship in a systematic, scientific manner. Each participant, by responding differently during different conditions of a single-case research study, provides experimental control (Hegde, 2003). Refer to Table 9–1 for a summary of differences between group and single-case research design.

Table 9–1. Differences Between Group Research Design and Single-Case Research Design

Components of Research	Group Research Design	Single-Case Research Design
Number of participants	Many; selected from a large pool of accessible participants	Few; as little as one and typically no more than four
Selection of participants	Through various processes employed to ensure randomization of participant selection and assignment	Any person fitting inclusion criteria is considered suitable for participation; often self-selected
Data collection	Identical pretest and posttest measures taken of the dependent variable	Ongoing collection of data; multiple data points for baseline and treatment conditions
Analysis of data (results)	Through statistical testing, to determine if there is a statistically significant difference between the average mean gains calculated based on pretest and posttest scores for the control and experimental groups	Through visual inspection of data points represented graphically; calculation of an effect size is also commonly conducted
Establishment of experimental control	Inclusion of a control group provides control over extraneous variables; if the experimental group shows change and the control group does not, control is assumed to have been established	Different response rates by the same participant to different conditions (e.g., baseline compared to treatment conditions) provides control, as does manipulation of the independent variable by the researcher

<table>
<tr><td>

Types of Single-Case Research Designs

The following sections describe a few of the most commonly used single-case research designs: ABA and ABAB reversal and withdrawal, multiple baselines, and alternating treatments. Data collected when researchers use any of these designs are analyzed through visual inspection. Each data point is charted and displayed on a graph, and effects are determined by the manner in which the dependent variable changes as a result of manipulation of the independent variable. Therefore, for each research design discussed, a graph depicting data collected for a hypothetical study will be provided and explained.

Countless cause-effect relationships between treatment methods and human behavior have been discovered through single-case research in the fields of psychology and applied behavior analysis. However, because this is a textbook relative to applying principles of behaviorism to the field of speech-language pathology, most of the examples given are specific to the verbal behaviors that are commonly treated by SLPs.

ABA Withdrawal or Reversal

The ABA research design is one of the earliest developed single-case research designs and certainly one of the most straightforward (Barlow, Nock, & Hersen, 2009). It can be used with one participant, but often researchers will run the same ABA design experiment on two or three participants concurrently, to add strength to their findings. Briefly, the researcher takes multiple baseline measures of the

</td><td>

dependent variable (the targeted behavior); this is the first A phase of the experiment. Then, the independent variable (the treatment method under investigation) is introduced; this is the B phase of the experiment. If the treatment is effective, the behavior should increase or decrease, depending upon whether the targeted behavior is desirable or undesirable. Treatment is given until a trend in the increase or decrease of the behavior has been established. Then, treatment is either discontinued (withdrawn) or applied to a behavior that is incompatible with the targeted behavior (reversed); this is the second A phase of the experiment.

Figure 9–1 depicts data for a hypothetical ABA study on the effects of positive reinforcement in the form of verbal praise on an 8-year-old female's attending behavior. The first five data points represent the first baseline (A) phase. Baseline measures were taken over the first five sessions held in the laboratory clinic room. The behavior was measured through whole-interval time sampling. The child was given a task to perform (e.g., putting together a puzzle, completing a worksheet, writing a paragraph, etc.) and then observed during 1-minute blocks of time. If the child was observed to attend to the task for the entire minute, then that was recorded as a plus sign; if not, then a minus sign was recorded. At the end of each session, a percentage was calculated by dividing the number of 1-minute intervals the child was observed to attend to task by the total number of minutes the child was observed. So, if the child was observed for 20 minutes and earned a plus mark for only 1 of those minutes, then the data point recorded on the chart was 5%. Visual inspection of the data during the first baseline phase indicates a steady baseline of 0% to 5%.

</td></tr>
</table>

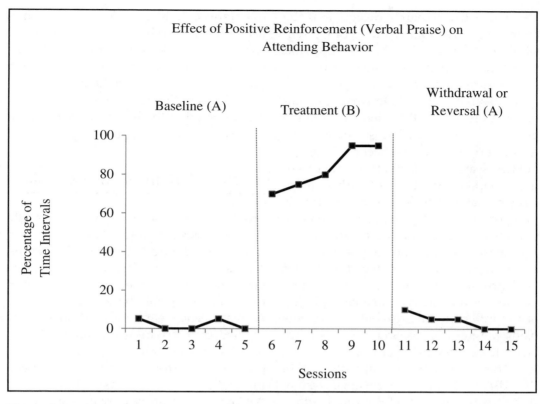

Figure 9–1. ABA single-case research design: Withdrawal or reversal.

After baseline data were collected, the treatment (B) phase began. The child was given a task to perform, and the researcher reinforced good attending behavior with verbal praise on a time interval schedule of 10 seconds (e.g., "You are really working hard!" or "Keep up the good work!"). The second five data points represent data collected through the same method of measurement used for the baseline sessions—whole-interval time sampling for 1-minute blocks of time. Visual inspection of the data during the treatment phase indicates an immediate and increasing improvement in attending behavior.

During the second A phase of the experiment, the researcher either withdraws the treatment (ABA withdrawal) or applies the treatment to a behavior that is incompatible with the targeted behavior (ABA reversal) to see if the behavior returns to baseline levels. For ABA withdrawal, treatment is simply withdrawn, and the child is observed performing a designated task in the absence of verbal praise to reinforce good attending behavior. Data are collected in the same manner as for the first baseline (A) phase. For ABA reversal, verbal praise is given for any behavior other than attending to task (e.g., "I like it when you ask me questions!" or "I sure like your stories!"). Visual inspection of the data for the second A phase indicates that the behavior returned to baseline levels at the conclusion of the experiment.

The ABA research design may be counterintuitive to a working SLP's sensibilities. Why, it might be asked, would a researcher sabotage a client's progress by withdrawing or, worse, reversing a good treatment effect? However, remember that the goal of the scientist is not the goal of the clinician. The scientist's goal is to determine a cause-effect relationship, not necessarily to effectuate improvement in participants. If it can be clearly demonstrated that a client's behavior responds in a positive way to the introduction of a treatment method and then reverts back to baseline levels when the treatment method is withdrawn or reversed, then that is solid evidence of the efficacy of that treatment method. With this type of manipulation of the independent variable, researchers using single-case research designs demonstrate experimental control.

There are, however, difficulties with the ABA withdrawal or reversal design. If the treatment method is strongly effective, then effects of treatment might carry over into the withdrawal or even reversal design, and the behavior might not return to baseline levels. This would be good news to the SLP performing routine clinical work but bad news for a scientist who is attempting to determine the effects of a treatment method. To minimize generalization of the effect, scientists using the ABA design treat during the B phase for only the amount of time it takes to document a trend in the behavior. They then quickly move on to the withdrawal or reversal A phase.

Another obvious problem with the ABA withdrawal or reversal research design is the fact that it ends with the participant no better off than when the experiment began. As discussed in Chapter 10, scientists are required to conduct themselves in an ethical manner during experimentation. It is questionable whether it is ethical to either passively, through withdrawal, or actively, through reversal, facilitate a return to baseline level without doing anything further to help the participant. The solution to this ethical dilemma can be found in the ABAB withdrawal or reversal research design.

ABAB Withdrawal or Reversal

The ABAB withdrawal or reversal research design consists of four phases. The first three are identical to the ABA withdrawal or reversal design. The scientist takes measures on the targeted behavior to establish a stable baseline; this is the A phase. The treatment method is then applied, and a trend is documented; this is the B phase. Treatment is then either passively withdrawn or actively reversed; this is the second A phase. However, in ABAB research design, treatment is reinstated in the fourth phase, or second B condition. If the behavior responds well to the treatment method during the first B phase, returns to baseline during the second A phase, and then again responds well when treatment is reinstated during the second B phase, the scientist has provided evidence of the efficacy of the treatment method.

Refer to Figure 9–2, which represents hypothetical data collected during an ABAB experiment regarding the effects of instructions coupled with demonstration on articulation of the phoneme /s/ in initial word position. During the first five sessions, the first A phase, the scientist took baseline measures of a participant's production of /s/ by presenting 20 pictured stimuli representing objects that begin with /s/ and asking the predetermined question, "What is this?" For

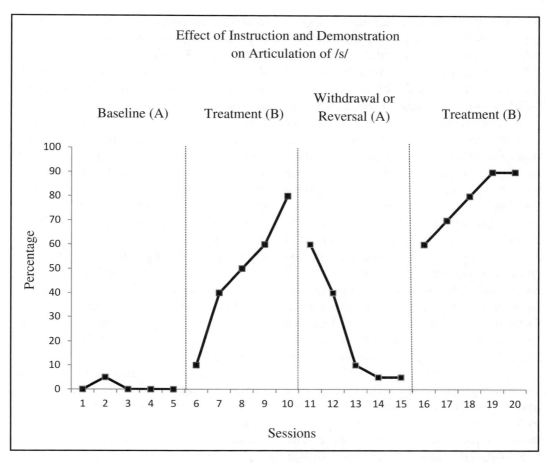

Figure 9–2. ABAB single-case research design: Withdrawal or reversal.

each discrete trial, correct productions of /s/ were recorded with a plus sign, and incorrect productions were recorded with a minus sign. Total correct productions were divided by the number of trials given (in this case, 20) and multiplied by 100 to determine a percentage correct. As indicated by the first five data points on the graph in Figure 9–2, baseline percentages were quite low.

After a stable baseline was established, the B phase, or treatment, began. The researcher gave instructions to the participant about how to make a good /s/ and demonstrated each step (e.g., the first

step might be explaining that the tongue belongs up on the alveolar ridge without touching the teeth and then showing the client how that is done). Discrete trials were then administered with pictured stimuli, as were presented during baseline trials, and each time the client made an incorrect production, the researcher repeated instructions and gave a demonstration. Data were collected for each session, and a percentage correct was calculated. The graphed data indicate a much improved percentage of correct /s/ production.

For the second B phase, the researcher might have either withdrawn treatment or actively reversed treatment by applying the method to a behavior incompatible with correct production of /s/. For ABAB withdrawal, instructions and demonstrations would be discontinued, and the researcher would repeat baseline trials. For ABAB reversal, the researcher would give incorrect instructions and demonstrations (e.g., telling the participant the tongue is placed between the teeth for production of /s/ and demonstrating a full frontal lisp). In either case, the researcher was looking for a return to baseline measures, which, as indicated by the data points for the second baseline (A) phase, occurred. The researcher then reinstated treatment—instructions and demonstrations for correct production of /s/ during discrete trial therapy. Again an improvement was documented, as indicated by the data points for the second B phase. Therefore, the researcher established evidence for the efficacy of giving instructions coupled with demonstrations in improving production of the /s/ phoneme. The ethical concerns involved with the ABA withdrawal or reversal design were avoided by providing the participant with further treatment after the experimental effect had been established.

So far, we have talked about experiments having to do with increasing a desirable behavior. Experimental designs might also be employed to decrease an undesirable behavior. Figure 9–3 presents hypothetical data generated by an ABAB experiment to investigate the effects of differential reinforcement of other behavior (DRO; see Chapter 8), a combination of extinction and positive reinforcement, on a 2-year-old child's tantrum behavior. Through functional behavior assessment (FBA), performed by a board certified behavior analyst (BCBA), the child's tantrum behavior was determined to be rein-

forced by the parents' attending behaviors (e.g., picking the child up, rocking the child, etc.). The first baseline (A) phase shows the number of tantrums the child had per day at high levels, as determined by the observations conducted by the researchers during the household's daily routine. In the first treatment (B) phase, DRO was applied. The parents were instructed to ignore the tantrum behavior but to reinforce every good behavior the child exhibits through verbal praise (e.g., "I like it when you're smiling!") and other positive attention (e.g., picking up the child or playing with the child when there is no tantrum behavior exhibited). The data depicted the expected extinction burst, or increase of the undesired behavior, as is expected with extinction, but the last two data points document a decided trend downward in the number of tantrums the child had each day. In the second baseline (A) phase, either withdrawal or reversal could have been employed. For withdrawal, the parents would be asked to go back to the manner in which they typically reacted to the child's tantrum behavior. For reversal, the parents would be asked to lavish even more attention on the child's tantrum behavior, to hasten the return to baseline levels. Finally, in the second treatment (B) phase, DRO was reinstated. The data depicted little in the way of an extinction burst, which is typical of a behavior that has previously been subjected to extinction, and tantrum behaviors went all the way to zero per day.

It might be argued that, because the ABAB research design documents the effect of a treatment method twice, rather than once as in the ABA research design, it provides stronger evidence of the effects of a treatment method. Therefore, the design is considered a powerful

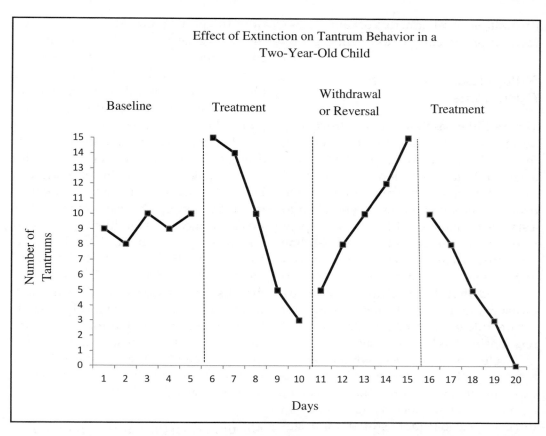

Figure 9–3. ABAB single-case research design: Withdrawal or reversal (undesired behavior).

experimental approach (Kazdin, 2011). Ethical concerns regarding the reversal or withdrawal of a desired effect, however, remain even though the ABAB design ends with the reinstatement of treatment.

Multiple Baseline Research Designs

Multiple baseline research designs avoid ethical concerns because they do not involve withdrawal or reversal phases that result in a return to baseline levels. Instead, a staggered number of baseline measures of the dependent variable, or targeted behavior, are taken for different partici-

pants, different target behaviors, or different settings before the introduction of the independent variable, or treatment method. If baseline levels remain the same and then change when the treatment method is introduced, it is demonstrated that the change in baseline levels is due to the introduction of the treatment method and not to extraneous variables (Kazdin, 2011). In this way, the researcher achieves experimental control and documents a cause-effect relationship between the treatment method, the independent variable, and the behavior, the dependent variable. The following sections explain and illustrate three variations of multiple baseline research design: (a) multiple baseline across participants,

(b) multiple baseline across behaviors, and (c) multiple baseline across settings.

Multiple Baseline Across Participants

The multiple baseline across participants design is appropriate for investigating the effects of a treatment method across a few individuals (often no more than four) who need intervention for the same behavior. Baseline measures are taken in a staggered manner, with each participant receiving a different number of baseline measures. Treatment is also introduced in a staggered manner. If it can be demonstrated that the participants' baseline measures remain stable and steady until the treatment is given, then a cause-effect relationship has been established.

Refer to Figure 9–4, which depicts hypothetical data generated from an experiment investigating the efficacy of response cost on increasing fluency in three 12-year-old male stutterers, designated Participants A, B, and C. The top chart represents data collected for Participant A. In the baseline phase, four baseline measures were taken by collecting and analyzing conversational speech samples to determine a percentage of fluent speech. Then, treatment was introduced by giving the participant a choice of reinforcing items to work for (e.g., small cars, baseball cards, yo-yos, action figures, etc.). The participant was then told that he must earn at least five poker chips in order to "buy" the chosen reinforcer at the end of the session. The researcher then engaged the participant in conversation, which was audiotaped, and administered poker chips on a 30-second time fixed-interval schedule of reinforcement for fluent speech. At the first sign of a dysfluency, a poker chip was withdrawn

from the participant. After each session, the researcher analyzed the audiotaped conversation to calculate a percentage of fluent speech. Each of the data points in the treatment phase, then, represents the percentage of fluent speech the participant exhibited for that treatment session.

The experiment was conducted in exactly the same manner for Participant B, whose chart is in the middle of Figure 9–4, and Participant C, whose chart is on the bottom. Notice, however, that 4 baseline measures for fluent speech were taken for Participant A, 7 baseline measures for Participant B, and 10 baseline measures for Participant C. Notice, also, that baseline measures for all participants were stable, steady, and at low levels until the treatment method, a token economy combined with response cost, was introduced. Therefore, the treatment method was shown to be effective in increasing fluency of speech in the three participants.

Multiple Baseline Across Behaviors

Unlike multiple baselines across participants, the multiple baselines across behaviors research design can be employed with just one participant, although, to add strength to an experimental study, scientists often repeat the design with more than one participant during the same study. The multiple baseline across behaviors design is suitable when a participant has more than one behavior that needs treatment, when those behaviors can be treated with the same method, and when there is a low likelihood of generalization of treatment across the behaviors. At least two or three markedly different behaviors are selected for treatment administered to the same individual. The number of baseline measures is staggered across behaviors, and treatment is introduced to each

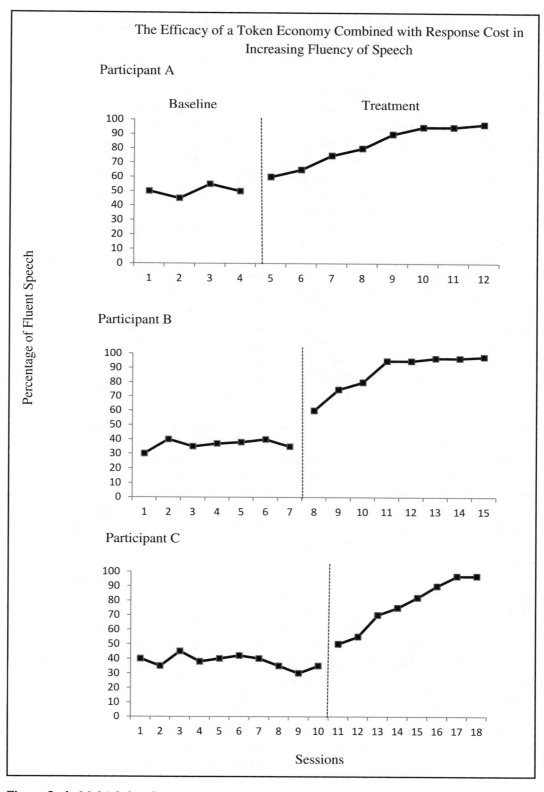

Figure 9–4. Multiple baselines across participants.

behavior after the baseline phase is complete. If the behaviors remain stable while in the baseline phase but show change when the treatment method is introduced, then a cause-effect relationship between the treatment method (the independent variable) and the behavior (the dependent variable) has been established, and scientific control has been demonstrated.

Refer to Figure 9–5, which represents hypothetical data generated from a multiple baselines across behaviors study on the efficacy of corrective feedback on correct articulation of phonemes in initial word position. Assessment results showed the 7-year-old female participant to have difficulties with production of the phonemes /s/, /l/, and /f/ in initial word position. The researcher took four baseline measures of all three phonemes and then began to treat the /s/ phoneme while continuing to take baseline measures of /l/ and /f/. To isolate corrective feedback as the independent variable, the researcher administered treatment only by letting the client know how to improve an incorrect production while just recording correct productions in a matter-of-fact manner. For example, the researcher might say, "You need to make sure your air comes straight out," or "I saw your tongue come out—make sure it's up and behind your teeth." After the second behavior, the /l/ phoneme, had received seven baseline measures, the same treatment was applied to the /l/ phoneme while treatment continued on the /s/ phoneme, and baseline measures of the /f/ phoneme continued to be taken. After the third behavior, the /f/ phoneme, had received 10 baseline measures, treatment was applied. Treatment for all three phonemes continued for as long as it took for the phonemes to reach a specified criterion measure—in this case, an accuracy level of at least 90%

over three consecutive sessions. Visual inspection of the data indicated that each of the targeted phonemes did not improve until after the introduction of the treatment method; therefore, a cause-effect relationship was established between corrective feedback, the independent variable, and correct articulation of phonemes in initial position, the dependent variable.

Multiple Baseline Across Settings

The multiple baselines across settings research design examines the effectiveness of a particular treatment method across two or more settings, such as the clinic setting, the home setting, the classroom setting, the job setting, and so forth. This design may also involve one participant, although, again, scientists may choose to repeat the experiment simultaneously with two or three participants to add strength to the study. A behavior is targeted as the dependent variable, and baseline measures of the behavior are taken in at least two settings. Again, the number of baseline measures is staggered across settings, as is the treatment method. If the behavior in each setting does not change until the treatment method is applied, then the efficacy of the treatment method has been demonstrated.

Refer to Figure 9–6, which represents hypothetical data gathered for a study on the efficacy of a speech-generating device (SGD) on appropriate requesting behavior, as defined by the researchers, in a nonverbal 5-year-old male child with intellectual disability. Three settings were selected: the school setting, the home setting, and the community setting. The child was observed in all three settings to determine the number of times in a day he made spontaneous appropriate requests in each setting. The number of baseline measures was staggered across settings,

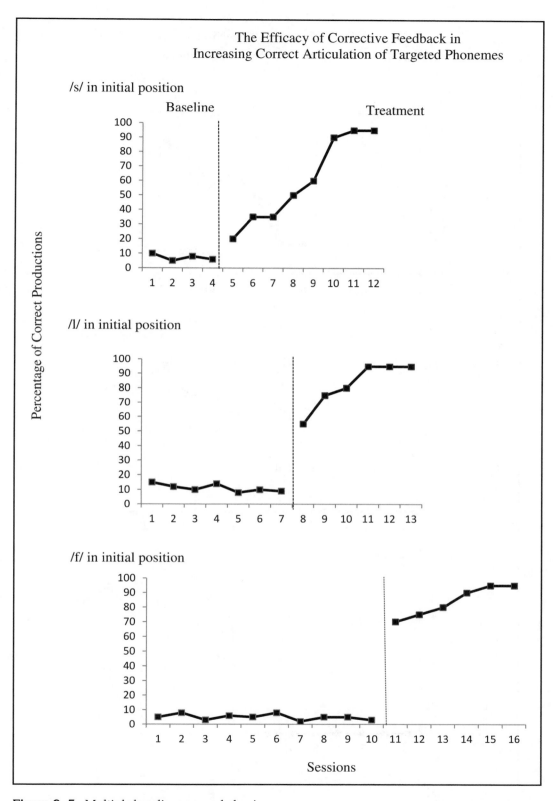

Figure 9–5. Multiple baselines across behaviors.

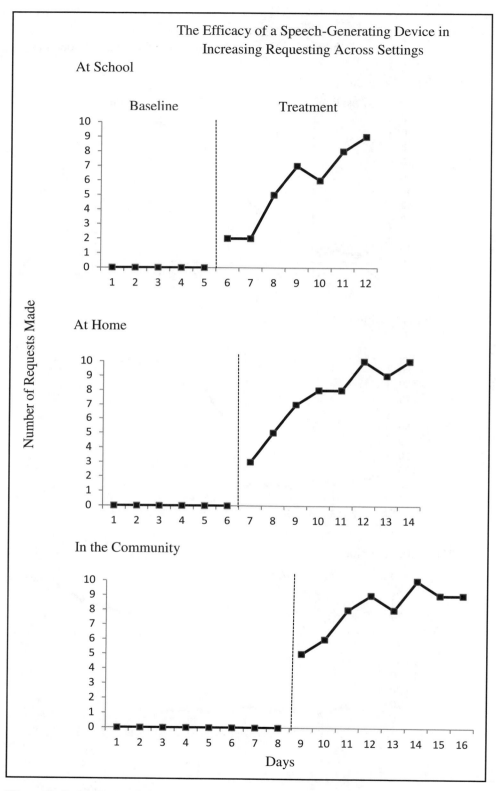

Figure 9–6. Multiple baselines across settings.

and baseline data indicated the child was not making appropriate requests in any of the three settings. He was then introduced to the SGD at school, while baseline measures continued to be taken in the remaining two settings. He was taught how to access the device to make requests such as "Help me, please," "Bathroom, please," and the carrier phrase, "I want _____" with icons representing various items for food and recreational activities. Data indicated a sharp increase in requesting behavior in the school setting.

After an additional two baseline measures, for a total of six, were taken in the home setting, the SGD was provided to the child at home, while baseline measures continued to be taken of his appropriate requesting behavior in community settings. Requesting behavior at home increased with the use of the SGD. Finally, after two additional baseline measures, for a total of eight, were taken in community settings (e.g., in the grocery store, at a restaurant, at the library, etc.), the SGD was provided to the child for those outings. Once again, appropriate requesting behavior in community settings increased with the use of the SGD. Because appropriate requesting behavior was not observed at all before the child was provided with an SGD in any of the settings observed, this is dramatic evidence that it was an effective approach in providing the child with the opportunity to make his needs and wants known.

Alternating Treatments Research Design

The alternating treatments research design is suitable for research questions having to do with the relative efficacy of two treatment methods that have a good evidence base regarding their effects. In other words, an alternating treatments experiment answers the question, "Which of two effective methods is most effective?" Unlike other single-case research designs, a baseline phase is not considered necessary, because the purpose of the study is simply to determine the relative efficacy of two methods that have already been shown to be effective.

Refer to Figure 9–7, which depicts hypothetical data collected from a study investigating the effects of discrete trial training (DTT) with stimulus cards versus DTT embedded in play-based activities in teaching irregular past tense verbs to a 5-year-old child diagnosed with an expressive language disorder. The researchers began by constructing two lists of 10 irregular verbs, one list for each treatment method. The order in which the treatment methods were introduced was determined in a semirandom fashion, perhaps by flipping a coin, making sure that one treatment did not always precede the other. The researchers then began to treat the child for production of irregular past tense verbs, following the semirandom order from session to session. Treatment with stimulus cards consisted of the child sitting at the clinic table, responding to picture and verbal stimuli (e.g., the researcher shows a picture of a girl running and says, "Today, she is running, but yesterday she _____"). Treatment with play-based activities consisted of engaging the child in play structured to evoke production of past tense verbs (e.g., pretending to have a birthday party and evoking productions of *blew* after the child pretends to blow out the candles and *ate* after the child pretends to eat the birthday cake). Data were taken for each session by calculating percentages of correct productions of past tense verbs. At the end of the

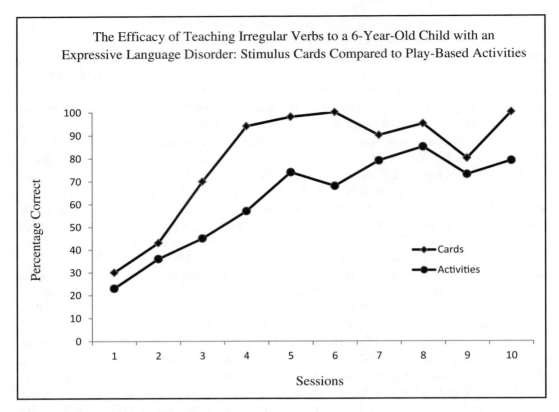

Figure 9–7. Alternating treatments design.

experiment, each data point was charted (see Figure 9–6). Visual inspection of the data indicates that DTT with stimulus cards resulted in higher percentages of correct productions of irregular past tense verbs than did DTT with play-based activities. This suggests that DTT with stimulus cards is a more effective method than DTT embedded in play-based activities.

There are some problems inherent in the alternating treatment design. Notice that, contrary to the name of the design, the two treatments are not presented to the participant in a systematically alternating way—first one, then the other, repeatedly. This is to guard against an extraneous variable that has been called the *order effect*. If the two treatments are simply alternated, with one treatment always preceding the other, the participant can anticipate which treatment is going to be presented each session, which might cause a variation in the manner in which the participant reacts to the treatment. If, on the other hand, the order in which the two treatments are presented is unpredictable, the participant is not so likely to be influenced by the order effect. Therefore, in alternating treatment design, the treatments are presented in a semirandom manner, perhaps by flipping a coin to determine the order in which the treatment methods will be presented throughout the experiment but making whatever adjustments might be necessary to ensure that one treatment does not always precede the other.

Another difficulty with alternating treatments research design has to do with *carryover effects*, which occur when the effects of one treatment method linger and affect the participant's performance in response to the second treatment method. If the first method is a particularly efficacious one, the second treatment method might appear to be more effective than it actually is. Conversely, if the first method is a particularly ineffective one, the second treatment method might appear to be less effective than it is, because the participant has been previously exposed to such a poor method.

Carryover effects can be minimized if the target behaviors are carefully selected so that one target behavior treated with one treatment method is distinct from the target behavior treated with the second treatment method. In the case of the hypothetical study presented in Figure 9–6, carryover effects have been guarded against by constructing different lists of irregular past tense verbs for each treatment method. Because each irregular past tense verb is a response class in and of itself, there should be no carryover effect between the two treatments.

External Validity in Single-Case Research

A common criticism made of single-case research is that results may lack **external validity**, a term that refers to the extent to which results of a study can be generalized, or extended to, a larger population. Because there is such a small number of participants involved in single-case research, results may not be widely applicable. The key to establishing external validity in single-case research is **repli-**

cation. Researchers must describe their treatment procedures in enough detail to make it possible for other researchers to replicate the experiment in other settings with other participants. If repeated experimentation yields similar positive results, the treatment method can be assumed to have generality across clients.

_____ _____ refers to the extent to which results of a research study can be extended to a larger population.

The key to establishing the external validity of results generated by a single-case research study is _____.

Chapter Summary

1. *Science*, a word derived from the Latin *scientia*, meaning knowledge, is a philosophy, a disposition, and a set of methods.
2. The scientific philosophy is characterized by:
   a. Determinism
   b. Empiricism
3. The scientific disposition is characterized by:
   a. Neutrality
   b. Objectivity
   c. Skepticism (particularly important for distinguishing pseudoscience from science)
4. The scientific method for experimental research consists of:
   a. Formulation of a research question

b. Researching background information
c. Constructing a hypothesis
d. Testing the hypothesis through experimentation
e. Analyzing results of the experiment and drawing conclusions
f. Disseminating results through peer-reviewed journals
5. In formulating a research question for investigation of the efficacy of a particular treatment technique, scientists define a **dependent variable**, the behavior that will be targeted for change, and an **independent variable**, the treatment method under investigation.
6. There are many similarities between what scientists do under laboratory conditions and what SLPs do in routine clinical work, but SLPs do not rule out **extraneous variables** that scientists carefully control for.
7. The evidence base for treatment techniques based on behavioral principles is derived mostly from single-case research conducted by scientists in the fields of psychology and applied behavior analysis.
8. Characteristics of single-case research, which distinguish this approach from group research design, include:
a. Small numbers of participants
b. No reliance on randomization for participant selection; participants are often **self-selected**
c. Ongoing data collection during baseline and treatment conditions
d. Data are analyzed through visual inspection
e. Experimental control is demonstrated through:
i. Manipulation of the independent variable
ii. Different responses of the same individual under

different conditions of the experiment
9. There are various types of single-case research designs scientists employ to establish cause-effect relationships, such as:
a. ABA withdrawal and reversal
b. ABAB withdrawal and reversal
c. Multiple baseline research designs
i. Multiple baseline across participants
ii. Multiple baseline across behaviors
iii. Multiple baseline across settings
iv. Alternating treatments
10. Because there are so few participants in single-case research, there is a question as to the external validity of results; replication is the key to establishing external validity in single-case research.

Application Exercises

1. You are a school SLP with an 8-year-old nonverbal boy with autism in a special day class on your caseload. The parents are determined to find a treatment that will help their child talk and on their own have resorted to several alternative methods you know to be **pseudoscientific**, such as auditory integration, chelation therapy, and a gluten-free diet. They have now decided they want you, the school SLP, to include an approach that you have never heard of in the boy's treatment plan. How would you investigate the efficacy of this approach?
2. Refer to Display Box 9–2. For each research question or statement of purpose, identify:

a. The dependent variable

b. The independent variable

c. Characteristics of the participants, if given

3. Go to http://www.scholar.google .com and enter the name of one of the single-case research designs described in this chapter. Many studies in which the researchers utilized the design you searched for will be referenced. Some of the references will have direct links to free-access articles that you can look at; for others, you will need to search your university journals to see if you can access them that way. Look at the articles and identify:

a. The research question

b. The independent and dependent variables

c. The inclusion and exclusion criteria for participants

d. The procedures described

e. Results obtained

4. In the discussion section of the article you located in response to Exercise 3, locate suggestions for future research. Formulate a research question based on one of those suggestions, making sure it contains an identifiable dependent and independent variable. Decide on a research design that would be suitable for answering your research question and devise a procedure for an experiment using that design.

References

American Speech-Language-Hearing Association. (1995). *Facilitated communication* [Position statement]. Retrieved from http://www.asha .org/policy

Barlow, D. H., Nock, M. K., & Hersen, M. (2009). *Single-case experimental designs: Strategies for studying behavior change* (3rd ed.). Boston, MA: Allyn & Bacon.

Dada, S., & Alant, E. (2009). The effect of aided language stimulation on vocabulary acquisition in children with little or no functional speech. *American Journal of Speech-Language Pathology, 18,* 50–64.

Finn, P., Bothe, A. K., & Bramlett, R. E. (2005). Science and pseudoscience in communication disorders: Criteria and applications. *American Journal of Speech-Language Pathology, 14,* 172–186.

Hegde, M. N. (1998). *Treatment procedures in communicative disorders* (3rd ed.). Austin, TX: Pro-Ed.

Hegde, M. N. (2003). *Clinical research in communicative disorders* (3rd ed.). Austin, TX: Pro-Ed.

Kazdin, A. E. (2011). *Single-case research designs: Methods for clinical and applied settings* (2nd ed.). New York, NY: Oxford University Press.

Kent-Walsh, J., Binger, C., & Hasham, Z. (2010). Effects of parent instruction on the symbolic communication of children using augmentative and alternative communication during storybook reading. *American Journal of Speech-Language Pathology, 19,* 97–107.

King, A. M., Hengst, J. A., & DeThorne, L. S. (2013). Severe speech sound disorders: A multimodal intervention. *Language, Speech, and Hearing Services in Schools, 44,* 195–210.

Maglione, M. A., Gans, D., Das, L., Timbie, J., & Kasari, C. (2012). Nonmedical interventions for children with ASD: Recommended guidelines and further research needs. *Pediatrics, 130,* S169–S178.

Morrow-Odom, K. L., & Swann, A. B. (2013). Effectiveness of melodic intonation therapy in a case of aphasia following right hemisphere stroke. *Aphasiology, 27,* 1322–1338.

O'Donnell, J. O., Armson, J., & Kiefte, M. (2008). The effectiveness of SpeechEasy during situations of daily living. *Journal of Fluency Disorders, 33,* 99–119.

Wambaugh, J. L., Nessler, C., Cameron, R., & Mauszycki, S. C. (2012). Acquired apraxia of speech: The effects of repeated practice and rate/rhythm control treatments on sound production accuracy. *American Journal of Speech-Language Pathology, 21,* S5–S27.

CHAPTER 10

Ethics in Scientific Research and Clinical Practice

A Brief History of Ethical Issues in Scientific Research

The pursuit of scientific inquiry has resulted in undeniable benefits to human society: conquered diseases, rapidly developing life-changing technology, and a world made smaller through increased air travel and instant communication. Scientific inquiry, however, has also been marked by ethical questions that have arisen as a result of scientists occasionally throughout history behaving badly. This chapter is concerned with those ethical questions and with the legal mandates now in place to address them. A distinction is made between ethical conduct of scientists engaged in experimentation and the ethical conduct of clinicians performing routine clinical work, and each is addressed separately, beginning with scientific experimentation.

World War II Atrocities

Perhaps more than any other event, the atrocities that took place during World War II, most notably in Nazi concentration camps, brought attention to the need to protect human participants in scientific research. Among many other horrors, some concentration camp prisoners were subjected to experiments designed to further the Nazi war effort or just to satisfy the sadistic curiosity of the infamous Nazi doctors who conducted them. As Wiesel (2005) eloquently and tragically stated:

> In Ravensbrück, Dachau, Buchenwald, and Auschwitz, German scientists operated on their victims without anesthesia. . . . The researchers let them die

of hunger, thirst, cold; they drowned them, amputated their limbs, suffocated them, dissected their still-living bodies to study their behavior and measure their stamina. (p. 1512)

According to Berger (1990), approximately 30 experimental projects conducted in Nazi concentration camps came to light shortly after the end of the war. Among them was a series of experiments conducted in Dachau to determine the most effective way of reviving human beings subjected to extreme cold, as were German pilots shot down over the North Sea and rescued. These experiments were investigated and described in a 228-page report detailing the methods used and data collected. Testimony included in the report indicated that some 280 to 300 individual prisoners were subjected to 360 to 400 experiments. The prisoners were immersed in an icy water tank for purposes of discovering how long they could live in such conditions and, for those who lived, what rewarming technique was most efficacious in reviving them.

The report indicated that immersing the victims in a warm bath was the most successful warming technique, which brought up a troublesome ethical question: Should these data, collected in such a heinous manner, be applied to treat people with hypothermia? Respondents in the scientific community offered answers ranging from an outright ban on utilizing such data to using the data without restriction. Berger (1990) addressed the controversy by analyzing the results of these experiments and concluding that "the Dachau hypothermia study has all the ingredients of a scientific fraud, and rejection of the data on purely scientific ground is inevitable" (p. 1440). Although

Berger (1990) acknowledged the value of ethical dialogue regarding such issues, he also stated that "continuing it [the ethical dialogue] runs the risk of implying that these grotesque Nazi medical exercises yielded results worthy of consideration and possibly of benefit to humanity. The present analysis clearly shows that nothing could be further from the truth" (p. 1440).

Discovery of the atrocities committed during World War II led to the prosecution of Nazi war criminals at the Nuremberg trials conducted from 1945 to 1946, including the prosecution of 20 Nazi doctors. Seven were acquitted, seven received a death sentence, and the remainder received prison sentences ranging from 10 years to life. Also resulting from the Nuremberg Doctor Trials was the Nuremberg Code (1949). Display Box 10–1 lists principles of research ethics set forth by the Nuremberg Code. The Nuremberg Code was the first international code of research ethics and stood alone until 1964, when the Declaration of Helsinki was adopted by the World Medical Association (Diekma, 2006). The Declaration of Helsinki was notable in that protections for children as research participants were set forth.

> The _____ _____
> was the first international code of
> research ethics.

Unethical Experimentation in the United States

Although the Nuremberg Code and the Declaration of Helsinki were international documents, many scientists in the United States did not view them as being particularly relevant to their scientific community (Diekma, 2006). However, investigative reporting in the 1960s revealed instances of scientific experimentation in the United States that clearly indicated the need for increased protection of human subjects. Among these questionable experimental projects were (a) the syphilis studies, (b) the Willowbrook hepatitis studies, and (c) the Human Radiation Experiments.

Syphilis Studies

The most well-known of the syphilis studies was the Tuskegee study, conducted by scientists working under the United States Public Health Service (USPHS), which in later years would become known as the Centers for Disease Control and Prevention (CDCP). Beginning in 1932, 600 African American men in Macon County, Alabama, were enticed to participate in a study regarding the natural course of syphilis; 399 of the men were syphilis positive, and 201 were healthy controls. The men were from a poor socioeconomic background, were mostly illiterate, and were not informed about the purpose of the study, about their own condition, or about available treatment. They were attracted by the promise of a free daily meal, free medical care, and a $50.00 insurance policy for funeral expenses.

In 1947, during the course of the study, penicillin became recognized as an effective treatment for syphilis. However, the researchers pressed on with the Tuskegee study, withholding treatment to continue observing the natural course of the disease. By the time the study was discontinued in 1972, 28 men had died of syphilis, 100 had died of complications from syphilis, 40 female partners had become infected

Display Box 10–1. The Nuremberg Code

1. The voluntary consent of the human subject is absolutely essential.
2. The experiment should be such as to yield fruitful results for the good of society, unprocurable by other methods or means of study, and not random and unnecessary in nature.
3. The experiment should be so designed and based on the results of animal experimentation and a knowledge of the natural history of the disease or other problem under study, that the anticipated results will justify the performance of the experiment.
4. The experiment should be so conducted as to avoid all unnecessary physical and mental suffering and injury.
5. No experiment should be conducted, where there is an a priori reason to believe that death or disabling injury will occur; except, perhaps, in those experiments where the experimental physicians also serve as subjects.
6. The degree of risk to be taken should never exceed that determined by the humanitarian importance of the problem to be solved by the experiment.
7. Proper preparations should be made and adequate facilities provided to protect the experimental subject against even remote possibilities of injury, disability, or death.
8. The experiment should be conducted only by scientifically qualified persons. The highest degree of skill and care should be required through all stages of the experiment of those who conduct or engage in the experiment.
9. During the course of the experiment, the human subject should be at liberty to bring the experiment to an end, if he has reached the physical or mental state, where continuation of the experiment seemed to him to be impossible.
10. During the course of the experiment, the scientist in charge must be prepared to terminate the experiment at any stage, if he has probable cause to believe, in the exercise of the good faith, superior skill and careful judgement required of him, that a continuation of the experiment is likely to result in injury, disability, or death to the experimental subject.

Source: Nuremberg Code (1949).

with the disease, and 19 children were born with congenital syphilis. There was never any attempt to cover up the study; indeed, published articles regarding the Tuskegee study enhanced the prestige of the USPHS in world health organizations (Cuerda-Galindo, Sierra-Valenti, Gonzalez-Lopez, & Lopez-Munoz, 2014). The study was discontinued only because the American press called attention to it.

Although the Tuskegee syphilis study has been called "arguably the most infamous biomedical research study in U.S. history" (Katz et al., 2006, p. 699), it was not the only unethical study conducted on syphilis in the United States. In the 1940s, inmates at Sing-Sing prison were injected with *Treponema pallidum*, a causative agent of syphilis (Cuerda & Lopez-Munoz, 2013). It was claimed that the inmates volunteered for the study.

Another syphilis study that recently came to light (Reverby, 2011) was conducted in Guatemala in 1946 to 1948 by Tuskegee researchers, working under the USPHS in partnership with Guatemalan scientists and an organization that would later come to be known as the Pan American Health Organization (Cuerda-Galindo et al., 2014). The goal of the Guatemalan study was to examine natural exposure to syphilis, confirm the efficacy of penicillin, and investigate the relative effectiveness of several strategies for prevention. The terrible difference between this study and the Tuskegee study was that USPHS scientists in Guatemala attempted to "deliberately infect poor and vulnerable men and women with syphilis in order to study the disease" (Reverby, 2011, p. 9). This proved to be difficult, however. Introducing syphilis inoculate into the cervixes of prostitutes to naturally infect the Guatemalan soldiers they serviced did not produce

the desired results. Moving on to attempt to infect psychiatric patients at a Guatemalan mental health facility also proved problematic, and the researchers abruptly gave up and terminated the experiments after the course of 2 years. Although the goal was purportedly to treat purposefully infected subjects with penicillin, it was determined that, out of 699 Guatemalans deliberately infected with syphilis, only 14% received "adequate treatment" (Reverby, 2011, p. 16).

The Willowbrook Hepatitis Experiments

Children with intellectual disabilities housed at the Willowbrook State School, since closed, on Staten Island in New York City were purposefully infected with the hepatitis virus during research conducted by Dr. Saul Krugman in the 1950s and 1960s. The stated goal of Dr. Krugman was to investigate whether inducing a mild form of hepatitis in children who had previously been injected with gamma-globulin would result in immunity; in essence, he was attempting to develop a vaccine (Robinson & Unruh, 2008). The experiments were highly controversial and the subject of much debate. Charges were made that Dr. Krugman coerced parents into giving consent by providing quick access to the facility, which had an extensive waiting list, and by housing participants in a more hygienic unit where better food was served compared to the rest of the facility. He was further criticized for putting children at risk during nontherapeutic experimentation, with little hope of the children realizing any benefit from the research (Diekma, 2006). Dr. Krugman and others defended his research as a legitimate way to investigate possible strategies to control the spread of hepatitis in institutionalized populations (Krugman, 1971). However, the Willowbrook experiments have historically been looked upon as a classic example of a captive, vulnerable group of participants exploited in the name of scientific research.

The Human Radiation Experiments

In 1994, President Clinton authorized the formation of the Advisory Committee on Human Radiation Experiments to investigate the conduct of scientists working for the U.S. government on projects designed to examine the effects of intentionally exposing human beings to ionizing radiation and also on the effects of the intentional environmental release of ionizing radiation on human health. The committee was charged with looking at experimentation conducted from 1944 through 1974, in a context of time that was marked by the Cold War and deep public anxiety over the threat of nuclear warfare.

What the committee painstakingly uncovered was disturbing. A large number of experiments, many of them conducted in secrecy, were performed by scientists working for various government agencies over the three-decade period of interest. The advisory committee randomly selected 125 of those experiments for closer scrutiny (Faden, 1996). Among those was an experiment conducted at the Fernald School in Waltham, Massachusetts, another school for intellectually disabled children. There, 74 male participants, belonging to a so-called Science Club were fed small amounts of radioactive calcium and iron mixed in oatmeal. The research was funded through a partnership with Quaker Oats Company, the National Institutes of Health, and the Atomic Energy Commission to determine the extent of mineral absorption from various dietary sources in the human body. Similarly, 70 children at the Wrentham State School, another facility in Massachusetts for the intellectually disabled, were given minute amounts of radioactive iodine "to test a proposed countermeasure to nuclear fallout" (Advisory Committee on Human Radiation Experiments, 1995, p. 320).

Vulnerable institutionalized children were not the only group to have been subjected to human radiation experimentation. The advisory committee took testimony from more than 200 people and described the stories they heard as follows:

> We heard from people or their family members who had been subjects in controversial radiation experiments, including the plutonium injections, total-body irradiation experiments. . . . We heard from people who lived "downwind" from nuclear weapons tests in Nevada and intentional releases of radioactive material in Washington state. We heard from Navajo miners who had served the country in uranium mines filled with radioactive dust, from native Alaskans who had been experimented upon by a military cold weather research lab, and from Marshall islanders, whose Pacific homeland had been contaminated by fallout after a 1954 hydrogen bomb test. (p. 9)

The advisory committee ended their report with recommendations for an official apology from the U.S. government and financial compensation for the victims of several of the more egregious experiments. In addition, there were numerous recommendations for the establishment of further protections for the human subjects in experimentation and of oversight agencies. However, the committee also emphasized that ethical conduct in scientific experimentation could not be achieved through policies, regulations, legislation, and oversight committees alone; rather, a humanitarian shift in perspective among the scientific community was necessary. As they so eloquently concluded, "The scientists of the future must have a clear understanding of their duties to human subjects and a clear expectation that the leaders of their fields value good ethics as much as they do good science" (p. 775).

> The _____ _____
> _____ _____ _____
> set forth guidelines to ensure ethical principles of scientific research would be upheld.

> Scientists must obtain approval from an _____ _____
> _____ before conducting research.

The National Research Act of 1974 and the Belmont Report

The reporting of unethical experimentation in the United States, particularly in regard to the Tuskegee study, led to the passage of the National Research Act of 1974, which established the National Commission for the Protection of Human Subjects of Biomedical and Behavioral Research (NCPHSBBR). The charge of the NCPHSBBR was to identify basic ethical principles of scientific research and to set forth guidelines to ensure those principles would be upheld. Their conclusions were published in the Belmont Report of 1979. Scientists are now required to submit their research proposals for approval by institutional review boards (IRBs) to determine that the proposal is in accordance with the guidelines set forth by the Belmont Report. Display Box 10–2 provides required elements of IRBs. Those guidelines include (a) informed consent, (b) consideration of the risk-to-benefit ratio, and (c) selection of participants.

Informed Consent

Individuals must give their informed consent to participate in scientific research. They are entitled to information detailing the procedures of the study, the possible risks that they may encounter, and the possible benefits that they may accrue. Participation must be entirely voluntary. Potential participants must be informed that if they decide not to participate in a study, they will experience no adverse effects. Furthermore, they must be informed that, if they choose to participate, they are free to leave the study at any point after it has commenced.

> Individuals must give their
> _____ _____ to participate in scientific research.

Consent forms should be written in layman's language, free of any professional jargon that may not be comprehensible to the average person. There are multiple steps in acceptable consent procedures. The initial contact with a potential participant should be through a person not involved with the study, such as

---

Display Box 10–2. Institutional Review Boards

Institutional review boards (IRBs) operate under the auspices of the Food and Drug Administration (FDA) and the U.S. Department of Health and Human Services (HHS). IRBs were established by the passage of the National Research Act of 1974. Scientists working at any institution receiving federal support for research (e.g., universities, hospitals, private clinics, etc.) must submit their proposals to their organization's IRB for approval before the research can be conducted. IRBs are required to be composed of at least five members, one of whom must be from the community and not affiliated with the represented organization and one of whom must be a nonscientist. The community member and the nonscientist can be the same person. The IRB is charged with determining that:

- Consent procedures are clearly stipulated and in accordance with ethical guidelines concerning informed consent.
- The method for participant selection is valid and in accordance with ethical guidelines concerning equity in participant selection.
- Possible risks to participants are disclosed and ways to minimize risk are described.
- Benefits that can reasonably be expected for the participants and for adding to the body of knowledge are considered in proportion to possible risks.

---

a member of an office staff. A letter and a consent to be contacted form should be sent to possible participants, asking them if they would like to be contacted by the researchers to learn the details of the study to be conducted. Display Box 10–3 provides a consent to be contacted form. People who return the consent to be contacted form can then be directly contacted by the researcher, who will explain in a neutral, noncoercive manner the purpose and procedures of the study. If a person then decides to participate in a study, a full consent form must be signed stating the nature of the study, the voluntary nature of the person's participation, and the person's right to leave the study at any point. Display Box 10–4 is an example of a full consent form. If the participant is a child, the parent or legal guardian of the child signs the consent form, but the child is also read a statement explaining the study in child-friendly language and detailing the child's rights as a research participant. Display Box 10–5 is an example of a script to be read to a child research participant.

There may be times when an IRB will approve a study that does not include

Display Box 10–3. Example of a Consent to Be Contacted Form

Consent to Be Contacted

You are being asked if you would like to learn about a study designed to evaluate the effectiveness of a potential treatment method in the area of childhood language disorders. The primary investigator in this study is [name]. You are being contacted because you have a child who has received services from [name of speech clinic] or you have a child on the waiting list for services. I am writing to ask your permission to contact you to offer information about the study. After information is provided, you will have the choice of whether or not you want to join the study. Please understand that you are under no obligation to send in your permission to be contacted, and no one will be angry with you if you do not send it in, and your child's services at the clinic will not be affected. If you would like to be contacted, please fill out the form below and mail it in the self-addressed envelope included with this letter.

If I may contact you by telephone and letter to explain the study, please sign below. By signing this form, you are not consenting to be in the research. You are only giving me permission to contact you.

- -

I would be interested in learning the details of the study conducted by [name of researcher] to evaluate the effectiveness of a potential treatment method in the area of childhood language disorders.

Name: _____

Address: _____

Daytime Tel.: _____ Evening Tel.: _____

Email address: _____

full disclosure of the details of the study to the participants. Some studies cannot be conducted in a valid way if participants know of the purpose of the study. A psychological study regarding how people react to elements of surprise, for example, would be impossible to conduct if people were expecting to be surprised.

Display Box 10–4. Example of a Consent Form

Consent Form

This is a study conducted by [name]. The purpose of the study is to evaluate the effectiveness of a potential treatment method in the area of childhood language disorders.

If you agree to participate, your child will be seen at [name of clinic]. Sessions will be held four times a week for 6 weeks, with each session lasting 35 minutes. Services will be provided free of charge to thank you for your participation.

There are risks in any study, and we have taken steps to protect you and your child. Children don't always enjoy participating in treatment sessions, so age-appropriate materials and activities will be used in treatment to make the sessions less aversive. Participant privacy will be maintained, and forms and files will only be seen by the researchers and clinic faculty.

The method used in this study is intended to teach grammatical structures to children diagnosed with language disorders. Therefore, it is possible that participants will benefit by improving their use of appropriate language skills. This may also provide a new treatment method for practicing speech-language pathologists, and it may lead to further research using this method.

Whether or not you choose to participate in this study is entirely your decision. You can decide not to be in the study, or you can drop out of the study at any time. If you have any further questions about the study, please email [name of researcher] at [email address].

This research project has been approved by the Committee on the Protection of Human Subjects Institutional Review Board, [name of institution]. Questions regarding the rights of research participants may be directed to the Committee on the Protection of Human Subjects at [telephone number].

If you would like to participate in the research study described in this form, please sign below. We will give you a copy of this form. Please remember that you can ask the researchers any questions that you may have.

_____   _____
Parent/Guardian Signature   Date

_____   _____
Researcher Signature   Date

Display Box 10–5. Example of a Script for Child Participants

Script to be Read to a Child Participant

Thank you for being part of our experiment. An experiment means that we have a question that we are trying to find an answer to. Our question is: "Can children learn about new ways of talking by answering questions about storybooks we read to them?" After we ask the question, then we look for people who can help us find the answer, and you are one of those people.

We are going to read some storybooks together, and I am going to ask you questions about the storybook. I will also ask you to tell me about the story. I think we will have some fun with this experiment, but if you ever feel sad or mad and want to stop answering my questions, you can. It is a rule about experiments that people who help us should be here because they want to be. You can tell me if you don't want to be here anymore, and I will understand, and I won't be mad, and you can stop being here.

Also, it may be important to the validity of a study for participants, and sometimes research assistants conducting the study, to be "blind" to the purpose or procedures of the study. This is to guard against possible experimenter bias or the placebo effect, which describes the tendency of people to believe they are benefiting from an administered treatment, even when the treatment consists of a placebo. In general, however, for most experimentation conducted today in the United States, the principle of informed consent for participants is upheld.

Risk-to-Benefit Ratio

Scientists applying to an IRB for approval of a research proposal must submit their assessment of the possible risks partici-pants may encounter during the course of the experiment. They then must weigh those risks against the ways in which the study might benefit the participants, the relevant body of research, the institutions they work for, and society in general. Researchers should ensure that the amount of potential risk to the participants is reasonable in proportion to the potential benefits; in other words, they must assess the **risk-to-benefit ratio**.

> Assessment of the risks in proportion to the benefits of a study is called the
>
> _____-____-_____
> _____.

Benefit can be defined as that which contributes something of value. In scientific research, the major goal is to realize benefit by contributing to an existing body of knowledge. Therefore, the first assessment a scientist might make in regard to benefit is to estimate the magnitude to which the study will increase what is already known about the phenomenon under investigation. Benefit on other levels, however, is also considered when assessing the risk-to-benefit ratio. Society at large may benefit from the results of the proposed research, such as when new treatments are found for various diseases. Benefits may also accrue to the institution at which the research is performed, in terms of increased prestige or the acquisition of grant money. Finally, there may be potential immediate benefit to the participants. If a new treatment under investigation proves to be effective, participants will benefit. Also, any compensation that participants might receive in terms of monetary rewards or free services given during the course of the study should also be considered a benefit.

Risk is usually described as *minimal risk* or *more than minimal risk* when the scientist submits a research proposal. A study is considered to put participants at minimal risk when procedures are not anticipated to result in harm or discomfort to the participant that is greater in magnitude than that encountered in daily life or routine medical procedures. If the study subjects participants to harm or discomfort that is more than would be encountered in daily life, then the study is considered to put participants at more than minimal risk. These descriptors are subjective to participant characteristics such as age and lifestyle. For example, if healthy athletic adolescents are required by a research study to run a lap around a track, then that would be a minimal risk activity for them. However, if the participants were over 60 years of age with a sed-entary lifestyle, requiring them to run a lap would put them at more than minimal risk.

Potential risk to participants consists of a variety of forms. Actual physical harm may occur in medical research evaluating a new treatment for cancer that proves to be ineffective, or in behavioral research evaluating a punishment technique, such as the stuttering experiments involving electric shock described in Chapter 1 (Flanagan, Goldiamond, & Azrin, 1958, 1959). Risks also involve psychological reactions that may occur. Participants may become upset in psychological studies requiring disclosure of difficult experiences such as suicidal thoughts or drug abuse. A participant who stutters may become anxious and embarrassed as a result of probes taken in different settings to measure levels of fluency established by an experimental technique. Risk also involves possible breaches of confidentiality, such as when a file is misplaced or left lying around for anyone to see.

The IRB may make suggestions to the researchers as to how to minimize risk to the participants. In regard to the previously described situations, the IRB might require psychological assistance to be available for participants in research studies investigating particularly sensitive issues such as suicide or drug abuse or to minimize the embarrassment the stutterer might experience in different settings by allowing the stutterer to choose the settings in which the probes would be taken. In the case of confidentiality issues, if the researcher has not adequately described security measures, the IRB might suggest that records be stored in a locked cabinet or that pseudonyms be used to identify participants. In other words, no study is entirely risk free, but every effort must be taken to minimize risk to the well-being of the participants.

The Belmont Report noted the subjectivity of risk assessment but firmly asserted the following principles:

1. Inhumane treatment of participants in research is never justified.
2. Risk should be minimized to the extent possible, while still achieving the research objective.
3. There should be ample justification for including participants from vulnerable groups (e.g., children, people with developmental disabilities, etc.).
4. Risks and benefits should be clearly described in consent documents as part of the informed consent procedure.

Participant Selection

Consider again the examples given of unethical, inhumane experimentation leading to the establishment of regulations protecting participants in scientific research. Recall that the participants in such research were often from groups that were captive, vulnerable, and easily exploited. Prisoners, members of minority groups, people from low socioeconomic strata, people who were institutionalized, and children with intellectual and developmental disabilities were subjected, without informed consent, to experimental procedures that put them at much more than minimal risk. The Belmont Report recognized the injustice that such experimentation inflicted on such groups and stated the following:

> Given their dependent status and their frequently compromised capacity for free consent, they should be protected against the danger of being involved in research solely for administrative convenience, or because they are easy

to manipulate as a result of their illness or socioeconomic condition. (NCPHS-BBR, 1979, last para.)

Today, special protections are in place for specified populations. Many IRBs automatically judge a research study to put participants at more than minimal risk if they include children or people with disabilities. Children must give affirmative assent to participate in research; this is why the child participation script is necessary. People who are institutionalized may no longer serve as participants in research just because they are conveniently accessible to researchers, especially when the research will not directly benefit them and has no bearing on their personal situation (U.S. Department of Health and Human Services, 1993).

The Distinction Between Scientific Research and Clinical Practice

So far in this chapter, ethical issues that surround conducting experimental scientific research have been discussed. There are similar issues that must be considered when conducting clinical practice, but there are distinctions that are made between scientific experimentation and clinical practice. These distinctions were succinctly explained in the Belmont Report, as follows:

> The term "practice" refers to interventions that are designed solely to enhance the well-being of an individual patient or client and that have a reasonable expectation of success. . . . By contrast, the term "research" designates an activity designed to test a

hypothesis, permit conclusions to be drawn, and thereby to develop or contribute to generalizable knowledge. . . . Research is usually described in a formal protocol that sets forth an objective and a set of procedures designed to reach that objective. (NCPHSBBR, 1979, Part A, Boundaries between Practice and Research, para. 2)

Speech-language pathologists (SLPs) applying behavioral principles during clinical work may modify their procedures in response to the individual needs of their clients. Routine modifications to intervention procedures do not constitute the type of experimentation that requires IRB approval. If, however, an SLP makes some major innovation to established procedures, it would be an ethical next step to conduct the type of formal experimentation that would require IRB approval to determine the efficacy of the innovation.

Although most routine clinical work is different from scientific experimentation, ethical considerations guide clinical practice just as strictly. The following sections discuss the attributes of professional people in general, leading to an examination of ethical conduct in specific clinical situations.

Ethical Issues in Conducting Treatment

Adults and children who seek the services of SLPs are real people experiencing real difficulties with their communicative skills. They may be upset; they may be frustrated. They may be so discouraged by past failures that they need help in realizing their ability to change and to reach their goals, however modest those

goals might be. Parents of children with communicative challenges are especially vulnerable. They need accurate information and education regarding techniques they can use to help their child. They need, in short, the support of an SLP who understands what it means to be an ethical professional person.

What Does It Mean to Be an Ethical Professional?

People who pursue career paths in professional occupations are distinguished in several ways from those who pursue other occupations. These distinctions include the pursuit of specialized education and membership in professional organizations, which set forth standards of professional performance, a scope of practice, and, most relevant to the topic of this chapter, a code of ethics.

Professionals attain a specific education that leads to a specialized body of knowledge and usually an advanced college degree. They then must submit themselves to a rigorous examination of their knowledge that leads to licensure, certification, or both, identifying them as qualified to practice in their field. For example, aspiring doctors take the medical board licensing exam, attorneys take the bar exam, SLPs take the national Praxis exam, and behavior analysts take the Behavior Analyst Certification Board exam. As a result of their rigorous training, professionals have a shared common knowledge of their profession and often use specialized terminology to communicate with each other.

Professionals belong to organizations that represent and advocate for their occupation, such as the American Speech-Language-Hearing Association (ASHA) for SLPs. These organizations set forth performance standards that members must uphold and also set forth requirements for continuing education. Professionals must consider themselves to be lifelong learners, must keep current in their field, and must complete a certain number of hours of continuing education in order to maintain licensure and certification.

> Continuing education requires professionals to be _____ learners.

The professional organization also sets forth a scope of practice that clearly defines the areas of practice that members are qualified to conduct. The scope of practice for SLPs is vast and continues to grow (ASHA, 2007). It is a dynamic instrument that has responded to trends leading to SLP involvement in dysphagia, in literacy, in neonatal intensive care, in the treatment and diagnosis of autism, and in the provision of augmentative and alternative communication systems.

> The _____ _____ _____ clearly defines areas of practice that professionals are qualified to conduct.

Finally, professionals are distinguished by adherence to a code of ethics. **Ethics** is a branch of philosophy that is concerned with distinguishing between human behavior that is right and human behavior that is wrong. Once that distinction is made, recommendations can be made regarding how people must conduct themselves in order to function as ethical individuals. Professionals are bound by the principles and rules that define ethi-

cal conduct formulated by their professional organization. For SLPs, the code of ethics sets forth broad principles that are characterized as "aspirational and inspirational in nature" (ASHA, 2010, p. 1). Refer to Display Box 10–6 for a website address leading to the ASHA code of ethics. Under each principle, there are several rules that are "specific statements of minimally acceptable professional conduct or prohibitions" (p. 1). The code of ethics is revised from time to time, to respond to societal changes that affect the profession of speech-language pathology. For example, the latest version of the code of ethics mentions "telecommunication (i.e., telehealth/e-health)" and states that SLPs can ethically deliver services via those means, when permitted by law to do so.

> _____ is a branch of philosophy that is concerned with distinguishing between human behavior that is right and human behavior that is wrong.

All professional organizations specify a code of ethics. For board certified behavior analysts (BCBAs), the Behavior Analyst Certification Board (BACB) currently has in place two documents referred to as "conduct guidelines" and "disciplinary standards" (BACB, 2014, para. 1). However, the organization is currently working to consolidate those two documents into one professional and ethical compliance code (to be released January 2016; go to http://www.bacb.com/Download files/BACB_Compliance_Code.pdf). The guidelines now in place emphasize several major areas. Behavior analysts must "maintain the high standards of professional behavior of the professional organization" (BACB, 2010, p. 1). They must

---

Display Box 10–6. The Code of Ethics (American Speech-Language-Hearing Association, 2010)

The Code of Ethics consists of four broad general principles with specific rules relevant to each principle. The Code of Ethics can be viewed in its entirety at: http://www.asha.org/Code-of-Ethics/

"operate in the best interest of clients" (p. 4). Other guidelines highlight the importance of consulting research to support practices such as conducting behavior assessment and devising and implementing plans for behavior change. The role of the behavior analyst in generating original research to add to the evidence base of the profession is also emphasized.

All ethical professionals conduct themselves according to the guidelines of their profession when delivering therapeutic services to clients and when conducting scientific research. To deliver the best service to clients who deeply need it, SLPs should keep in mind the following ethical issues in conducting treatment: (a) informing the client regarding the nature of treatment methods, (b) maintaining confidentiality, (c) considering the client's preferences, and (d) upholding the client's right to effective treatment.

to use in place of technical terms. Similarly, behavioral principles should be explained in plain language, going into enough detail to let clients know what to expect during treatment. For example, clients should be told that there will be many opportunities to practice skills they are trying to learn and that there will be feedback given to them regarding the correctness of their productions. Prompts and cues designed to evoke correct responses should be described, along with the method of data collection. If a token economy is to be used, clients need to know what they must do to earn tokens and how many tokens they need to turn in for what kind of back-up reinforcers. Changes made to the original treatment plan should be discussed with the client, along with the rationale for making those changes. This type of information should be given throughout the therapeutic process.

Informing the Client

The client has the right to be fully informed regarding the treatment procedures the clinician recommends. Information should be given in a forthright manner, and the clinician should avoid using professional jargon, which may not be at all understood by the client. Table 10–1 provides some examples of client-friendly language

Confidentiality

The word *confidentiality* does not appear in the Code of Ethics, but Principle I, Rule N states the following:

Individuals [SLPs] shall not reveal, without authorization, any professional or personal information about identified persons served profession-

Table 10–1. Examples of Client-Friendly Language

Instead of . . .	Say . . .
Articulation	The way sounds are made when you talk
Discrete trials	Opportunities to practice the client's stated goals
Dysfluency	Stuttering
Fluency	The way we speak when the words come out smoothly, with no struggle
Morphemes	The small structures we add to the beginning or ending of words that affect the meaning of the word; for example, the *–ed* we add to the end of verbs to talk about something we did in the past
Phonological processes	Common patterns of mistakes children make when they talk; if those mistakes persist for too long, they need some help
Pragmatic language skills	What we learn to do when we talk to other people; for example, during a conversation, we take turns, we give eye contact, and we stick to the same topic of conversation for a while
Prosody	Intonation when you speak; for example, we raise our pitch when we ask a question and lower it when we make a statement
Semantics	The meaning of the words we speak
Syntax	How we put words together to make correct sentences
Target behaviors	The skills the client will learn during therapy
Vocal intensity	The loudness of your voice
Vocal frequency	The pitch of your voice; everyone has a range of how high and low pitch ranges when we talk

ally or identified participants involved in research and scholarly activities unless doing so is necessary to protect the welfare of the person or of the community or is otherwise required by law. (ASHA, 2010, p. 2)

There are some key phrases in this rule that indicate the exceptions to the SLP's responsibility to keep confidential information about the client and about the treatment the client is receiving. The phrase "without authorization" indicates that information may be shared about a client when the client authorizes, in writing, release of information. Clients may authorize clinicians to release information regarding their speech and language diagnosis and treatment objectives to medical personnel who are also providing care for the client. Similarly, school SLPs may receive authorization from a student's parents to release information regarding the student's Individual Education Plan (IEP) to other SLPs in private practice or to the student's pediatrician. Most organizations that SLPs work for have specific forms prepared for clients and clients' parents, guardians, or caregivers to sign specifying exactly what information may be released.

The rule also stipulates that clinicians may release information when it is necessary to do so for the welfare of the person or of the community. Although situations such as these are probably more common for psychologists, it is still possible that clients may, for example, express to clinicians suicidal thoughts or plans for aggressive actions against teachers or students in a public school. In these cases, SLPs have the responsibility to bring this information to the attention of authorities who may be able to help the client and protect society.

Finally, the phrase "otherwise required by law" indicates that there are also circumstances in which SLPs must share information about clients because there are legal obligations to do so. There are at least two instances in which disclosure of client information is required by law. SLPs, as are other professionals, are mandatory reporters of child neglect and child abuse. Display Box 10–7 provides a list of professionals who are mandatory reporters. Requirements for mandatory reporters vary slightly, according to which state the SLP works in, but the ultimate mandate is firm. When a professional person has reason to suspect that a child has been subjected to abuse, neglect, or, in many instances, both, it must be reported to law enforcement agencies, child protection services, or hotlines available in many states. The law in most states is clear regarding the responsibility of professional people to report directly to these agencies, rather than abide by policies of the organizations they work for that may suggest first reporting to supervising administrators or internal entities, such as a school district police department (Child Welfare Information Gateway, 2014).

SLPs may also from time to time receive a subpoena requiring them to release what would otherwise be confidential client information. A subpoena orders the recipient to testify in person, or to provide specified documents to the court or attorneys issuing the subpoena. Often, an SLP is asked to both testify and to provide specified documents. When a subpoena is received, there is no choice

---

Display Box 10–7. Mandatory Reporters of Child Abuse and Neglect

This list is from the laws of the state of California, which is one of the most inclusive lists in the nation. Two states, New Jersey and Wyoming, state only that "all persons" must report child abuse and neglect. Mandated reporters include the following:

- Teachers, teacher's aides, administrators, and employees of public or private schools

- Administrators or employees of day camps, youth centers, or youth recreation programs
- Administrators or employees of licensed community care or child daycare facilities; Head Start program teachers
- Public assistance workers
- Foster parents, group home personnel, and personnel of residential care facilities
- Social workers, probation officers, and parole officers
- Employees of school district police or security departments
- District attorney investigators, inspectors, or local child support agency caseworkers
- Peace officers and firefighters, except for volunteer firefighters
- Physicians, surgeons, psychiatrists, psychologists, dentists, residents, interns, podiatrists, chiropractors, licensed nurses, dental hygienists, optometrists, marriage and family therapists, or social workers
- State or county public health employees who treat minors for venereal diseases or other conditions
- Coroners and medical examiners
- Commercial film and photographic print or image processors; computer technicians
- Child visitation monitors
- Animal control or humane society officers
- Clergy members and custodians of records of clergy members
- Employees of police departments, county sheriff's departments, county probation departments, or county welfare departments
- Employees or volunteers of a Court-Appointed Special Advocate program
- Alcohol and drug counselors
- Employees or administrators of public or private postsecondary institutions
- Athletic coaches, athletic administrators, or athletic directors employed by any public or private schools
- Athletic coaches, including, but not limited to, assistant coaches or graduate assistants involved in coaching at public or private postsecondary institutions

Source: Child Welfare Information Gateway (2014).

but to relinquish whatever information has been asked for, with or without the client's permission. Display Box 10–8 presents a situation involving an SLP receiving a subpoena.

Considering Clients' Preferences

The exchange of information between clients and clinicians should not be a one-way process. As previously discussed in Chapter 7 on generalization and maintenance, clinicians need to actively seek out and consider input from clients when devising assessment and treatment plans. Clients' preferences and values are integral to the concept of evidence-based practice, which, according to ASHA (2004),

consists of three elements: (a) analysis and consideration of clinical scientific evidence, (b) the expertise of the clinician, and (c) the client's values, interests, and choices.

A clinician who practices evidence-based behavioral methods may come into conflict from time to time with clients who express different choices. As mentioned in Chapter 1, behaviorism has been the subject of intense controversy in the past and, to a lesser extent, currently. Some clients may have objections to a behavioral approach based on their own beliefs and values that may be more in agreement with positions of spirituality and mentalism—concepts that are not supported by behavioral principles. Some might also just not like behavioral approaches, which can be at least mildly

---

Display Box 10–8. Relinquishing Information Required by Law

Consider the following situation:

An SLP at the Get-Well Rehab Center has been subpoenaed to appear in court. The SLP had been treating Mr. Jones for a couple of weeks as part of his rehabilitation stay in the hospital. The SLP had to stop seeing Mr. Jones (whose diagnosis was moderate apraxia of speech) because his insurance would no longer pay for his services, despite documented daily improvement in his communication skills. Mrs. Jones, his wife, was outraged by the insurance company and decided to sue. The SLP was called as an expert witness. As part of these court proceedings, the SLP was required to make public Mr. Jones's speech diagnosis, her documentation of his improvement, his case history, and so forth.

- Is there any unethical behavior on the part of the SLP in this case?
- Is there anything that the SLP could have done differently?

aversive, even to those who seek them out. For example, time-out is a very well-researched behavioral method for treating undesirable behaviors; in the field of communicative disorders, it is especially applicable to the treatment of stuttering. Clinicians employ the time-out procedure when working with dysfluent clients by holding a hand up at the first sign of the client's dysfluency and turning away briefly from the client before allowing the client to continue. Although this has been shown to be effective, some clients may object to the procedure as awkward or uncomfortable for them, even after the clinician has explained the method and described the research base that supports it. In that case, the clinician will need to find another effective way to treat the client's dysfluency.

Another conflict might arise when clients demand to be treated using a method that lacks a scientific research base or, worse, has been shown through scientific research to be ineffective; in other words, a method that is pseudoscientific (see Chapter 9 for a more thorough discussion of pseudoscientific treatment methods). Parents of children with autism may be especially vulnerable to the claims made by pseudoscientific "experts" who advocate for methods that lack scientific evidence of efficacy. SLPs may need to explain that they deliver services only using methods that are well supported by scientific research. SLPs should discuss with clients the research base for the behavioral approach and the lack of scientific evidence for the desired treatment method. If the clients still wish to seek treatment through pseudoscientific methods, they may be referred elsewhere.

Another interesting phenomenon occurs when people with communicative disorders reject altogether seeking treatment through scientifically supported methods. For example, some people who stutter may become discouraged and angry over failed treatment methods and simply decide, often with the help of support groups, to accept themselves as lifelong stutterers (Yaruss et al., 2002). Similarly, people who are deaf may have been subjected to a great deal of speech and language therapy as young children, in deference to their families' wish for them to use oral speech. Some may grow up to reject oral speech in favor of American Sign Language, embracing the Deaf culture. These are choices that people have a right to make; SLPs should not foist their services on people who do not want them. The majority of people with communicative disorders, however, want effective treatment—and they have the right to have it.

The Client's Right to Effective Treatment

Most clients want to improve and will therefore embrace effective treatment. All people who need it should have access to effective treatment; indeed, it has been suggested that access to effective treatment is a fundamental right. In the field of behavior analysis, van Houten et al. (1988) described the client's right to effective treatment and systematically set forth components comprising effective treatment. Although their article is directly relevant to service delivery by behavior analysts, their description of effective treatment can be extended to the field of speech-language pathology. Components of effective treatment, as described by van Houten et al. (1988), that are applicable to SLPs include (a) provision of an effective therapeutic environment, (b) delivery of services that promote the personal welfare of the client, (c) clinical competency, and (d) an emphasis on functional skills.

The Therapeutic Environment

Clinicians working in private practice are perhaps in the best position to control the therapeutic environment they provide for the client. Clinic rooms should be roomy enough for at least two people to work in comfortably. The physical layout of a private clinic room should provide maximum opportunities for interactions between the clinician and the client. Seating arrangements should be well thought out and determined according to the needs of the client. For example, the clinician may sit across the table from an adult, on the floor with a small child, or side-by-side with an older child who needs some additional support in attending to treatment tasks. Furniture should be suitable for the age and size of the client. Materials available should be geared toward client preferences and appropriate for evoking the targeted behaviors.

Not all clinicians, of course, are private practitioners. Sometimes, SLPs working for other types of agencies, such as schools, hospitals, and skilled nursing facilities, find themselves in environments that are less than ideal. Anecdotes from school SLPs in particular have indicated that sometimes space in public schools is hard to come by. For example, they may be required to work in a converted maintenance closet, backstage in the school auditorium (sometimes during band practice), or in a portable classroom located a distance away from the other classrooms. Fortunately, a therapeutic environment is more than the physical layout and materials available. Clients also need to feel that they are safe and supported in the clinic room and that they are being treated by a competent, caring clinician. Clients will work hard when there is a warm rapport between client and clinician based on trust, respect, and collaboration, no matter how imperfect the physical environment might be. The therapeutic environment can also be extended to include supportive parents at home, teachers in the classroom, and caregivers in medical settings.

The Personal Welfare of the Client

Principle I of the ASHA Code of Ethics states clearly that clinicians must "hold paramount the welfare of persons they serve professionally" (ASHA, 2010, p. 1). This would seem to be an obvious statement; however, sometimes SLPs work for organizations that may require them to adhere to policies that are more for the good of the organization than for the good of the client. These are policies that are often driven by limited funding for necessary services or lack of a sufficient number of programs to meet the needs of all clients the organization serves. Display Box 10–9 gives examples of policy conflicting with client interests. When SLPs encounter such situations, they need to remember that they are independent professionals bound by a code of ethics that takes priority over policies that hamper their ability to serve and advocate for their clients.

Clinical Competency

Clients have the right to receive treatment from competent clinicians. Principle I, Rule A of the Code of Ethics states simply that "individuals [SLPs] shall provide all services competently" (ASHA, 2010, p. 1).

Display Box 10–9. When Policy Conflicts With Client Interests

Consider the following situations:

An SLP working in the public schools has succeeded in obtaining funding for a voice output communication aid (VOCA) for a nonverbal kindergarten child with autism. She strongly feels that the child should also have access to a VOCA in the home and community settings. However, school district policy prohibits the child from taking the VOCA home. The SLP would like to suggest obtaining a second VOCA for the child to use at home and in the community, but she has been firmly told that she should not make such a recommendation, because the school district might be held responsible for funding the second device.

An SLP has been employed by a hospital, and, as part of her duties, she is assigned to the neonatal intensive care unit (NICU) where she is expected to provide evaluation and intervention in the areas of infant communication and feeding and to provide counseling and education to parents and staff. She immediately notices, however, that the hospital does not have a policy supportive of developmental care. The NICU is noisy and brightly lit. Developmentally supportive practices such as swaddling, kangaroo care, and nesting are not in place. Parent involvement in decision making is minimal.

An SLP working with children with autism in the public schools has been asked to assess the speech and language skills of a 5-year-old boy to help in determining proper placement. Her assessment reveals emerging expressive language with difficulties in pragmatic language skills commonly encountered in children with autism. The Individual Education Program (IEP) team has recommended placement for this child in a functional skill classroom for low-functioning special needs children, with minimal opportunities for mainstreaming, because that is the program in which the district has space available for the child. The SLP strongly feels that this is an inappropriate placement for the child because of his higher functioning skills. She is prohibited from expressing this opinion, however, because

> of an unwritten school policy that emphasizes the importance of being a "team player."
>
> ■ How can the SLPs in these situations uphold their ethical obligation to "hold paramount the welfare of persons they serve professionally" (ASHA, 2010, p. 1)?

SLPs go through rigorous undergraduate and graduate programs of study and serve a clinical fellowship year (CFY) under the supervision of a licensed and certified SLP before becoming licensed and certified themselves. In addition, they have stringent continuing education requirements that they must fulfill to keep current in the field. In other words, by virtue of their past and continuing education, SLPs strive to uphold high standards of clinical competency.

However, the Scope of Practice for SLPs is quite broad, and SLPs may switch populations and settings from time to time, in response to their intellectual curiosity and life situations. This is certainly permissible, but Principle II, Rule B of the Code of Ethics states that "individuals shall engage in only those aspects of their professional practice and competence, considering their level of education, training, and experience" (ASHA, 2010, p. 3). Therefore, SLPs who make a drastic shift in the emphasis of their practice need to seek out continuing education, and they need to seek out the help of fellow SLPs who have experience in the desired setting, populations, or both for consultation and job shadowing. Ideally, SLPs who change settings, with populations they have not previously served, will receive training and support from the organizations they are entering. Display Box 10–10 presents a scenario describing an ethical dilemma for an SLP changing her practice setting.

An Emphasis on Functional Skills

van Houten et al. (1988) stated, "The ultimate goal of all services is to increase the ability of individuals to function effectively in both their immediate environment and the larger society" (p. 382). Clients therefore have the right to access services that will result in measurable improvements in those aspects of communication that affect their quality of life, including increased skills in (a) gaining access to desired objects and activities, (b) entering into satisfying social interactions, (c) improving occupational performance, and (d) increasing access to educational curriculum.

The targeted communicative behaviors SLPs teach, then, should be directly relevant to the ability of the client to function effectively within client-specific environments. Including client input is critical in devising these types of highly specific functional goals and requires SLPs and other professional people to enter into collaborative partnerships with clients. For example, Ingham, Ingham, and Bothe (2012) stated that in order to deliver treatment services to people who stutter (PWS) that "result in personally significant outcomes, the decisions need to be made by clients. In other words, treatment should incorporate speaking tasks or situations that the person who stutters selects as being personally significant" (p. 267). To illustrate this point, two case studies

---

Display Box 10–10. Changing Practice Settings

Consider the following situation:

Sally has been working in the state of California in a school setting ever since she graduated with her master's degree in speech-language pathology 10 years ago. Her master's program was well balanced, including coursework in treating communicative disorders in school-aged children and in treating adults with neurological and swallowing disorders. She holds her credential issued by the California Commission on Teacher Credentialing and her California license, and she maintains her Certificate of Clinical Competence issued by the American Speech-Language-Hearing Association. She has recently experienced a significant increase in living expenses, due to her daughter's admittance to a private university with high tuition in another state. Sally has always received phone calls from health care providers looking for SLPs to work in skilled nursing facilities. She has been offered as much as $60.00 per hour for per diem work in medical settings. She is now thinking very seriously about taking an offer of part-time employment from an agency that contracts out to medical settings. Her duties will include assessment and treatment for cognitive function, swallowing disorders, and feeding issues. The contracting agency has told her that, because she is a fully licensed SLP, they do not feel it is necessary for her to receive formal training through their organization.

- What ethical issues are involved with this scenario?
- Is there any way in which Sally can ethically accept this offer of employment?

---

were described; one client learned to fluently produce her name in front of more than one person, and one client learned to fluently produce his name and the name of his company while making business telephone calls (Ingham et al., 2012). Other stutterers might select personally significant speaking tasks such as ordering food in a restaurant, asking a person to go out on a date, or speaking in front of an audience.

Clients and their significant others should be consulted regarding devising target behaviors that, when taught, will result in such personally and socially significant outcomes. Adults with intellectual disabilities, for example, may need to learn phrases that will be useful for them in their jobs, such as, *I'm done, What can I do now?, Can you help me with this?*, and so forth. Parents of children who use systems of augmentative and alternative communication might want their children to learn to ask for objects or activities or to respond to yes/no questions. Adolescents who have experienced a traumatic brain injury may need functional target behaviors that will allow them to return to school, such as learning to organize an academic schedule, to attend to academic tasks, or to improve recall of information. Treatment provided by SLPs to address such functional skills will result in improvement to clients that is personally and socially significant, thereby contributing to an increased quality of life for clients, for their significant others, and for society in general.

Chapter Summary

1. Atrocities committed in Nazi concentration camps during World War II brought the world's attention to the treatment of individuals subjected to unethical, inhumane scientific experimentation.
2. As a result of the uncovering of unethical experimentation conducted in the United States, the National Research Act of 1974 was enacted to put into place legally mandated protections for participants in scientific research funded by U.S. government agencies.
3. As a result of the National Research Act of 1974, the National Commission for the Protection of Human Subjects of Biomedical and Behavioral Research (NCPHSBBR) was established to identify basic ethical principles of scientific research and to set forth guidelines to ensure those principles would be upheld.
4. In 1979, the NCPHSBBR published the Belmont Report, detailing their conclu-

sions. Applications of principles of the ethical conduct of scientific research included guidelines regarding:
   a. Informed consent
   b. Assessment of the risk-to-benefit ratio
   c. Participant selection
5. Scientists must now submit proposed research for approval by institutional review boards (IRBs) to determine if the proposed research is in conformance with principles of the ethical conduct of scientific research.
6. There are strict ethical considerations to be made when conducting clinical practice, but there are distinctions that are made between scientific experimentation and clinical practice.
7. Modifications made to treatment plans during routine clinical work do not require review by IRBs; however, if a significant departure from established clinical procedures is made, the ethical next step would be to conduct the type of formal experimentation that would require IRB approval to determine the efficacy of the innovation.
8. A professional person is defined by the following characteristics:
   a. An education that leads to a specialized body of knowledge and usually an advanced college degree
   b. Membership in professional organizations that represent and advocate for their occupation, such as the American Speech-Language-Hearing Association for SLPs
   c. Adherence to a scope of practice that clearly defines the areas of practice that members are qualified to conduct
   d. Adherence to a professional code of ethics

9. Further issues to be considered when conducting ethical clinical practice include:
   a. Keeping the client informed regarding treatment procedures, in language that avoids the use of professional jargon, which may not be understood by the client
   b. Maintaining client confidentiality
   c. Considering the client's preferences
   d. Upholding the client's right to effective treatment
10. The client's right to effective treatment includes the following components:
    a. An appropriate therapeutic environment
    b. Service focused on the personal welfare of the client
    c. Service delivered by a competent clinician
    d. Treatment that emphasizes functional skills that are socially significant to the client

Application Exercises

1. Go to http://psyc604.stasson.org/Milgram2.pdf for yet another example of a study conducted before the advent of legally mandated protections for participants in scientific research. Consider how the study relates to the following concepts regarding the ethical conduct of scientific experimentation:
   a. Risk-to-benefit ratio
   b. Informed consent
   c. Participant selection
2. Go to http://www.asha.org and search for the Code of Ethics. Look at the broad principles and specific rules under each principle. Look for rules that apply to the following three scenarios:

Scenario 1

Angela is the mother of a 4-year-old minimally verbal boy who has recently been diagnosed with moderately severe intellectual disability. She is, understandably, distraught, and she rejects the findings of those professionals. She consults with various other professionals, all of whom agree with the diagnosis of mental retardation. Then she goes to consult with John, a speech-language pathologist in private practice. John listens to what Angela has to say and interacts with her son for approximately 15 minutes. Then, he tells her with great confidence that her child most certainly does not have mental retardation. "Just enroll him in speech therapy with me," John tells Angela, "and within 6 months, he will just explode with speech and language." Angela happily agrees to bring her child to John, and she is charged $80.00 for each 40-minute session, twice a week.

Scenario 2

You are an SLP working for a skilled nursing facility in town for a well-known for-profit organization. You have been treating Mrs. Gonzales, who has Wernicke aphasia with severely impaired auditory comprehension and verbal expression deficits. In the course of treatment, Mrs. Gonzales has shown no improvement in any of the areas you are targeting in treatment (despite your many attempts at modifying your approach). You discuss this case with the director of rehab, and in the course of your discussion, it is apparent that the director of rehab wants you to continue seeing Mrs. Gonzales because you must maintain a certain number of units to be considered a "productive therapist." In a subtle way, she hints that maybe you should "document a little bit differently."

Scenario 3

You are a school SLP with an 8-year-old nonverbal boy with autism in a special day class on your caseload. The parents are determined to find a treatment that will help their child talk and on their own have resorted to several alternative methods that are not evidence based. They have now decided they want you, the school SLP, to include an approach that you have never heard of in the boy's treatment plan. How would you ethically address this situation?

References

Advisory Committee on Human Radiation Experiments. (1995). *Final report of the Advisory Committee on Human Radiation Experiments*. Washington, DC: U.S. Government Printing Office.

American Speech-Language-Hearing Association. (2004). *Report of the Joint Committee on Evidence-Based Practice*. Retrieved from http://www.asha.org/Members/ebp/intro/

American Speech-Language-Hearing Association. (2007). *Scope of practice in speech-language pathology* [Scope of practice]. Retrieved from http://www.asha.org/policy

American Speech-Language-Hearing Association. (2010). *Code of ethics* [Ethics]. Retrieved from http://www.asha.org/policy

Behavior Analyst Certification Board. (2010). *Guidelines for responsible conduct for behavior analysts*. Retrieved May 2, 2015, from http://www.bacb.com/Downloadfiles/BACBguidelines/BACB_Conduct_Guidelines.pdf

Behavior Analyst Certification Board. (2014). *BACB Newsletter: Special Edition on Ethics*. Retrieved May 2, 2015, from http://www.bacb.com/newsletter/BACB_Newsletter_09-14.pdf

Berger, R. L. (1990). Nazi science—The Dachau hypothermia experiments. *The New England Journal of Medicine, 322*, 1435–1440.

Child Welfare Information Gateway. (2014). *Mandatory reporters of child abuse and neglect*. Washington, DC: U.S. Department of Health and Human Services, Children's Bureau. Retrieved from https://www.childwelfare.gov/systemwide/laws_policies/statutes/manda.cfm

Cuerda, E., & Lopez-Munoz, F. (2013). Ethical considerations of the human research: Syphilis experiments and denial of drug therapy. *Clinical Experimental Pharmacology, 3*. Retrieved from http://dx.doi.org/10.4172/2161-1459.1000e124

Cuerda-Galindo, E., Sierra-Valenti, X., Gonzalez-Lopez, E., & Lopez-Munoz, F. (2014). Syphilis and human experimentation from World War II to the present: A historical perspective and reflections on ethics. *ACTAS Dermo-Sifiliograficas, 105*, 847–853.

Diekma, D. (2006). Conducting ethical research in pediatrics: A brief historical overview and review of pediatric regulations. *The Journal of Pediatrics, 149*, S3–S11.

Faden, R. (1996). The Advisory Committee on Human Radiation Experiments: Reflections on a presidential commission. *Hastings Center Report, 26*, 5–10.

Flanagan, B., Goldiamond, I., & Azrin, N. (1958). Operant stuttering: The control of stuttering behavior through response-contingent consequences. *Journal of the Experimental Analysis of Behavior, 1*, 173–177.

Flanagan, B., Goldiamond, I., & Azrin, N. (1959). Instatement of stuttering in normally fluent individuals through operant procedures. *Science, 130*, 979–981.

Ingham, R. J., Ingham, J. C., & Bothe, A. K. (2012). Integrating functional measures with treatment: A tactic for enhancing personally significant change in the treatment of adults and adolescents who stutter. *American Journal of Speech-Language Pathology, 21*, 264–277.

Katz, R. V., Kegeles, S. S., Kressin, N. R., Green, B. L., Wang, M. Q., James, S. A., & Claudio, C. (2006). The Tuskegee Legacy Project: Willingness of minorities to participate in biomedical research. *Journal of Health Care for the Poor and Underserved, 17,* 698–715.

Krugman, S. (1971). Experiments at the Willowbrook State School [Letter to the editor]. *The Lancet, 1*(7706), 966–967.

National Commission for the Protection of Human Subjects of Biomedical and Behavioral Research. (1979). *The Belmont report: Ethical principles and guidelines for the protection of human subjects of research.* Washington, DC: U.S. Department of Health and Human Services. Retrieved from http://www.hhs.gov/ohrp/humansubjects/guidance/belmont.html

Nuremberg Code. (1949). *Trials of war criminals before the Nuremberg Military Tribunals under Control Council Law No. 10* (Vol. 2, pp. 181–182). Washington, DC: U.S. Government Printing Office.

Reverby, S. (2011). "Normal exposure" and inoculation syphilis: A PHS "Tuskegee" doctor in Guatemala, 1946–1948. *Journal of Policy History, 23,* 6–28.

Robinson, W. M., & Unruh, B. T. (2008). The hepatitis experiments at the Willowbrook State School. In E. J. Emanuel, C. Grady, R. A. Crouch, R. K. Lie, F. G. Miller, & D. Wendler (Eds.), *The Oxford textbook of clinical research ethics* (pp. 81–84). New York, NY: Oxford University Press.

U.S. Department of Health and Human Services. (1993). *Institutional review board guidebook: Chapter 5. Special classes of subjects.* Retrieved May 13, 2015, from http://www.hhs.gov/ohrp/archive/irb/irb_chapter6.htm

van Houten, R., Axelrod, S., Bailey, J. S., Favell, J. E., Foxx, R. M., Iwata, B. A., & Lovaas, O. I. (1988). The right to effective behavioral treatment. *Journal of Applied Behavior Analysis, 21,* 381–384.

Wiesel, E. (2005). Without conscience. *The New England Journal of Medicine, 352,* 1511–1513.

Yaruss, J. S., Quesal, R. W., Reeves, L., Molt, L. F., Kluetz, B., Caruso, A. J., . . . Lewis, F. (2002). Speech treatment and support group experiences of people who participate in the National Stuttering Association. *Journal of Fluency Disorders, 27,* 115–134.

Glossary

A-B-C- contingencies. The relationship between antecedent stimuli (the "A"), behaviors (the "B"), and consequence stimuli (the "C"); often referred to as three-term or S-R-C (i.e., stimulus-response-consequence)

ABC recording. Collecting data during direct observations conducted within FBAs to discover the antecedents and consequences of an observed behavior

Antecedent. Stimuli that evoke behaviors

Antecedent interventions. Attempts to reduce undesirable behaviors by altering the environmental events that occur prior to the response in order to decrease the occurrence of the behavior

Antecedent manipulations. Altering the stimuli that occur prior to a behavior being exhibited

Applied behavior analysis. A science in which interventions based on principles of behaviorism are applied to increase socially significant behavior, and variables affecting behavior are discovered through experimentation

Assertive autoclitics. Autoclitics define the relationship between causal variables and responses in such a way that they move the listener in a positive direction or intensify behavior

Autoclitic mands. Verbal behaviors that are controlled by a specific motivating operation and are produced to mand the listener to react in some specific way to the primary verbal operant

Autoclitics. Secondary verbal operants that include morphological structures and other elements of grammar, as well as any part of the verbal behavior that provides additional information about what the speaker has said and the circumstances under which the person is speaking

Automatic reinforcement. Occurs when a behavior itself produces sensory stimulation that automatically reinforces the undesirable response; not dependent upon the mediation of another person

Avoidance. Occurs when a client engages in specific behaviors to keep from coming in contact with an aversive stimulus

Backward chaining. The clinician initially teaches the last component of a target behavior, and once this task has been established, the client is then expected to perform the last and second to last steps in succession prior to receiving reinforcement; this process is continued until the target behavior in its totality is produced

Baselines. Measures of the target behavior in the absence of treatment

Behaviorism. An approach to psychology that combines elements of philosophy, methodology, and theory

Behavior modification. The application of well-researched, empirically based principles of behaviorism by a person or persons to either increase or decrease a specified human behavior in another person

Board certified behavior analyst (BCBA). A professional person who conducts descriptive and systematic behavioral assessments, including functional analyses, and provides behavior analytic interpretations of the results

Chaining. Reinforcing successive components of a target behavior

Classical conditioning. A process of behavior modification in which a reflexive response to an unconditioned stimulus is given to a previously neutral stimulus; achieved by repeated pairings of the neutral stimulus and the unconditioned stimulus that eventually becomes a conditioned stimulus

Conditioned reinforcers. Over time, individuals learn the reinforcing value of certain stimuli based on their previous pairing with other reinforcers

Conditioned response. The learned response (reflexive behavior) to a conditioned stimulus

Conditioned stimulus. A formerly neutral stimulus (e.g., a bell ringing), which, when paired with an unconditioned stimulus (e.g., food), elicits a conditioned response (e.g., salivation)

Contingency. The correlation between a behavior and various other environmental stimuli

Contingency priming. A technique that involves clients asking for reinforcement when significant others in their natural environment fail to give it

Continuous schedules of reinforcement. The client receives a reinforcer after every correct response

Convergent intraverbal control. Occurs when several verbal stimuli evoke a single intraverbal response

Conversational probe. A procedure conducted to determine if the correct response is produced in the presence of only new, untaught stimuli during conversation

Corrective feedback. A positive punishment procedure that involves providing clients with information that describes why a response was in error

Dependent variable. In scientific research, the event examined to determine how it changes when the independent variable is introduced

Derivative measures. Involve combining two sets of data obtained during an observation session, as in calculating a percentage

Descriptive autoclitics. Autoclitics that describe the primary verbal operant; they tact the controlling variables of the verbal operant they accompany

Determinism. The belief that everything that happens in the world is the result of cause-effect relationships and that there is a systematic order in which phenomena relate to each other

Dictation. A type of transcription where a written response is controlled by a vocal stimulus

Differential reinforcement. A treatment method that involves placing one behavior on extinction while concurrently providing reinforcement for another

Differential reinforcement of alternative behaviors (DRA). Involves putting the undesirable behavior on extinction and reinforcing a defined alternative behavior that serves the same function

Differential reinforcement of incompatible behaviors (DRI). Involves placing undesirable behaviors on extinction while reinforcing responses that cannot be produced at the same time as the undesirable behavior

Differential reinforcement of low rates of responding (DRL). Involves providing reinforcement contingent on the client exhibiting the undesirable response at a lower rate

Differential reinforcement of other behaviors (DRO). Involves placing an undesirable response on extinction while reinforcing all other desirable behaviors, as long as the targeted undesirable behavior is not exhibited

Discrete trial. An instructional unit designed to teach a specific skill

Discrete trial teaching (DTT). An intensive behavioral approach to teaching specific skills in which massed discrete trials are presented

Discrimination. The process of responding to different antecedent stimuli in different ways

Discriminative stimulus (S^D). A stimulus in the presence of which a particular response will be reinforced

Divergent intraverbal control. A single verbal stimulus evokes several intraverbal responses

Durational measures. Used to quantify the amount of time a client engages in a target behavior

Echoics. Verbal operants that are imitations of another person's verbal behavior

Effect size. A measure of the magnitude of the effect seen in scientific experimentation, determined through statistical testing

Elopement. Occurs when a client attempts to physically leave the therapeutic environment

Empiricism. The belief that knowledge can be derived only from sensory experiences—from that which can be seen, heard, touched, tasted, or smelled

Environmental contingency. Occurs when there is a consistent relationship between environmental stimuli and a behavior

Environmental manipulations. Antecedent changes made to treatment and/or naturalistic settings that serve to decrease the undesirable behavior

Equivalency. In group research design, the similarity between the control and experimental groups; assumed to be achieved when participants are randomly selected for a group research design experiment and then randomly assigned to experimental and control group

Escape. Occurs when the client initially comes in contact with the aversive situation and then engages in a behavior that serves to terminate the nonpreferred stimulus

Ethics. A branch of philosophy that is concerned with distinguishing between human behavior that is right and human behavior that is wrong

Evocative effect. Motivating operations that change the frequency of behaviors that were previously reinforced by a specific activity, object, or event by creating multiple opportunities for that behavior to occur (more than might naturally occur in that environment)

Exclusion criteria. Set forth those characteristics that would preclude participation in a research study

Extended stimulus control. Occurs when mands are evoked even though the characteristic reinforcement of the behavior is unlikely or impossible, but the listener or situation is similar enough to ones in which the behavior was previously reinforced that it controls the response

Extended tact. A tact that is generalized to a novel item with similar properties

External validity. A term that refers to the extent to which results of a study can be generalized, or extended to, a larger population

Extinction. Reducing a behavior by removing the consequences that reinforce the behavior

Extinction burst. A sudden increase in the client's use of an undesirable response in the initial stages of using extinction

Extraneous variable. In scientific research, an event that may contribute to the effect seen in a dependent variable and thereby confound the results of the study

Fading. The gradual reduction of the special stimulus control of target behaviors provided by the clinician, so that the response is maintained in the presence of more natural stimuli

Fixed interval (FI). A schedule of reinforcement providing an opportunity to earn a reinforcer for the first correct response after a set amount of time

Fixed ratio (FR). A schedule of reinforcement during which a clinician provides a reinforcer after a predetermined number of correct responses

Formal. A term used to describe intraverbal clusters where the stimuli and responses are linked together because they sound similar (e.g., rhyming)

Forward chaining. The clinician initially teaches the first component of the target behavior and then gradually includes subsequent components of the terminal response

Fragmentary tacts. Autoclitics that appear as grammatical tags, bound morphemes, or inflections

Frequency measures. Counting the number of times a client exhibits a target behavior during a specific time frame

Functional analysis. The process of experimentally testing hypotheses about the functions of undesirable behaviors

Functional behavior assessments (FBA). The primary set of procedures used by BCBAs in the field of ABA to determine potential functions of behaviors

Functional communication training (FCT). A specific type of differential reinforcement of alternative behavior that involves teaching the use of communicative responses that serve the same function as the undesirable behavior

Functional units. Verbal behaviors grouped by their cause and effect. Functional units of verbal behavior include mands, tacts, echoics, intraverbals, autoclitics, and textuals

Generalization. Occurs when, without specific teaching, target behaviors are exhibited in new settings, with new people, in response to new antecedent stimuli, or in new ways

Generalized conditioned reinforcement. Conditioned reinforcers that can be effective in a myriad of situations because they can provide an individual access to a wide variety of other reinforcers and are not dependent upon a state of deprivation

Group research design. Commonly employed experimental designs, which involve much greater numbers of participants

Hierarchy of prompts. A planned and systematic presentation of prompts

High-probability (high-p) request sequences. The presentation of several requests that the client is likely to comply with (the high-p requests) prior to introducing the target antecedent stimulus (the low-p request)

Imitation. As applied to treatment, occurs when the client repeats the model provided by the SLP

Impure verbal operant. A verbal operant under the control of multiple controlling relations (i.e., it results from a combination of multiple antecedents and/or consequences)

Inclusion criteria. Set forth required characteristics of participants for a research study

Independent variable. In scientific research, the cause the scientist investigates to see what kind of effect it has on a dependent variable, if any

Informative feedback. Reinforcing a correct response by giving clients information regarding their performance of a target behavior

Interfering behaviors. Behaviors that disrupt the provision of speech-language services

Intermittent schedules of reinforcement. Only some correct responses receive reinforcement

Intermixed probe. A procedure to check for generalization by the clinician presenting two sets of stimulus items; a set that has been used during treatment (the "taught" items) and a set consisting of new stimulus items the client has not previously seen (the "untaught" items)

Intertrial interval. A brief pause, between 1 and 5 seconds, after one discrete trial has been presented and before another begins

Interval measures. Counting the number of times a behavior occurs during a repeated specified block of time

Interval schedules of reinforcement. Delivering reinforcers according to interval periods of time

Intraverbal chain. When an intraverbal response has a fixed order upon which the delivery of reinforcement is contingent

Intraverbal clusters. When groups of verbal operants evoke each other in the absence of a unidirectional relationship

Intraverbals. Verbal operants generated by a speaker's own verbal behavior or by the verbal behavior of others

Lag schedule of reinforcement. Reinforcement is given only when the client's response varies in some way from previous responses; used to increase the variability of a target behavior

Latency. Refers to the amount of time between an antecedent stimulus and the client's response

Least-to-most. Initially providing the least intrusive prompting method and then moving through a hierarchy of cues until the response is evoked

Level. In regard to data displayed on a line graph, describes a data point in reference to its placement on the y-axis

Mands. Verbal operants motivated by a state of deprivation or aversive stimuli that typically specify the reinforcing consequence (e.g., commands, requests, and questions)

Manual guidance. Physically manipulating the client's motor movements through production of a target response

Measurement. Assigning numerical values to observed phenomena

Mentalism. Emphasizes assumed internal processes such as thought and perception as the key to understanding why human beings behave the way they do

Metaphorical extension. When a tact is extended to an object in a different stimulus class with similar properties

Metonymical extension. When generalization of a tact accounts for a verbal operant that seems to have no controlling stimuli

Model. The stimulus for imitation

Modeling. The clinician's production with required imitation; a frequently

employed antecedent manipulation used in the field of speech-language pathology

Most-to-least. Providing more invasive prompting methods such as manual guidance and modeling in the initial stages of treatment and then moving through a hierarchy of cues that become gradually less invasive

Motivating operations (MO). Variables that affect the probability that a specific verbal behavior will occur

Negative autoclitics. Autoclitics that qualify or cancel the verbal behavior they accompany and may signal the cessation or weakening of a behavior

Negative punishment. The process of removing a desirable stimulus in order to decrease the frequency of a behavior

Negative reinforcement. Increases a behavior by removing or postponing an event that a person finds to be aversive

Neutrality. In regard to the scientific method, requires scientists to have no preconception as to the results of their inquiries

Neurophysiologic contingencies. The medical variables that may underlie an observed behavior

Noncontingent reinforcement. An antecedent intervention procedure that involves providing time-based reinforcement that is unrelated to the client's responses

Objectivity. In regard to the scientific method, obtained when scientists explain an experiment in enough detail so that other scientists in other settings with other participants can replicate the experiment

Obtrusive. An assessment can be described as obtrusive if a person is aware of the fact that he or she is being observed and measurements are being taken

Operant. A unit of verbal behavior that is functionally related to one or more independent variables

Operant conditioning. A process through which behavior is shaped and maintained by the consequences that immediately follow the behavior

Operational definitions. Descriptions of behaviors that lend themselves to observation and measurement of the defined behavior

Overgeneralization. In language acquisition, the application of a grammatical rule to words that are exceptions to that rule (e.g., *foots* instead of *feet* and *goed* instead of *went*)

Palilalia. Self-echoics that are excessive, uncontrolled, or pathological in other ways

Partial echoic. Repetition of only a portion of what is heard

Partial-interval recording. A variation of interval measurement in which the behavior is scored as present if it occurs at any time during the interval

Phonemic cues. A type of verbal prompt in which clinicians provide their clients with the first phoneme of the target response to evoke the desired behavior

Positional prompts. Physically moving the antecedent stimuli that clients are expected to engage with closer to them

Positive behavior support. Strategies that result in the reduction of undesirable behavior, including differential reinforcement, rather than punishment

Positive punishment. Occurs when a stimulus is delivered right after a behavior is exhibited, resulting in the decreased frequency of that behavior

Positive reinforcement. Occurs when a reinforcer is presented right after a behavior has occurred, resulting in the increase of that behavior

Preference assessments. Procedures conducted to identify a pool of stimuli that the client prefers and may serve as good reinforcers for targeted behaviors

Premack principle. Based on the concept that high-probability behaviors can serve as reinforcers for low-probability behaviors

Priming. Conducted prior to a given situation in order to familiarize the client with the setting, materials, and/or information involved in a given activity

Probability of response. The likelihood that an operant will occur again given the same or similar circumstances

Probe procedures. Conducted to determine if correct response rates are maintained in the presence of untrained stimuli

Prompt dependent. Describes a client who over discriminates and produces the correct response only in the presence of the special S^D presented during DTT

Prompts. The hints that a clinician gives a client to increase the probability of a correct response

Pseudoscience. Refers to treatment methods that have no empirical evidence to support them but are promoted by those who falsely claim them to be effective

Punishment. A contingency placed on a behavior resulting in a *decrease* of a specified behavior

Pure probe procedure. A procedure conducted to determine if the correct response is produced in the presence of only new, untaught stimuli

Pure verbal operants. Verbal operants associated with a single controlling variable (antecedent) or consequence

Qualifying autoclitics. Autoclitics that qualify the verbal behaviors they accompany in such a way that the intensity or direction of the listener's behavior is modified; most often achieved through assertion or negation

Quantifying autoclitics. Autoclitics that indicate the numerical properties of the controlling stimuli that prompted the primary verbal response

Randomization. Occurs when participants are randomly selected from a large population of accessible participants and then again randomly assigned to either a control group or experimental group

Ratio schedules of reinforcement. Based upon the number of correct responses exhibited by the client

Ratio strain. Occurs when the correct response rate decreases as a result of too abruptly thinning a reinforcement schedule

Reactivity. A behavioral term referring to the extent to which an observation or assessment procedure results in a modification in the usual behavior of the person being observed or assessed

Reinforce. To strengthen the probability of a response to a given stimulus by giving or withholding a reward

Reinforcement. The process of strengthening and increasing the frequency of a behavior

Reinforcer. An event that follows a behavior and results in increasing that behavior

Reinforcer-establishing effect. Motivating operations that momentarily alter the reinforcing effectiveness of a stimulus, as might occur by creating a state of deprivation or introducing an aversive stimulus

Replication. Occurs when other researchers repeat a study in other settings, with other participants

Respondent conditioning. Pairing a neutral stimulus to an unconditioned stimulus to eventually elicit an unconditioned response by presentation of the neutral stimulus alone

Response classes. Sets of behaviors that occur under highly similar or identical antecedent and consequence conditions

Response cost. A negative punishment technique that involves the removal of reinforcers contingent upon a behavior, resulting in the decrease of that behavior

Response function. The consequence an individual receives for engaging in a response

Response generalization. The effects of treatment transferring to untaught, through typically similar, forms of the target response

Risk-to-benefit ratio. In scientific research, the assessment of the risks to participants in proportion to the benefits expected to be achieved

Scatterplot. A data collection method that may be used to collect information during direct observation sessions to determine the times of the day when the behavior is most likely to occur

Schedules of reinforcement. Specify either the number of correct responses, amount of elapsed time, or number of different responses needed prior to earning a reinforcer

Science. The behavior of scientists who act according to a certain philosophy, display characteristics of a certain disposition, and follow a set of procedures

Scientific method. A method of research in which a problem is identified, relevant data are gathered, a hypothesis is formulated from these data, and the hypothesis is empirically tested

Self-monitoring. Involves clients learning to systematically observe and record their own behavior

Self-selection. Occurs when individuals volunteer to participate in scientific experiments; acceptable in small *n* research design

Setting generalization. Occurs when clients exhibit taught skills in new locations, outside of the clinic room (e.g., at home, in the classroom, etc.)

Shaping. Successively reinforcing approximations of a target behavior over time, until the target behavior is correctly produced

Single-case research design. A procedure in scientific research involving the intensive study of one participant continuously or repeatedly across time; also called small *n* research design

Skepticism. A mental attitude that results in questioning everything (especially those notions that are commonly taken for granted) and preferring no explanation to a poor one

Small n research design. A procedure in scientific research involving only one or a few participants, with the *n* standing for the word *number*

Social reinforcement. A type of conditioned reinforcement that is mediated by a listener

Social validity. Established when treatment goals, procedures, and results are deemed to be acceptable and socially significant by the client, therapist, and significant others

Stimulability testing. Evoking correct productions of identified possible target behaviors through any necessary prompt

Stimulus generalization. Occurs when the client produces a target behavior in response to untaught, although typically similar, antecedent stimuli

Strength. As applied to verbal behavior, the relative probability of a behavior being emitted given a specific set of circumstances

Strength-based assessment. A set of assessment procedures emphasizing a description of capabilities of the client and of the client's support systems, such as the family, in order to devise a treatment plan that capitalizes on those capabilities

Successive approximation. Shaping a behavior through reinforcement of a series of initial and intermediate responses until a terminal response is achieved

Tactile-kinesthetic prompts. The use of physical contact to help the client engage in a target behavior

Tacts. Verbal operants evoked by a particular object or event, or property of an object or event. They often name, comment on, or describe objects or events in the environment

Task analysis. The process of defining each of the sequential steps included in a complex target behavior

Textual behavior. Verbal behavior under the control of nonauditory verbal stimuli such as written text, phonetic transcription, or musical notes (i.e., reading)

Textual prompts. Written and printed stimuli, such as sentence strips, written instructions, scripts, checklists, and other similar methods, that serve as cues for desired verbal behavior

Thematic. A term used to describe intraverbal clusters where the stimuli and responses are linked together because they share a common meaning or have shared similar reinforcement contingencies

Time-out. A negative punishment procedure terminating an individual's ability to earn positive reinforcement for a set time period following an undesirable behavior

Token economy. A specific technique that makes use of generalized conditioned reinforcement with three primary components: the target behavior, the generalized conditioned reinforcer, and the backup reinforcer

Topography. Refers to the form and structure of a given response

Transcription. Nonvocal verbal behavior (i.e., writing)

Trend. In regard to data displayed on a line graph, the direction of the data set

Unconditioned reinforcers. Consequences that follow a behavior and increase the behavior that are not dependent upon prior learning, because they support the survival of a species (i.e., food)

Unconditioned stimulus. Elicits a reflexive response without any prior learning

Undesirable communicative behaviors. The primary responses SLPs attempt to reduce during treatment

Variability. In reference to data displayed on a line graph, the distance between data points on the *y*-axis

Variable interval (VI). A schedule of reinforcement in which the opportunity to earn a reinforcer is provided after a predetermined average amount of time

Variable ratio (VR). A schedule of reinforcement in which reinforcement is provided after a predetermined average number of correct responses

Verbal behavior. Behavior that involves interactions between the speaker and listener, whereby the speaker gains access to reinforcement and controls the environment through the behavior of the listener

Verbal episode. The combined behaviors of the speaker and listener

Verbal interaction sampling. A specific measurement technique that can be used to collect data on the communicative behavior of at least two individuals during a social interaction

Verbal prompts. Spoken words, or parts of words, used to help an individual produce a target behavior

Verbal repertoire. A collection of verbal operants that can be assigned to an individual

Visual prompts. Anything that clients can see which increases the probability that they will produce a target response

Whole-interval recording. A variation of interval measurement in which a behavior is scored as occurring only if it is exhibited throughout the entire interval

Index

Note: Page numbers in **bold** reference non-text material.